MENTAL HEALTH NURSING

MENTAL HEALTH NURSING

K. Madhav Naidu

genNEXT Publication

Mental Health Nursing

Rs. 890

ISBN: 978-81-908675-3-5

Published in 2010 in India by
Gennext Publication
23 Main Ansari Road, Darya Ganj,
New Delhi-110002
E-Mail:GenNextpublication@hotmail.com
Phone: 23282060

Printed at: Singhal Print Media, Delhi

Contents

Preface *viii*

1. **Introduction** 1

2. **Principles and Concepts of Mental Health Nursing** 49

Classification of Mental Disorders, Personality Defence Mechanisms, Maladaptive Behaviour, Etiology: Bio-psycho-social Factors, Psychopathology of Mental Disorders, Principles of Mental Health Nursing, Standards of Mental Health Nursing Practice, Theoretical Models and the Role of Nurse, References

3. **Assessment of Mental Health Nursing** 71

History Taking, Mental Status Examination, Mini Mental Status Examination, Neurological Examination, Investigations, Psychological Tests, Role and Responsibilities of Nurse, References

4. **Therapeutic Communication** 91

Types, Techniques & Characteristics, Interview Skill, Types of Relationship, Ethics and Responsibilities, Elements of Nurse Patient Contract, IPR-Johari Window, Goals, Phases, Tasks, Therapeutic Techniques, Phases of Therapeutic Relationship, Therapeutic Impasse and its Intervention, References

5. **Treatment Modalities and Therapies** 117

Psycho Pharmacology, Psychological Therapies, Alternative System of Medicine, Occupational Therapy, Physical Therapy: Electroconvulsive Therapy, Geriatric Considerations, Role of Nurse in Mental Health Therapies, References

6. **Management of Psychotic Disorders** 135

Classification: ICD, Nursing Assessment, Treatment Modalities, Geriatric Considerations, Follow-up and Home Care and Rehabilitation, References

7. Management of Mood Disorders **153**

Nursing Assessment of Depression, Treatment Modalities of Patients with Mood Disorders, Geriatric Considerations, Follow up and Home Care Rehabilitation, References

8. Management of Neurotic Disorders **179**

Etiology, Diagnosis, Nursing Assessment, Treatment Modalities, Geriatric Consideration, Follow-up and Home Care and Rehabilitation, References

9. Management of Patients with Substance Use Disorders **195**

Generally Used Psychotropic Substance, Etiology of Dependence, Nursing Assessment, Treatment, Geriatric Considerations, Follow-up and Home Care and Rehabilitation, Rehabilitation, References

10. Management of Personality, Sexual and Eating Disorders **207**

Classification of Disorders, Etiology, Psychopathology, Characteristics, Diagnosis, Nursing Assessment, Nursing Diagnoses, Treatment Modalities, Geriatric Considerations, Follow up and Home Care and Rehabilitation, References

11. Management of Childhood and Adolescent Disorders **241**

Classification of Disorders, Etiology, Psychopathology, Characteristics, Diagnosis, Nursing Assessment, Treatment Modalities, Follow-up and Home Care and Rehabilitation, References

12. Management of Organic Brain Disorders **259**

Classification: ICD, Etiology, Psychopathology, Clinical Features, Diagnosis and Differential Diagnosis, Nursing Assessment, Treatment Modalities, Geriatric Considerations, Follow-up and Home Care and Rehabilitation, References

13. Psychiatric Emergencies **271**

Types of Psychiatric Emergencies and their Management, Stress Adaptation Model, Grief, Types of Crisis, Crisis Intervention, Geriatric Considerations, Role and Responsibilities of Nurse, References

14. Legal Issues in Mental Health Nursing **289**

The Mental Health Act, 1987, Indian Lunacy Act. 1912, Rights of Mentally Ill Clients, Forensic Psychiatry, Acts Related to Narcotic and Psychotropic Substances and Illegal Drug Trafficking, Admission and Discharge Procedures, Role and Responsibilities of Nurse, References

15. Community Mental Health Nursing **339**

Growth of Community Mental Health Services, National Mental Health Programme, Institutionalization Versus Deinstutionalization, Model of Preventive Psychiatry, Levels of Prevention, Primary, Secondary, Tertiary Levels, Mental Health Agencies, Mental Health Nursing Issues for Special Population, References

Bibliography **361**

Index **365**

Preface

This new textbook prepares qualified mental health nurses and those in training with the information and grounding necessary to question practice, contribute to decision making in multi-disciplinary care teams, and draw upon research-based knowledge in the delivery of care and development of mental health services. This textbook will be essential reading for pre-registration mental health nursing students, post-qualifying mental health nurses and other health care professionals working in mental health services.

This book is a practical guide to developing the skills essential for mental health nursing in the twenty-first century. It aims to provide an easily comprehensible structure for understanding the essential aspects of mental health nursing and their application in practice. Now a days mental health nursing is a complex matrix of theoretical concepts, models, frameworks, competencies and policies. This barrage of ideas and perspectives can seem bewildering for a student nurse trying to learn his or her role in practice. The aim of this book is to help the student develop the skills needed for the practice environment. It identifies the skills essential for the mental health nurse and provides an easy to understand guide to what and how to do it. The book draws on the policy and theoretical underpinnings of mental health nursing but concentrates in the essential skills and their application in practice.

This book provides an easy to understand and practical framework for the development and use of the skills essential to mental health nursing. It is designed to be taken with you to practice environment so that you can easily refer to it when you are learning a skill. You should always be supervised by a registered nurse until you are competent at a particular skill.

1

Introduction

Psychiatric nursing or mental health nursing is the specialty of nursing that treats people of all ages and groups with mental disease or mental distress, for example schizophrenia, bipolar disorder, psychosis, depression or dementia. Nurses in this field obtain additional education in psychological therapies, building a therapeutic bond, dealing with challenging behaviour, and the administration of psychiatric medication.

PERSPECTIVES OF MENTAL HEALTH AND MENTAL HEALTH NURSING

Mental health nursing deals with the analysis and management of human reactions to genuine or possible mental health problems. It is a dedicated field of nursing practice that employs theories of human behaviour as its scientific model and calls for the meaningful use of self as its art of expression. It is related with encouraging optimal health for the public. Complete services concentrate on avoidance of mental sickness, health maintenance, management of and recommendation for mental and physical health problems, diagnosis and management of mental disorders, and rehabilitation.

Though there is no general meaning of mental health, people in the assisting professions seem to agree that mental health is a positive state in which one is dependable, exhibits cognizance, is self-directive, is rationally tension free, and can deal with usual daily worries. Such people function well in the public, are accepted within a group, and are in general satisfied with their lives. Other definitions refer to the capability to resolve problems; accomplish one's capability for love and work; deal with crisis without aid beyond the support of family or friends; and keep a state of wellbeing by enjoying life, setting aims and practical boundaries, and becoming independent, interdependent, or dependent as the need arises without eternally losing one's independency.

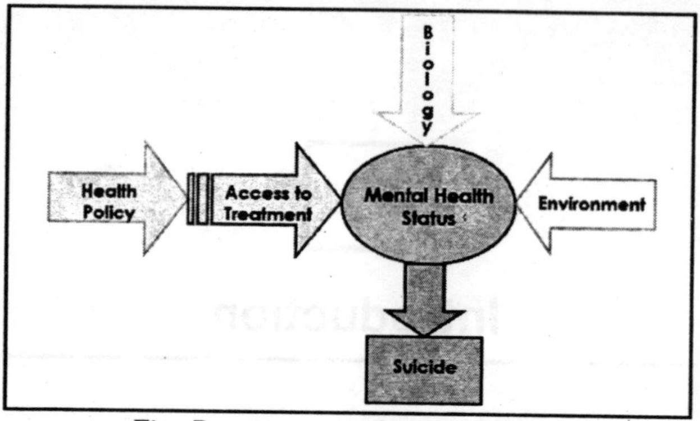

Fig. Perspectives of Mental Health

Cultural notions influence how mental health and mental sickness are decided. For example, acceptable behaviour in one cultural group may or may not be tolerated in some other group.

HISTORY OF PSYCHIATRY

Psychiatry is a medical area of expertise which is there to analyze, avert, and treat mental disorders in human beings. Psychiatric judgment basically involves a mental status assessment and taking a case history, and psychological tests may be done. Physical examinations may be conducted and some times neuroimages or other neurophysiological measurements taken. Diagnostic procedures differ but official standards are scheduled in different manuals, the most common being the ICD from the World Health Organization and the DSM from the American Psychiatric Association. Psychiatric medication is a fundamental treatment alternative, which is for the most part distinctive to psychiatry along with rarer procedures such as Electroconvulsive therapy. Psychotherapy is also a major treatment alternative in psychiatry, though it is also the speciality of other mental health professions. Psychiatric services may be provided on an in-patient or out-patient base. In several authorized cases this may be done on an involuntary basis. Both the research and clinical application of psychiatry are regarded as interdisciplinary. Due to this, various subspecialties and theoretical approaches exist. Psychiatrists can be regarded as doctors who specialize in the physician-patient relationship using some of medicine's latest classification systems, diagnostic tools and treatments.

Psychiatry can be said to have started in the fifth century BC, although the first hospitals for the mentally sick were made in the Middle Ages. The eighteenth century saw the growth of psychiatry as a accepted discipline and mental health organizations came to employ more intricate, as well as some more humane, treatments. The nineteenth century saw a massive increase in patient populations. The twentieth century saw a Renaissance of a biological understanding of mental disorders besides the introduction of disease classifications and psychiatric medications. An anti-psychiatry drive came forth in the 1960s and a shift led to the discontinuing of state psychiatric hospitals in favour of community treatment. There have been modifications in psychiatric diagnoses and treatments and in the equilibrium between the biological and social sciences. Research has continued investigating the origins, classification, and treatment of mental disorders.

Those professionals who practice psychiatry are unlike other mental health professionals and doctors in that they must be knowledgeable about both the social and biological sciences. The field is interested in the operations of different organs and body systems as classified by the patient's subjective experiences and the objective physiology of the patient. Psychiatry exists to treat mental illnesses which are conventionally classified into three very broad classes; mental sickness, intense learning disability, and personality disorder. Even though the spotlight of psychiatry has changed little during time, the diagnostic and treatment processes have developed dramatically and continue to do so. Since the late twentieth century, the discipline of psychiatry has proceeded to become more biological and less conceptually detached from the discipline of medicine.

Even though the medical specialty of psychiatry employs research in the discipline of neuroscience, psychology, medicine, biology, biochemistry, and pharmacology, it has in general been regarded as a middle ground between neurology and psychology. Unlike other doctors and neurologists, psychiatrists specialize in the physician-patient relationship and are educated to varying degrees in the use of psychotherapy and other therapeutic communication techniques. Psychiatrists also differ from psychologists in that they are doctors and the entirety of their post-graduate training is focused around the discipline of medicine. Psychiatrists can thus prescribe medication, order laboratory tests, employ neuroimaging in a clinical setting, and carry on physical examinations.

HISTORICAL DEVELOPMENT OF MENTAL HEALTH

An evaluation of the social changes taking place before 1773 is essential to appreciate the growth of psychiatric mental health nursing. The origins of most of psychiatry's concepts begin with prehistoric times when primitive people believed spirits possessed the body and had to be driven out to cure. Before the fifth century BC, the Greeks, Romans, and Arabs thought that emotional illnesses were an organic dysfunction of the brain.

Hippocrates (460-375 BC) reported a range of personalities, or temperaments, and suggested that mental sickness was a disturbance of four body fluids, or "humors." Aristotle (382-322 BC) concluded that the mind was linked with the heart, even though Galen (130-200 AD), a Greek physician, said that emotional or mental illnesses were linked with the brain. Treatment approaches during this time-frame included the use of sedation, good nutrition, good physical hygiene, music, and leisure activities such as riding, walking, and listening to the sounds of a waterfall. Fresh air, sunshine, and pure water were believed to promote curing for the mentally sick.

MIDDLE AGES TO 1773

During the middle Ages, humanitarian treatment of mentally sick people suffered a setback as mentally sick people were barred from the public and confined in asylums or organizations. Various theories pertaining to demonic possession also were advanced. Especially, individuals who displayed abnormal behaviour were regarded as lunatics, witches, or demons possessed by evil spirits. Superstition, mysticism, magic, and witchcraft persisted as patients were locked away in asylums, whipped, starved, tortured, or submitted to bloodletting. Beheading, hanging, and burning at the stake were general occurrences. Exorcism was exercised in some monasteries.

Throughout this same period, doctors described symptoms of depression, paranoia, delusions, hysteria, and nightmares. Individuals exhibiting such symptoms were believed to be incompetent and potentially dangerous. The first mental hospital, Bethlehem Royal Hospital, opened in England in 1403. Pronounced "Bedlam," the name came to symbolise the inhumane treatment of individuals who were put on public exhibit. Harmless inmates looked for charity on the streets.

In contrast, the eighteenth century is considered a period of reason and observation. As per Peplau (1956), the historical growth of psychiatric nursing started in 1773. Peplau distinguished five periods, or phases in the founding of psychiatric nursing, both as an aspect of all nursing and as a specialty in nursing. Phenothiazines and other main tranquilizers were introduced in the United States in the early 1950s to treat the primary symptoms of psychoses, allowing patients to be more reactive to therapeutic care. During this same time period, open-door policies were applied in big mental organizations, permitting patients to leave the units or wards under supervision.

In 1963, the Community Mental Health Act allowed funding for the formation of community health centres to furnish the following services to the public: emergency mental health care, such as crisis centres and telephone hotlines; patient care or hospitalization, such as day-care centres and therapeutic communities; aftercare, together with halfway houses and foster homes; and consultation services, as provided in counselling centres. This act encouraged the specialization of psychiatric nursing services as the provision of care shifted to the community. Nurse practitioners or clinical specialists could supply direct care to psychiatric patients in different settings. The deinstitutionalization of patients from state mental hospitals to community living was regarded as a positive move; nevertheless, insufficient funding resulted in growth in the number of homeless mentally sick people.

As observed, during the twentieth century, psychiatric nursing started to develop as a clinical specialty. Nurses were formerly involved as managers and coordinators of activities as they supplied therapeutic care based on the medical model. With advanced study and clinical practice received in a master's program in psychiatric nursing, clinical specialists and nurse practitioners acquired expert knowledge in the care and prevention of psychiatric illnesses.

PHILOSOPHY, PRINCIPLES OF MENTAL HEALTH AND PSYCHIATRIC NURSING

Effective mental health nursing involves the practice of the following principles, in recognition of which the knowledge of psychology is of enormous help.

1. Nursing the whole patient
2. Right psychological methodology to the individual patient
3. Ample sympathetic understanding of patient
4. Effective health teaching
5. Successful, personnel and professional adjustments

An adept nurse will give thoughtfulness to these intellectual and emotional factors in addition to the physical significances of the specific sickness. A physical sickness is accompanied by mental and emotional disturbances, which can't and shouldn't be dismissed in scheme of effective nursing. Jessie Williams remarks in psychology for students' nurses, it is essential to recognize that each individual patient is a distinctive personality who reacts to sickness, with his body, mind and emotions in his own personal way.

A child has to be operated for septic tonsils. Adept nurses will not prepare the child only physically or medically for this imminent operation. She will see that the child does not get panicky or frightened at the idea of operation. Fears or concerns if not relieved may aggravate the child's physical condition or slow down the process of his recovery. The correct methodology of the nurse will accomplish a complete bonding with the patient and put him at ease in the unfamiliar set up of the ward. The nurse

1. Receives the patient as though he or she is her guest. Receive him/her with warmth and gentleness.
2. Orients the patient to the ward, its environment, the physical facilities available, the different people who work in and the different responsibilities allotted to them in a sympathetic way.
3. The patient may be nervous or tensed due to his sickness. He may have several questions and as such may ask several immaterial questions.
4. Tries to answer his questions as well as she can. Always give the right information. Better postpones an answer instead of giving wrong information.
5. Talks to the patient and his relatives compassionately. Clarify things distinctly and in plain language at the level of the patient's intellect. Sympathy means feeling with the patient, dignified kindness and thoughtfulness without excessive and sentimental concern.
6. Tries to lessen the uneasiness of over moderate patients by deviating their attention to impersonal topics.
7. Listens to the patient. Let him relate to his own words exactly what is that bothers him. When he finds that he is being listened to with underlying attention, he will speak liberally and without embarrassment. In short the nurse should see that nursing remains as it always used to be, the art of personal service to the sick.

UNDERSTANDING OF PATIENT

Right psychological methodology results in good bonding with the patient. A very significant aspect of understanding the patient is to recognize and accept the fact of personal differences among patients. Some patients are helpful, friendly and react in an amiable manner, even though there are others who remain distant and in some extreme cases antagonised.

Some patients are self-interested and demanding asking for nurse's care and presence all the time. Some patients understand swiftly, respond to nurse's instructions readily, even though there are others, who don't seem to follow nurse's instructions. No two patients are alike. They are different from one another intellectually, emotionally, socially, culturally, socioeconomically and hereditary These elements contribute to their differences and it is these differences, which make nursing interesting.

A nurse, to whom the nursing care of infant is allotted, should recognize that the infant demands security, love, affection and understanding. This has to be furnished by the nurse through patting and tendering the baby. An adept nurse can minimize the danger by meeting his or her needs in a right manner.

The following suggestions are useful.

1. See that the child's environment is joyful and pleasing.
2. The child needs to have visitors especially the members of his or her family. Meet their needs gracefully.
3. Establish an amiable rapport with the young patients by talking to him at his own level by knowing his pet name and his likes and dislikes.
4. Allow him toys that can be taken to bed. Play in his natural usage.
5. Play spirit can be used in getting the plans of treatment carried out and seeking the child's co-operation. It is no use pushing him into compliance. The use of force will increase his resistance.
6. Furnish love and tenderness that he is not able to get from his parents, who are not present.
7. Exercise patience. Don't allow oneself to be upset by whims and fancies.
8. It is suitable that the child acts independently and does not remain in dependent status too long. Encourage him to do things for himself.

9. See that the child does not remain worried, strained, moody or distressed on account of being subject to new, sudden and harsh changes.
10. The nurse needs to guard herself against becoming personally involved with a child patient. This may happen when a child has developed very short attachment to a specific nurse resulting in his rejection of all other nurses, who attend to him. Let the nurse recognize this situation and limit the attention she gives him.

Parents of sick children need to be helped. They may not act normally due to their severe nervousness. An adept nurse should use poise, sympathy, tolerance and tactfulness when dealing with their questions of nervousness. The teenage patients can be helped better if his growth patterns and needs are suitably realized. Adolescents are used to the boundless energy that they find difficult to slow down and take it easy. The nurse plays a function of a counsellor. The teenager should be treated as a grown up and matured individuals. He feels secured if he is handled as equal in age and experience, if difficulties are talked about with him and his feelings are respected

The adult patient may lose his common emotional control may be bothered by the fear of the unknown and of possible death. He might find to withdraw or he may make excessive demands. The ward restrictions may infuriate him and this may lead to non-cooperative behaviour.

The rationale of good nursing care of an adult is that he shouldn't be allowed to regret. He should be encouraged to partake in recreational activities personally and with the group. The aged patients present their own problems. Age brings about several physical, intellectual and emotional changes in the person, which cause the general insecurity. Depression and feelings of loneliness frequently set in. The nurse should be equipped with the knowledge of old age. She should pay close attention at first to his physical hygienic and should see that the utmost physiological health is maintained through diet, rest and exercise. The understanding of patients will be helped if the nurse possesses knowledge of the general effects of sickness and hospitalization on their behaviour reactions.

CHARACTERISTICS OF MENTAL HEALTH

Health is a state of being hale, sound or whole in body, mind or soul. Mental health today is recognized as a significant facet of ones total health status is basic factor that contribute to the maintenance of physical health in addition to social effectiveness. In the words of John, Sutton and Webster is a positive but relative quality of life. It is a condition, which is a feature of the average individual who needs the demands of life on the basis of his own capacities and restrictions. By the word relative we imply that the level of mental health, which a person enjoys at a time, is continuously changing.

It is not mere absence of mental sickness that constitutes mental health. Then again it is a positive active quality of the person's daily living. This quality of living is evidenced in the conduct of a person whose body and mind are working together in the same direction. His thoughts, feelings, actions, functional harmony is oriented towards the general end. It means the capability to equilibrium feelings, derives ambition and ideals in ones daily living. It means the capability to face and accept realities of life. It connotes such habits of work and attitudes towards people and things that bring greatest satisfaction and happiness to the person. But the person gets this satisfaction and happiness without any friction with the social order or group to which he or she belongs.

From these one can conclude that mental health has two significant facets. It is both personal and social. The personal aspect connotes that the person is informally adjusted. He is self confident, adequate and free from internal conflicts and worry or in consistencies. He is skilled enough to be able to adjust to new situations. But he attains this internal adaptation in a social setup. Society has several value system, customs and traditions, by which it governs itself and promote the general welfare if its members. It is in this the social frame work that the internal adaptation has to be built up only then the person becomes an individual who is acceptable as a member of society.

It is an understandable fact that social forces are in constant flux. They are regularly moving and changing. Likewise our internal adaptation is also affecting various stresses. As such mental health is a process of adaptation, which involves compromise and adjustment, development and continuity. Due to the significance of personal and social facets some psychologists have defined mental health as the capability of the individual to make personal and social adjustments. If one can establish an acceptable relationship between himself and his environment, between his needs, desires and those of other people or if one can meet the demands of a situation he has achieved adaptation.

Adaptation results in happiness because it implies that emotional conflicts and worries have been solved and relieved.

Keeping this standard in mind one can say that a mentally healthy nurse will be able to make successful adjustments that are needed by the nature of her job adaptation to her arduous life to work and study toward duties to night duty and to a residential life away from her home. Other definitions of mental health refer to such powers as of making decisions, of accepting duties in accordance with ones capacities, of finding satisfaction, success and happiness in the accomplishment of everyday tasks of living effectively with others of showing socially considerate conduct.

MENTAL DISORDERS

Various mental illnesses have enabled psychiatrists and psychologists to discover some general symptoms of mental illnesses. These symptoms pertain to various distinguishable facets of the mind. They have been produced by several needs and meaningful situations in the life of the person. Several of these symptoms have been produced by the operation of our mental mechanism.

THEORETICAL APPROACHES TO PSYCHIATRIC NURSING

Psychiatric nurses are being encouraged to consider the value of biomedical explanations of serious sickness, such as schizophrenia, and to accommodate these theories and models in the practice of nursing.

By unfolding the growth of our theoretical past, we gain insights that improve our understanding of our current progress, and we are empowered to accomplish our disciplinary aims. By looking at our theoretical present, we see shadows of our past in addition to visions of our future. Reconstructing our theoretical heritage is a process that involves reconstructing our present reality. Prior to the 1950s, the medical model dominated psychiatric mental health nursing practice. Physicians and psychiatrists assessed, diagnosed, and planned care for people with psychiatric disorders. Nurse practitioners were taught and supervised mainly by physicians and psychiatrists who incorporated the theories of people such as Freud, Sullivan, Skinner, Bowen, or Erikson into their practice. Nevertheless, during this same period, nursing leaders started to emerge to furnish impetus for the growth of psychiatric nursing as an independent field.

Theoretical models were developed by theorists such as Hildegard Peplau in 1952, Virginia Henderson in 1955, Martha Rogers in 1970, Imogene King in 1971, Dorothea Orem in 1971, and Sister Callista Roy in

1971. These models provided a foundation and strategy for theory growth by introducing orderliness into the research process and providing ideas for statements of theoretical hypotheses (i.e., predicted relationships among variables under investigation). Hypotheses lead to empirical studies that seek to affirm or discredit predictions.

Theoretical hypotheses eventually lead to the growth of theories, which are abstract generalizations that present systematic explanations about the relationships among variables. Early theorists centred on interpersonal relationships between patient and nurse, behavioural reactions to stress and the environment, and approaches to self-care deficit. The phrase systems-oriented theory also developed at this time. For instance, in systems-oriented theory the person is regarded as part of the family system. Stress in one part of the system (e.g., family) affects other parts of the system. Changes in family structure contribute to changes in the behaviour of people.

Since the 1970s, nursing theories have emerged based on caring, cultural care diversity and generality, modelling and role modelling, energy fields, and human becoming. Theory is regarded as a branch of science dealing with theoretical principles that describe, explain, and predict a class of phenomena. Meleis (1997) defines theory as an organized, coherent, and systematic articulation of a set of statements related to important questions in a field that is communicated in a meaningful whole. It is a symbolic portrayal of facets of reality that are discovered or invented to describe, explain, predict, or prescribe reactions, events, situations, conditions, or relationships.

Johnson (1997) noted that theory is essential for the further growth of nursing as a profession. Many nurse theorists, such as Hildegard Peplau, Dorothea Orem, Sister Callista Roy, and Rosemarie Parse, have centred on concepts especially related to psychiatric nursing. Other theorists are discussed in the text where relevant.

PEPLAU'S INTERPERSONAL THEORY

Hildegard Peplau was responsible in part for the emergence of theory-based psychiatric nursing practice. She considered that the nurse functions as therapist, counsellor, socializing agent, manager, technical nurse, mother surrogate, and teacher. Her Interpersonal theory integrates communication and relationship concepts from Harry Stack Sullivan's Interpersonal theory. Her theory concentrates mainly on the nurse-patient relationship in which problem-solving skills are developed. Four phases occur during this interactive process: orientation, identification, exploitation, and solution:

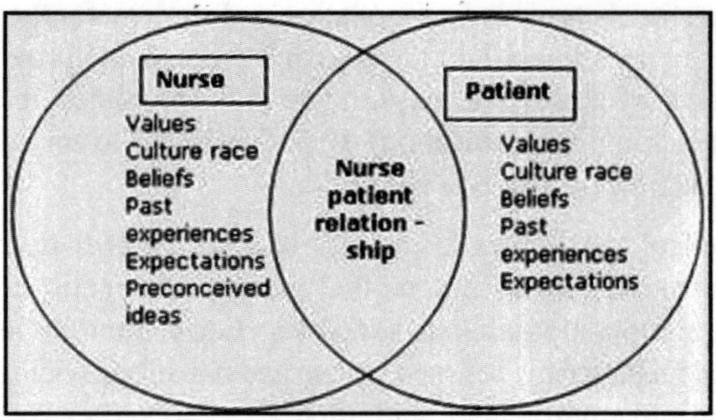

Fig. Peplau's Interpersonal Theory

Analysis of this theory reveals that it is effective in long-term care, home health, and psychiatric settings where time allows for the growth of a nurse-patient relationship and, hopefully, a solution to promote health. Nevertheless, the theory's usefulness is limited in short-term, acute care nursing settings, where hospitalizations last for only a few hours or a few days. It is also ineffectual when the patient is regarded as to be a group of people, a family, or a community.

OREM'S BEHAVIOURAL NURSING THEORY

Orem's Behavioural Nursing theory concentrates on self-care deficit. It proposes that the recipients of nursing care are individuals who are unable of continuous self-care or independent care due to health-related or health-derived restrictions. Human beings are described as integrated wholes functioning biologically, symbolically, and socially. Due to a person's self-care deficits, a nurse, family member, or friend may educate or consult with the person to improve the deficit. This theory is used in the psychiatric setting, where people may neglect self-care needs such as eating, drinking, rest, personal hygiene, and safety due to their underlying disorder.

ROY'S THEORY OF ADAPTATION

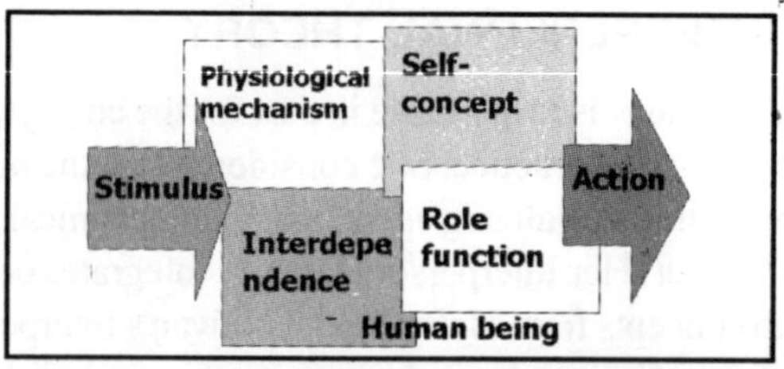

Fig. Roy's Theory of Adaptation

Roy's theory of Adaptation, modelled from a behavioural theory, states that human beings use coping mechanisms to adjust to both internal and external stimuli. Two main internal coping mechanisms are the regulator and the cognator. The regulator mechanism refers to a person's physiologic response to stress, whereas the cognator mechanism pertains to perceptual, social, and information-processing functions.

Coping behaviour occurs in four adaptive modes: physiologic, self-concept, role function, and interdependence. People sustain health through the integration of the four modes of adaptation. This theory is used in the psychiatric setting as the nurse evaluates patient behaviour and stimuli and develops a plan of care to assist the patient in adaptation in the four modes contributing to health, quality of life, and dying with dignity.

PARSE'S THEORY OF HUMAN BECOMING

Parse's theory of Human Becoming demonstrates an alternative to both the traditional biomedical methodology and the bio-psycho-social-spiritual methodology of most other theories of nursing. Parse first published this theory in 1981. It posits quality of life from each person's own perspective as the goal of nursing practice. Putting differently, the function of the nurse is to guide the patient or simply be with him or her to bear witness to the patient's experiences. Three themes are noted: meaning, rhythmicity, and transcendence.

The first theme, meaning, refers to patients coparticipating in creating what is real for them through self-expression in living their values in a chosen way rather than because of the expectation of others. The second theme, rhythmicity, explains that in living moment to moment, one determines whether to show or not to show facets of one's self as opportunities and restrictions emerge in moving with and apart from others. The third theme, transcendence, explains that moving beyond the now moment is forging a distinctive personal path for oneself in the midst of ambiguity and continuous change.

Parse's theory is regarded as by some modern practitioners to be an excellent model for community psychiatric nursing in which the nurse focuses on the patient's experiences, not problems; bears witness to the patient's experiences; respects the person's capacity for self-knowing; and assists the patient in cocreating a worthful space for the patient to voice the lived experience of health. Humanly lived experiences such as loss and grief are believed to react well to interventions based on Parse's theory. Patients with mood disorders and psychotic disorders also have benefited from interventions promoting independence and empowerment.

APPLICATION TO PRACTICE

Meleis discusses the application of nursing theory to psychiatric nursing practice. Utilizing nursing theory, nurses concentrate on various facets of care depending on identified needs or presenting problems of psychiatric patients. Many approaches may be used: needs oriented; interaction oriented; outcome oriented; and eclectic methodology.

Needs-Oriented Approach: With a needs-oriented approach nurses are dynamically doing and functioning. They problem-resolve, perform physiologic and psychosocial activities for the patient, supplement knowledge, and may become provisional selfcare agents for patients with selfcare deficits.

Interaction-Oriented Approach: The interaction-oriented approach is employed by nurses who rely on interactions and comprise themselves in the sphere of other actions. They view themselves as a therapeutic tool and assess their actions as per the patient's response. They counsel, guide, and teach patients, helping them to find meaning in their situations. They appear to be process oriented.

Outcome-Oriented Approach: The outcome-oriented approach is employed by nurses who are viewed as goal setters. They are referred to as controllers, conservators, and healers without touch. They concentrate on asserting and promoting energy and harmony with the environment. They don't view themselves as therapeutic agents as they concentrate on enhancing the growth of health environments.

Self-Awareness Prompt: Do you consider yourself mainly centred on a needs-oriented, interaction-oriented, or outcome-oriented approach to patient care? How would each of these fields of focus be used in psychiatric nursing?

Eclectic Approach: The eclectic approach is an individualized style that incorporates the patient's own resources as a distinctive person with the most suitable theoretical model. Therapists may specialize in one specific theoretical model or combine facets of different ones. The therapist realizes there is no one way to cope with all of life's stresses or problems of living and is open to new ideas and approaches as the need arises.

AGREEMENT AMONG NURSING THEORISTS

Though nursing theorists differ in their beliefs and concepts, they do agree on some points. The following are some of the statements of agreement that guide student nurses as they enter the field of psychiatric nursing:

- Nursing theories furnish descriptions of how to help patients become comfortable, how to deliver treatment with the least damage, and how to improve high-level wellness.
- Nursing theories offer a beginning general language and a beginning agreement about who the nursing care recipients are.
- We shouldn't view the recipients only through biologic glasses or psychological glasses, but rather through holistic glasses.
- Recipients have needs and nursing assists them in meeting those needs.

Nurses furnish care for patients who are in constant interaction with their environment. They may have unmet needs, may be unable to care for themselves, or may be unable to adjust to the environment because of interruptions or potential interruptions in health. The function of nurses is to furnish therapeutic care so that patients are able to adjust to the environment and meet identified needs related to selfcare capability, health, and well-being.

PREVALENCE AND INCIDENCE OF MENTAL HEALTH PROBLEMS AND DISORDERS

It is difficult to know exactly how several people experience mental health problems as not everyone experiencing such difficulties will seek or receive treatment. Episodes of mental sickness can come and go throughout an individual's life. Some people experience their mental sickness only once and then fully recover. Unfortunately, only about half of those affected by mental sickness receive treatment. Mental sickness is a general term that refers to a group of illnesses that affect the brain, in the same way that heart disease refers to a group of illnesses that affect the heart. Mental illnesses can be separated into two main classes:

- Depression and anxiety disorders - for instance, pertinacious feelings of depression, sadness, worry or fear that are so disturbing they affect the person's capability to deal with day-to-day activities. Conditions that can cause these feelings comprise: anxiety disorders (for instance, phobias and obsessive compulsive disorder), eating disorders and depression.
- Psychotic sickness - for instance, schizophrenia and bipolar disorder (formerly called manic depressive sickness). Psychosis

affects the brain and causes changes in an individual's thinking, emotions and conduct. People who experience an acute psychotic episode lose contact with reality and may develop delusions or hallucinations.

EPIDEMIOLOGY

About twenty-five percent adults all over the world are affected by mental sickness at some time in their life. Some are affected by more than one condition. The most commongeneral forms of mental sickness are:

- Depression - around sixteen per cent of adults are affected by depression at some point in their life.
- Anxiety disorders - around ten per cent of adults are affected by anxiety disorders at some point in their life.

The balance of people with mental sickness are affected by psychotic illnesses (for instance, schizophrenia or bipolar disorder) and by other conditions.

Three per cent of adults are seriously affected by mental sickness. The more seriously disabling 'low prevalence' mental illnesses comprise:

- Schizophrenia - this disorder affects approximately one per cent of Australians at some point in their life.
- Bipolar disorder - this condition affects up to two per cent of Australians at some time during their life.
- Other forms of psychosis - for instance, drug-induced psychosis.
- Some chronic forms of depression.

Most people with mental sickness don't have family members with the sickness. For some mental disorders, there does not seem to be a link at all. Though an inclination to schizophrenia and bipolar disorder can be inherited, this is only one of many elements that contribute to the growth of the sickness. It is likely that these mental disorders also involve a chemical imbalance and are triggered by:

- Stressful life events
- Drug misuse
- Hormonal changes.
- Nevertheless, the causes are still not fully understood. Families of those affected need support too.

Up to one in ten people affected by mental sickness commit suicide, compared to an average of one in a hundred for the whole population. Effective, ongoing treatment is necessary to minimize the danger of suicide.

RECOVERY

Provided they receive appropriate ongoing support and treatment, most people with mental sickness recover well and are able to lead fulfilling lives in the community. With appropriate support and treatment, the most likely outcomes for specific conditions are:

- Anxiety disorders - the bulk of people will improve over time.
- Bipolar disorder - about eighty per cent of people will improve.
- Schizophrenia - about sixty per cent of people with schizophrenia will improve and can live independently with support. About twenty per cent of those diagnosed with schizophrenia will have an episode or two, and then never experience symptoms again. For another twenty per cent, symptoms are more pertinacious, treatments are less effective and greater support services are needed.

MENTAL HEALTH ACT

The aim of the Law of Mental Health in India is to solidify and amend the law relating to the treatment and care of mentally sick person, to make better provisions with respect to their property and affairs and for matters connected therewith or incidental thereto. It has 10 chapters:

Chapter I: Preliminary

Chapter II: Mental Health Authorities

Chapter III: Psychiatric Hospitals and Psychiatric Nursing Homes

Chapter IV: Admission and Detention in Psychiatric Hospital or Psychiatric Nursing Home

Chapter V: Inspection, Discharge, Leave of Absence and Removal of Mentally Sick individuals.

Chapter VI: Judicial Inquisition Regarding Alleged Mentally Sick person Possessing Property, custody of his Person & Management of his Property.

Chapter VII: Liability to meet cost of maintenance of Mentally Sick individuals detained Psychiatric Hospital or Psychiatric Nursing Home.

Chapter VIII: Protection of Human Rights of Mentally Sick Individuals.

Chapter IX: Penalties and Procedure.

Chapter X: Miscellaneous.

I. It is called the Mental Health Act 1987 & came into force with effect from 1.4.93 in all the States and Union Territories.

II. Mental Health Authorities:

   i. Central Authority for Mental Health Services: - established by the Central Government.

   ii. State Authority for Mental Health Services - established by the State Government.

Authority shall:

1. Be in charge of regulation growth, direction and Coordination with respect to Mental Health Services under the Central Government and all other matters Concerning Central Government/authority/subordinate to Central Government.
2. Supervise Psychiatric Hospital/Psychiatric Nursing Homes/other Mental Health Service agencies under the Control of Central Government/State Government respectively.
3. Advice the Central Government/State Government in all matters relating to Mental Health.
4. Discharge such other functions with respect to matters relating to mental health as the Central Government/State Government may call for.

III. Psychiatric Hospitals and Psychiatric Nursing Homes:

   i. Establishment or maintenance of psychiatric hospital/nursing home by the Central Government/State Government. Within the limits of its jurisdiction for the admission, treatment and care of mentally sick individuals at such places as it may think fit.

   ii. Establishment or maintenance of psychiatric hospital/nursing home only with license under this Act.

   iii. Application for license:

      1. Every person holding a license under this act; if wishes to continue after the expiry of person the nursing home/hospital should apply at least one month before the date of expiry to issue a fresh license.

2. An individual who intends to establish or maintain such nursing home/hospital shall apply to the licensing authority for the grant of license.
3. Every application should be of the prescribed format with the prescribed fee.

iv. Grant or refusal of license:

The licensing authority should be satisfied in matters relating to

1. Establishment/maintenance
2. Minimum facilities provided which are proscribed for the admission, treatment and care for mentally sick individuals &
3. The hospital/nursing home should be under the control of medical officers.

If not satisfied on the above facets the licensing authority can cancel the orders after giving a reasonable chance for hearing.

Duration of renewal of license:

The psychiatric hospital/nursing home shall be maintained in accordance with conditions laid down in the Act.

The licensing authority can revoke the license by an order in writing if it is satisfied that the hospital/nursing home is not maintained in accordance with the Act. If it is against the moral, mental or physical well being of the inpatients thereof after giving a reasonable opportunity of being heard.

An appeal can be made on such revocation with such period of time.

The appeal can be made in a prescribed format with a prescribed fee.

IV. It has got 3 parts. The first part being admission

a. On voluntary basis - Requisition by major for admission as voluntary patient. So any person who considers himself as mentally sick can apply to a medical officer-in-charge for being admitted as voluntary patient in the hospital/ nursing home.
b. Requisition made by the Guardian for admission of a ward whom he considers as mentally sick to be admitted in a hospital or nursing home. In both the cases the medical officer on receipt of such application conduct an enquiry within a period of 24 hrs may admit such an applicant.

The patient should abide by the regulations made by the medical officer.

I. Admission under special circumstance: So if a mentally sick person is unable to express his willingness for admission, he may be admitted on an application made by a relative of such an individual in a prescribed format accompanied by two medical certificates by two medical practitioners.

II. Reception orders on application - A medical officer in charge of a hospital/nursing home, husband, wife or any relative of such person shall apply to the magistrate for the detention of such an individual and a reception order.

Chapter V deals with inspection, discharge, leave of absence and removal of mentally sick person.

The State government/Central Government shall appoint not less than five visitors for the inspection of hospital/nursing home. Not less than 3 visitors shall make a joint inspection of every part of the hospital/nursing home at least once in every month. If such a visitor does not partake in such an inspection for 3 consecutive months, he shall cease to hold the office.

In case of inspection of mentally sick prisoners all the 3 visitors should visit at least once in three months in the place where he is detained.

Part II deals with discharge of mentally sick person.

The medical officer in charge may direct the discharge of any person other than a voluntary patient by an order in writing based on the recommendations made by two medical practitioners. In case if an individual is admitted by the application made under this Act, shall be discharged only if an application is made to the medical officer by the pertained person.

Any person not being sick prisoner who feels that he has recovered from his mental sickness may make an application for his discharge.

Part III deals with leave of absence of medically sick person from a psychiatrist hospital may be made by an application by the husband or wife or relatives or any other person related to the medical officer. If the medical officer refuses to grant leave of absence, the applicant may apply to the magistrate within the local limit.

The application should be of the prescribed format.

Chapter VI deals with the property of the mentally sick person.

If a mentally sick person possess a property, it can be taken care of by any of his relatives or by public curator or by the advocate general of the state related or by the collector of the district in case the property is a land, by means of an application to the district court which shall pass order after examining the related mentally sick person personally. If the district court finds the mentally sick person incapable of maintaining his property may appoint a guardian to take care of the person and a manager for his property who shall within a period of six months from the date of appointment gives a statement of all claims due and all debts and liabilities due by such mentally sick person. He should also within a period of three months from the close of the financial year an account of property, sums received and disbursed.

Chapter VII deals with the cost of maintenance of a mentally sick person.

The cost of maintenance unless otherwise provided by the law should be borne by the state. In case of a mentally ill person having an estate or the person bound to maintain a mentally sick person has a means to maintain shall apply to the related government or to the district court for a direction to tear the cost of maintenance of such mentally sick person.

Chapter VIII deals with the protection of human rights of mentally sick person.

No mentally sick person should be treated with indignity or cruelty during the treatment. No mentally sick person shall be used for research unless otherwise for the benefit of such person or with the acceptance of such person in writing. In case of the person is incompetent due to minority or otherwise, with the consent of the guardian.

Chapter IX deals with penalties and procedures:

Any person establishes or maintains such nursing home or hospital in contravention of the Act, shall be punishable with an imprisonment of 3 months or with fine or with both.

Any person who detains mentally sick person otherwise than in accordance with the Act, shall be punishable with imprisonment for two years or with a fine of Rs. 1000/- or with both.

Any other person who contravenes any of the provision of the Act for which no penalty is expressly provided shall be punishable with an imprisonment for a period of 6 months or with a fine of Rs. 500/- or with both.

NATIONAL MENTAL HEALTH POLICY

OBJECTIVES

The main objective of this policy is to accomplish an acceptable standard of good health amongst the general population of the country.

1. Goals to be Achieved by 2000-2015

1. Eradicate Polio and Yaws by 2005.
2. Eliminate Leprosy.
3. Eliminate KalaAzar.
4. Eliminate Lymphatic Filariasis.
5. Achieve Zero level growth of HIV/AIDS by 2007
6. Reduce Mortality by 50 % on account of TB, Malaria, and other vector and water borne diseases by 2010
7. Reduce prevalence of blindness by 0.5% by 2010
8. Reduce IMR to 30/1000 and MMR to 100/Lakh by 2010.

Policies under NHP-2002 and the Problems Tackled

Financial Resources: The public health investment in the country over the years has been comparatively low, and as a percentage of GDP has declined from 1.3 percent in 1990 to 0.9 percent in 1999. In this frame work, it has been the expectation that the main contribution for the funding of public health services will be from the resources of the States, with some supplementary input from Central resources.

Equity: In the period when centralized planning was accepted as a main instrument of growth in the country, the attainment of an equitable regional distribution was regarded as one of its main objectives. In spite of this conscious focus in the growth process.

Access to, and benefits from, the public health system have been very uneven between the better endowed and the more vulnerable sections of society. This is especially true for women, children and the socially disadvantaged sections of society.

Delivery of National Public Health Programmes: It is self-apparent that in a country as big as India, which has a wide variety of Socio-economic settings, national health programmes have to be designed with enough flexibility to permit the State public health administrations to craft their own programme package as per their needs. Because, for various reasons, the responsibility of the Central Government in funding additional public health services will continue over a period of time. Over the last decade or so, the Government has relied upon a 'vertical' implementation structure for the main disease control programmes. Through this, the system has been able to make a substantial dent in reducing the burden of specific diseases. Nevertheless, such an organizational structure, which calls for independent manpower for each disease programme, is extremely expensive and difficult to sustain.

The State of Public Health Infrastructure: For the out door medical facilities in existence, funding is in general insufficient; the presence of medical and Para-medical personnel is frequently much less than that required by prescribed norms; the availability of consumables is often negligible; the equipment in several public hospitals is frequently obsolescent and unusable; and, the buildings are in a dilapidated state. In the indoor treatment facilities, again, the equipment is frequently obsolescent; the availability of necessary drugs is minimal; the capacity of the facilities is grossly inadequate, which leads to over-crowding, and consequentially to a steep deterioration in the quality of the services. As a result of such inadequate public health facilities, it has been estimated that less than 20 percent of the population, which seek OPD services, and less than 45 percent of that which seek indoor treatment, avail of such services in public hospitals. This is in spite of the fact that most of these patients don't have the means to make out-of-pocket payments for private health services except at the cost of other necessary expenditure for items such as basic nutrition.

Extending Public Health Services: Even though there is a general shortage for medical personnel in the country, this shortfall is disproportionately impacted on the less developed and rural areas. No incentive system attempted so far, has induced private medical personnel to go to such areas and even in the public health sector, effort to deploy medical personnel in such underserved areas, has normally been a losing battle.

India has a vast reservoir of practitioners in the Indian systems of medicine and homoeopathy, who have undergone formal training in their own fields. The possibility of utilizing such practitioners in the implementation of State or Central government public health programmes, in order to increase the basic health care in the country is addressed in the NHP-2002.

Role of Local Self- government Institutions: Some states have adopted a policy of devolving programmes and funds in the health sector through different levels of the Panchayati Raj Institutions. In general, the experience has been an encouraging one. The adoption of such an organizational structure has enabled need- based allocation of resources and closer supervision through the elected representatives. The policy examines the need for a wider adoption of the mode of delivery of health services, in rural in addition to urban areas, in other parts of the country.

Norms for Health Care Personnel: It is observed that the deployment of physicians and nurses in both public and private institutions will follow a policy of specific recommendation.

Education of Health Care Professionals: Medical and Dental colleges are not evenly spread across the country. Apathy from the uneven geographical distribution of medical institutions, the quality of education is highly uneven and in many instances even sub- standard. Syllabus is excessively theoretical, making it difficult for the fresh graduate to effectively meet even the primary health care needs of the population. There is a general reluctance on the part of graduate physicians to serve in areas distant from their native place.

Several medical fields, such as molecular biology and gene manipulation, have be3come relevant in the period after the formulation of the previous National health Policy. Also, several specialty fields- anaesthesiology, radiology and forensic medicine are currently very scarce, resulting in critical deficiencies in the package of available public health services.

Need for Specialists in Public Health and Family Medicine: In any developing country with inadequate availability of health services, the requirement of expertise in the fields of public health and family medicine is markedly more than the expertise required for other clinical specialties. Also, the current curriculum in the graduate and post-graduate courses is outdated and unrelated to contemporary community need. The more talented medical graduates in general seek education in clinical fields, even though the remaining goes into general practice. Even though the availability of postgraduate educational facilities is 50 percent of the total number of qualifying graduates each year, and case regarded as adequate, the distribution of the fields in the postgraduate training facilities is overwhelmingly in favour of clinical specializations.

Nursing Personnel: The ratio of nursing personnel in the country vis. a physician is very low as per professionally accepted norms. There is also an acute shortage of nurses trained in super specialty fields for deployment in tertiary care facilities.

Use of Generic Drugs and Vaccines: India enjoys a relatively low cost health care system due to the widespread availability of indigenously manufactured generic drugs and vaccines. There is an apprehension that globalization will lead to growth in the cost of drugs, thereby leading to rising trends in overall health costs, this policy recommends measures to ensure the future Health Security of the country.

Urban Health: In most of the urban areas public health services are very meagre. To the degree that such services exist, there is no uniform organizational structure. The urban population in the country is presently as high as 30 percent and is likely to go up to around 33 percent by 2010. The bulk of the increase is likely to take place through migration, resulting in slums which are available don't percolate to such unplanned habitations forcing people to avail of private health care through out of pocket expenditure.

Health Research: Over the years, health research activity in the country has been very limited. In the government sector such research has been confined to the research institutions under the Indian Council of Medical Research and other institutions funded by the states and central government. Medical research in the country needs to be centred on the therapeutic drugs and vaccines for tropical diseases, which are normally neglected by international pharmaceutical companies on account of their limited profitability potential. The thrust will need to be in the newly emerging frontier fields of research based on genetics, genome based drug and vaccine growth, molecular biology etc.

Role of the Private Sector: Considering the economic restructuring under way in the country, and over the globe, in the last decade, the changing function of the private sector in providing health care will also have to be addressed in this policy. Also, the private sector contributes significantly to secondary level care and some tertiary care. It is a widespread perception that private health services are very uneven in quality, sometimes even sub standard.

Private health services are also perceived to be financially exploitative and the observance of professional ethics is noted only as an exception. With increasing function of private health care, the implementation of statutory regulation and the monitoring of minimum standards of diagnostic centres of medical institutions become imperative.

Mental Health: Mental health disorders are actually much more prevalent than is evident on the surface. Even though such disorders don't contribute significantly to mortality, they have a serious bearing on the quality of life of the affected individuals and their families. Sometimes based on religious faith, mental disorders are treated as spiritual affliction.

This has led to establishment of unlicensed mental institutions as an adjunct to religious institutions where reliance is placed on faith cure. Serious conditions of mental disorder call for hospitalization and treatment under trained supervision.

Information, Education and Communication: A substantial component of primary health care consists of initiatives for disseminating to the citizenry, public health related information. Public health programmes especially, need high visibility at the decentralized level in order to have an impact. This task is difficult as 35 percent of our country's population is illiterate. The present IEC strategy is too fragmented, relies too heavily on the mass media and does not address the needs of this segment of the population. It is widely accepted that school and college students are the most impressionable targets for imparting information relating to the basic principles of preventive health care. The policy will attempt to target this group to improve the general level of awareness in regard to health promoting behaviour.

Currently, non-governmental service providers are treating a big number of patients at the primary level for main diseases. Nevertheless the treatment regimens followed are various and not scientifically optimum, leading to growth in the incidence of drug resistance. This policy will address itself to recommending arrangements, which will eliminate the risks arising from inappropriate treatment.

Role of Civil Society: Historically, it has been the practice to implement main national disease control programmes through the public health machinery of the state and central governments. It has become increasingly evident that several components of such programmes can't be efficiently applied merely through government functionaries. A considerable change in the mode of implementation has come about in the last two decades, with the increasing involvement of NGO's and other institutions of civil society. It is to be recognized that widespread debate on various public health issues has, in fact, been initiated and sustained by NGO's and other members of the civil society. Also, such institutions in the delivery of different components of public health services are making an increasing contribution. Several disease control programmes call for close inter action with the beneficiaries for regular administration of drugs, periodic carrying out of pathological tests, dissemination of information regarding disease control and other general health information.

National Disease Surveillance Network: The technical network available in the country for disease surveillance is extremely rudimentary and to the degree that the system exists, it extends only up to the district level. Disease statistics are not flowing through an integrated network from the decentralized public health facilities to the state or central government health administration. Such an arrangement only provides belated information which at best serves a limited statistical purpose. The absence of an efficient disease surveillance network is a main handicap in providing a prompt and cost effective health care system. The efficient disease surveillance network set up for polio and HIV or AIDS has demonstrated the enormous value of such a public health instrument. In order to be able to use an integrated disease surveillance network for operational purposes, real time information is essential at all levels of the health administration.

Health Statistics: The absence of a systematic and scientific health statistics database is a main deficiency in the current scenario. The health statistics collected are not the product of a rigorous methodology. Statistics available from different parts of the county, in respect of main diseases, are frequently not obtained in a manner, which make aggregation possible or meaningful. NHP2002 address itself to the programme for putting in place a modern and scientific health statistics database as well as a system of national health accounts.

Women's Health: Social, cultural and economic factors continue to inhibit women from gaining ample access even to the existing public health facilities. This handicap does not merely affect women as people; it also has an adverse impact on the health, general well being and growth of the entire family, especially children. This policy recognizes the catalytic function of empowered women in improving the overall health standards of the community.

Medical Ethics: Professional medical ethics in the sector is a field, which has not received much attention. Professional practices are perceived to be grossly commercial and the medical profession has lost its elevated position as a provider of basic services to fellow human beings. In the past, medical research has been conducted within the ethical guidelines notified by the Indian Council of Medical Research. The first document containing these guidelines was released in 1960 and was comprehensively revised in 2001. With the rapid developments in the approach to medical research, a periodic revision will no doubt be more often required in future. Also the new frontier fields of research impinge on visceral issues relating to the sanctity of human life and the moral dilemma of human intervention in the designing of life forms. Besides this, in the emerging fields of research, there is the uncharted danger of creating new life forms, which may irreversibly damage the environment, as it exists today.

Enforcement of Quality Standards for Food and Drugs: There is an increasing expectation and need of the citizenry for efficient enforcement of reasonable quality standards for food and drugs. Recognizing that this policy will make an appropriate policy recommendation on this issue.

Regulation of Standards of Standards in Para Medical Disciplines: It has been observed that a large number of training institutions have mushroomed especially in the private sector for Para medical personnel with various skills- Lab technicians, radio diagnostic technicians, Physiotherapists, etc Currently, there is no regulation or monitoring, either of the curricula of these institutions, of the performance of the practitioners in these fields. This policy will make recommendations to ensure the standardization of such training and the monitoring of actual performance.

Environmental and Occupation Health: The ambient environmental conditions are an important determinant of the health risks to which a community is exposed. Unsafe drinking water, unhygienic sanitation and air pollution significantly contribute to the burden of disease, especially in urban settings. The participants conventionally undertake the initiatives in respect of these environmental factors, whether private or public, in the other growth sectors. Work conditions in many sectors of employment in the country are sub standard. As a resist, workers engaged in such employment become especially vulnerable to occupation-associated ailments. The long-term danger of chronic morbidity is especially marked in the case of child labour.

Providing Medical Facilities to Users from Overseas: The secondary and tertiary facilities available in the country are of good quality and cost effective compared to international medical facilities. This is true not only of facilities in the allopathic fields, but also of those belonging to the alternative systems of medicine, especially Ayurveda.

There are some apprehensions about the possible adverse impact of economic globalization on the health sector. Pharmaceutical drugs and other health services have always been available in the country at extremely inexpensive prices. India has established a reputation around the globe for the innovative growth of original process patents for the manufacture of a wide range of drugs and vaccines within the ambit of the existing patent laws. The address to the future imperatives of health security in the country will be looked after.

Sectoral policy documents are meant to serve as a guide to action for institutions and individual participants operating in that sector. Consistent with this role, NHP2002 limits itself to making recommendations for the participants operating within the health sector.

Population Growth and Health Standards: Efforts made over the years for improving health standards have been partially neutralized by the rapid growth of the population. It is well recognized that population stabilization measures and general health initiatives, when effectively synchronized, synergistically maximize the socio-economic well being of the people. Government has separately announced the National population policy-2000. The main general features covered under the National population policy 2000and NHP2002 relate to the prevention and control of communicable diseases, giving priority to the containment of HIV/Aids infection, the universal immunization of children against all main preventable diseases addressing the unmet need.

Alternative System of Medicine: Under the overarching umbrella of the national health model the alternative systems of medicine- Ayurveda, Unani, Siddha and Homeopathy. Due to the inherent advantages such as diversity, modest cost, low level of technological input and the growing popularity of natural plant based products, these systems are attractive, especially in the underserved, remote and tribal areas. The alternative systems will draw upon the substantial potential of India as one of the eight significant global centres for plant diversity in medicinal and aromatic plants.

NATIONAL MENTAL HEALTH PROGRAMME

The National Mental Health Programme was started in 1982 for providing community based mental health care utilizing the existing public health infrastructure. The WHO report on Global Burden Diseases has projected mental sickness to be the fourth main cause of morbidity. In the Meta analysis of epidemiological studies in India the prevalence rate of mental and behavioural disorder for urban sector is 80.6 percent and rural sector 48.9 percent.

The District Mental Health Programme is a centrally sponsored scheme launched in 1996 and involves extending psychiatric services at the community level. The District Mental Health Programme is currently under implementation in 102 districts throughout the country. The National Mental Health Programme also comprises strengthening of medical college department of psychiatry (under which 70 medical colleges have been covered), modernisation of mental hospitals (under which 23 mental hospitals have been funded), focusing on IEC and public education, research and training. A sum of Rs. 70 crore has been earmarked for implementation of the National Mental Health Programme during the year 2007-08.

Medical ethics examines not only violations of individual integrity in clinical practice but also the sanction that available policies and legislation grant to questionable medical practices. The ethical issues in psychiatry are to be examined in the context of the liaisons between the practices of medical and paramedical institutions, our recent national policy on mental health care and the narrowly construed Mental Health Act (1987) currently in effect.

OBJECTIVES

Current mental health practice in the country is regulated by the National Mental Health Programme (1982) (NMHP). The main objectives of the NMHP are: (i) to ensure availability and accessibility of minimum mental health care for all in the foreseeable future, especially to the most vulnerable and underprivileged sections of the population; (ii) to encourage application of mental health knowledge generally health care and in social growth; (iii) to promote community participation in the mental health service growth and to stimulate efforts towards self- help in the community.

As such, the NMHP is in tune with the Alma Ata Declaration. More importantly, we must also see it as being in line with the politics of health policies in the emerging (third) world order organised mainly by the WHO, with nation states by-and-large relinquishing their welfare functions to private enterprises or to community practice. The salient features of the community package of the NMHP are: (i) tying up mental health care with the existing general health infrastructure, such as the public health centres and the district hospitals, and training the existing staff, (ii) tying up mental health care with already existing community growth programmes and promoting culture friendly cures. Although the NMHP says nothing specific about the use of purely medical techniques like drug therapy and electroconvulsive therapy, it seems to imply that it favours non- invasive techniques of treatment. The NMHP states: 'There is good evidence to say that about 15- 20% of all patients who seek help generally health services both in developed and developing countries, do so for emotional and psychosocial problems. Current medical methods of dealing with these problems by unnecessary investigations and costly medicines are not only inadequate and ineffective but produce widespread frustration to both the seeker and the provider of these health services'.

The NMHP also has a place for the practitioners of the Indian systems of medicine, who should play their 'unique role in the discipline of health. The agenda of the NMHP is then to humanise mental health practice by articulating the 'proper' mental health principles, that is, the principles of community care.

The NMHP has been proclaimed a historical landmark document in our national health policy. Given the fact that we didn't have any document at all till 1982 on mental health policy, this proclamation is excusable. Community care philosophy, which the NMHP embodies, is probably also a more humane alternative for the mentally sick to the highly restrictive and regulative mental hospital services. Nevertheless, the NMHP is at best ineffective, and at worst it promotes the dehumanised models of cure that it explicitly rejects.

MENTAL HEALTH PRACTICE

Mental health practice, like other types of social practices, can be used as tools of social control, because practitioners implicitly or explicitly resource social stereotypes to assess, diagnose and cure. The criteria of cure, such as 'socialisation', 'adaptation', 'becoming socially useful', 'inner happiness' etc., frequently contain moral assumptions, preferred social values and stereotypes. Broverman et. al. showed that psychiatric practice is informed by 'highly consensual norms' about gender stereotypes. Their study showed that the notions of mental health the professionals used were 'more influenced by the greater social value of masculine stereotypic characteristics than by the lesser valued feminine stereotypic characteristics'.

Later studies in the West showed that this trend is probably changing. For instance, clinicians are now reported to show positive attitudes towards homosexuals. Nevertheless, the West has had a long history of feminist and anti- psychiatric dissent and effective social planning altering mainstream consciousness, which we have not had. Till studies are initiated, we can only conjecture about how professionals' attitude would colour their psychiatric evaluations, and consequently, the treatment options for their patients.

All interpersonal negotiations in social practice must inevitably involve the use of stereotypes, increasing one's vulnerability to social control. Choosing to cope with the system of health is already to accept the possibilities and liabilities of such control. This is even more descriptive of health systems that seek to modify human conduct. But whether one retains one's dignity within the system depends on the power one has in these negotiations.

The point of choice one has over what happens to one within the mental health systems arguably reduces with psychotherapy, psychopharmacology, electroconvulsive therapy and psychosurgery, in that order. One has very little lay information about the changes linked with drug use and other body techniques. Often, one experiences irremediable bodily changes, such as tardive dyskinesia, taking place with long term use of neuroleptics or anti- psychotics. The shock of having to cope with a pair of abruptly crippled limbs can be an added trauma to someone already suffering from a intense mental sickness. The sense of betrayal one feels at not having been informed before by her physician of the likely consequences of the drugs she has been utilizing is understandable.

NEED FOR STUDIES

Studies abroad show that the marginalised and the vulnerable (especially women) are more likely to be given more prescriptions for psychoactive drugs. We have no comparable studies of psychoactive drug use patterns in our country. Such a study is a dire need. Prescriptions for drugs may have more to do with the stereotypes that the psychiatrist is processing in his dealings with the patient, rather than any 'objective' knowledge about the healing potential of chemicals.

ELECTRO-CONVULSIVE THERAPY

The use of ECT or 'shock therapy', as it is frequently called, has gone up by 20 times in the last twenty years, as per one study done at KEM Hospital, Bombay. Studies show that ECT is what everybody wants, the professionals as well as the 'close relatives' of the mentally sick. Boral, Bagchi and Nandi reported that an overwhelming 70% of relatives of patients favoured ECT treatment, and an equally large 75% of relatives favoured drug treatment, as against 77% of relatives who were doubtful about the efficiency of psychotherapy. Professionals will swear by the humaneness of the treatment and maintain that it has no long term adverse effects. But cognitive deficits have been consistently associated up with ECT use. And even professionals will admit that the administration of ECT in the country is far from humane. Agarwal in an editorial note, wrote that surveys in the West showed 'remarkable deficiencies' in the administration of ECT. Agarwal warns that 'as a developing country, the situation in India is bound to be more disappointing'. Murthy cautions soberingly against the widespread and unconditional use of ECT in the case of depression and suicide.

Even if one grants that the knowledge base we have on ECT justifies its use, the ethical basis of ECT depends upon how closely the practical conditions of administering ECT conform to several standards of medical care; whether clear diagnostic criteria are practised (not just prescribed in the treatment manuals) in the use of the treatment; and whether informed consent is obtained, and whether such consent comprises information about possible cognitive deficits following ECT. Agarwal, above, in listing the problems about abuse of ECT techniques in the country, notes that the question of patient's consent is rarely looked into by practitioners. The problem, here, as with the prescriptions and use of drugs, is that no information is available.

The NMHP commits itself to non- invasive cures by resourcing 'proper' principles of community care. But it does not specify policies for the use of the medical cures. Even though the policy prescribes generally terms the administrative structure of mental health care through the community, it remains silent on the nature of 'proper' principles and practices. Does the silence on these issues imply a sanction of these widely practised medical cures?

MENTAL HEALTH CARE FOR ALL

The NMHP promises 'availability and accessibility of mental health care for all'. Nevertheless, it prioritises epilepsy, mental retardation and psychoses. This prioritisation takes away all the promised benefits of the policy. These debilities are what are called 'intense' illnesses. Studies show that intense illnesses in the community is of the order of 1%. The frequency of epilepsy, MR and psychoses is probably less than this. There is nevertheless, a whole range of psychological problems (developmental, psycho-social, etc.) which contribute to the other 10 to 15% recorded as morbidity rate in Indian communities. Especially among the vulnerable sections of society, such as the elderly, the women, people in cultural or geographic transition, disaster struck people, the divorced, widowed, etc., the morbidity rate of the general mental disorders is very high. Thus the NMHP limits itself to only a very small target population by prioritising the intense mental disorders.

More significantly, the use of the medical models- drug therapy or ECT for cure is almost inevitable in the case of these sickness. In treating psychotic disorders, mental retardation or epilepsy, a practitioner is almost never called upon to invent non- invasive techniques or forms of psychotherapy. If drug use or ECT can be justified at all, it is justified all the more easily in the case of these endogenous types of mental disorders than other general types. So even though the NMHP seems to pledge its philosophy on the side of non- invasive and community close techniques, it prioritises illnesses in such a way that the use of medical models of cure is inevitable.

There are of course economic reasons for the studied ineffectiveness of the NMHP to serve community needs. Covertly adopting the medical model ensures that no additional resources are spent on mental health. The very terms of the NMHP state this quite emphatically.

APPROACHES

The NMHP has been designed to have the following approaches:

- Integration of the mental health care service with the existing general health services;
- To utilise the existing infrastructure of health services and also to deliver the minimum mental health care services;
- To furnish appropriate task oriented training to the existing health staff;
- To link mental health services with the existing community growth programme.

The design of the programme is such that we make do with existing infrastructure and personnel, ensuring that no extra expenditure is incurred in implementing the mental health programme. The medical practitioners can be 'trained' to address mental health issues also, and also the PHC staffers. Psychotherapy, which works in the more frequent general disorders, calls for expert training, institutional and organisational investments. If the state wanted to implement the mental health policy in principle, it would call for to spend much more than if it simply associated up mental health with existing health facilities. This attitude to minimize resources spent on mental health care is completely consistent with the recent trends of the dimunition of state funding for health care generally.

Thus, even though the NMHP openly proclaims a community care philosophy, it works by prioritisations which will ensure that the medical model will persist, also ensuring that no additional costs will be expended for mental health care. By remaining silent on the nature of treatment options to be made available in community care, it does not call into question or debate the widespread medical models of mental health cure.

MENTAL HEALTH TEAM

Mental health teams can help people with a mental health sickness live in the community with support. This could be on a day-to-day basis or support at times when an individual may need it. These teams may comprise:

- Social workers
- Community mental health nurses
- Occupational therapists
- Psychiatrists
- Psychologists
- Counsellors
- Community support workers, like home helps for instance

Community mental health teams can take care of your health and social needs.

Care co-ordinators: If someone has different elements to care, for instance then the patient can see a psychiatrist, counsellor, physician and social worker, where he or she may have access to a care co-ordinator, sometimes known as a keyworker or case manager.

This person will talk to all the different professionals and be a single person for patient to talk to and support the patient. Care co-ordinator will be a member of the community mental health team and will draw up a care plan with the patient. The patient should be given a copy of your care plan.

Community mental health nurses: Community mental health nurses are registered nurses who are trained in mental health and can:

- Talk to the patient about ways to cope
- Give long-term support to the patient in the community
- Give some medication

Community mental health nurses can specialise in working with older people, children or people with drug or alcohol problems.

Counsellors: Counsellors furnish a 'talking therapy' where the patient will be invited to talk about his or her thoughts and feelings; the counsellor will then discuss with the patient ways of coping. Counselling can also be provided by:

- Community mental health nurses
- Psychotherapists
- Psychologists
- Social workers
- Occupational therapists

There is in general a waiting list for counselling services on the National Health Service (NHS) but there are voluntary organisations that also offer talking treatments - the patient should ask his physician (GP) or community mental health team for details.

Health visitors: Health visitors are qualified nurses with specialist training who work in the community. They help people with a mental sickness to continue to live in their home. Health visitors can:

- Help you stay healthy by talking to you about diet and exercise
- Be someone to talk to
- Offer practical advice about food, hygiene and day-to-day living
- Tell the patient about other services that may be useful to him.

NATURE AND SCOPE OF MENTAL HEALTH NURSING

Psychiatric nursing or mental health nursing is the speciality of nursing that cares for people of all ages with mental sickness or mental distress, such as schizophrenia, bipolar disorder, psychosis, depression or dementia. Nurses in this field receive additional training in psychological therapies, building a therapeutic alliance, dealing with challenging behaviour, and the administration of psychiatric medication.

As with other fields of nursing practice, psychiatric mental health nursing works within nursing models, using nursing care plans, and seeks to care for the whole person. Nevertheless, the emphasis of mental health nursing is on the growth of a therapeutic relationship or alliance. In practice, this means that the nurse should seek to engage with the person in care in a positive and collaborative manner that empowers them to draw on their inner resources in addition to any other treatment they may be receiving. Growth of the therapeutic relationship can be challenging, not just because of the nature of the person's mental sickness or distress, but also because the person may be detained in a psychiatric hospital and be receiving treatment against their will under mental health law.

ROLE AND FUNCTIONS OF MENTAL HEALTH NURSE IN VARIOUS SETTINGS

The need for psychiatric mental health nursing has its roots near the end of the 19th century when it was believed that patients in mental hospitals should receive nursing care. Psychiatric mental health nursing has since come a long way, with psychiatric-mental health content incorporated into all diploma and baccalaureate nursing programs. As new needs for services developed in the health care arena, the role and function of the psychiatric-mental health nurse expanded, leading to modern practice registered nurses in psychiatric-mental health nursing. Psychiatric-mental health nurses are a rich resource as providers of psychiatric-mental health services and patient care partners for the consumers of those services.

The clinical practice of psychiatric nursing occurs at two levels - basic and advanced. At the basic level, registered nurses work with people, families, groups, and communities to assess mental health needs, develop diagnoses, and plan, implement, and assess nursing care. Basic level nursing practice characterized by interventions that promote and foster health, assess dysfunction, assist patients to regain or improve their coping abilities, and prevent further disability. These interventions concentrate on psychiatric-mental health patients and comprise health promotion, preventive management of a therapeutic environment; assisting patient with selfcare activities; administering and monitoring psychobiological treatment regimens; health teaching; together with psychoeducation; crisis intervention and counselling and case management.

Registered nurses who seek additional education and obtain a masters or doctoral degree can become advanced practice nurses in the specialty. After post-master's supervised clinical practice, they can become certified as specialists in adult, or child and adolescent psychiatric-mental health nursing. In addition to the functions performed at the basic level, these advanced practice nurses assess, diagnose, and treat psychiatric disorders and potential mental health problems. They furnish the full range of primary mental health care services to people, families, groups and communities, function as psychotherapists, and in some states they have the authority to prescribe medications. Psychiatric-mental health nurses in advanced practices are qualified to practice independently to offer direct care services in settings such as agencies, communities, homes, hospitals, and offices. Some psychiatric-mental health clinical nurse specialists practice consultation/liaison nursing, delivering mental health services to physically sick patients or consultation to staff generally medical settings. Due to their broad background in biological, pharmacological, sociological, and psychological sciences, psychiatric-mental health nurses are a rich resource as providers of psychiatric-mental health services and patient care partners for the consumers of those services.

FACTORS AFFECTING THE LEVEL OF NURSING PRACTICE

Historically, research into problematic work environments has centred on levels of stress experienced by employees, since the mid 1970's, burnout, in various occupations has been the topic of several research projects. One occupation that has not been extensively researched but that indicated a high level of burnout was nursing. Many studies have concluded that health care staff are more prone to experience an increased incidence of stress and depression related to workplace experiences than are those in other occupations.

Murray and Snyder (1991) noted that nurses experience a range of complications related to workplace assaults together with physical, social, family, and emotional reactions. Following critical workplace incidents, psychiatric nurses have been found to manifest avoidance behaviours with family and others as well as to withdraw from severe relationships. Also, they experience a heightened sense of anger and vulnerability and tend to subsequently view the world as unpredictable and unjust.

Patient suicide and violence against psychiatric staff have been recognized as contributing factors to the types of behavioural and cognitive changes seen in post- traumatic stress disorder. These changes affect the capability of individual nurses to function both in and out of the workplace. The long term implications are burnout and dysfunctional conducts resulting in compromised patient care and increased conflicts between psychiatric nurses and their families and co-workers. Eventually, several people may develop symptomatology indicating elevated levels of both PTSD and depression further compromising professional and personal relationships.

Another compounding factor is the level to which secondary or vicarious traumatic stress impacts on psychiatric staff, claims that secondary traumatic stress is a response of the initial, or primary, victim that generates a resulting secondary response in the caregiver. Anxiety and depression are generally recognized reactions to such stress. Valet further proposes that care givers attempt to nullify their reactions through survival strategies.

A study of ambulance personnel who were exposed to critical incidents revealed that approximately one third had symptoms of burnout and PTSD culminating in lower job satisfaction. This type of level was also observed in personnel working in other jobs where trauma exposure is not unusual such as firefighting, emergency room nursing, police work, military combat and military nursing.

DEMOGRAPHIC AND PERSONALITY FACTORS

A number of demographic variables have been found to be predictors of stress and depression in psychiatric nurses. Gender, which has frequently been identified as playing a significant role in the rate of occurrence of various types of psychopathology, has also surfaced as a factor in disorders in psychiatric nurses. Female psychiatric nurses exhibit slightly more psychological distress than male psychiatric nurses. Females generally also exhibit a greater prevalence of PTSD than males in virtually all studies. An exception was a meta-analysis of a military sample which found no important difference between genders as a risk factors for developing PTSD.

Psychopathology if left untreated may have serious consequences for the affected individual regardless of gender. For instance, even though nurses generally are reported as being at higher risk for suicide, there is no difference in numbers of attempted suicides between the sexes.

Low levels of personality hardiness and self-esteem have also been found to be predictors of both anxiety and depression. Personality hardiness is described as the inter-relatedness of three factors practiced by the individual in their lifestyle: control of environment, commitment to self-fulfilling goals and reasonable levels of challenge in daily life. These traits serve as buffers and seem to protect the individual from the psychological repercussions of stress.

Other studies utilizing personality scales have examined the function of personal disposition in psychological symptomatology. The personality trait of neuroticism has been positively correlated with increased levels of numerous psychiatric pathologies together with physical and psychological distress, anxiety, depression, and PTSD. Piedmont (1993), using the Maslach Burnout Inventory, found that emotional exhaustion and depersonalization are strongly correlated with neuroticism and may predispose the individual to burnout. High scores on neuroticism have also been reported to intensify the individual's perception of psychological and physical symptoms.

WORK ENVIRONMENT

Some of the factors which influence workers level of stress are: the environment itself, interpersonal relationships, level of employer responsibility for a positive work environment, and availability of support programs for employees. Moreover, work related stress in hospital nurses was found to increase both the reported incidence of emotional exhaustion reports of poorer health.

Cooper's (1995) meta analysis identified employer reactions to critical incidents such as psychiatric patient suicide and assault of psychiatric staff as key in facilitating or impeding the integration of the incident. The employer frequently failed to furnish support on behalf of employees when, for instance, psychiatric nurses face a suicide on the ward. Institutional reactions comprise panic, denial, and the blaming of staff victims for incidents such as assault. Even though the staff member involved may react by manifesting PTSD symptoms, the employer compounds the problem through their reaction. A further difficulty arises when staff attempt to deal with such incidents themselves and to preserve a good worldview and sense of personal invulnerability. This psychological coping can lead to a tendency to "blame the victims" and in incidents of assaults "the victims blame themselves." Lack of management support and role problems are serious considerations within the hospital milieu.

CONCEPTS OF NORMAL AND ABNORMAL BEHAVIOUR

Abnormality is an elusive concept. It does not conform to statistical or normative criteria for abnormality, and may differ in social groups and cultures. Its traditional nature can lead to bias in psychiatric diagnosis. It is regarded as to be one of the main problems in dealing with diagnosis and classification to actually define what is normal in order to define what is not. Nevertheless, there are several factors involved in a definition of 'normality', e.g. social and cultural norms and a satisfactory model has not yet been established.

There are no plain solutions to distinguishing between normal and abnormal conduct, and though there are quite a few methods of trying to establish abnormality, no single method is 'foolproof'.

Frequently, a decision about whether or not an individual's conduct is abnormal depends on a series of value judgements based on subjective impressions, and it must be remembered that, unlike in other branches of medicine, there are normally no tests or exploratory operations to guide the clinician in making a diagnosis. Basically, there are in general restrictions in definitions of normality.

In the following, some main approaches to definitions will be summarised and briefly evaluated. Some of the criteria mentioned to define abnormality are the following: the mental health criterion, abnormality as personal distress, the statistical criterion, abnormality as mental sickness etc.

Definitions of 'normality' are part of the diagnostic process, and this is why it is regarded as to be significant to establish some objective criteria. Another issue related to this is the debate about whether mental illnesses have somatogenic or psychogenic origins. No matter what, several uncertainties remain about how to best define dysfunctional conduct in terms of abnormality. At present, there is a tendency to rely on a combination of the criteria, each of limited value, and on the subjective assessments of clinicians in combination with the diagnostic tools of classification systems.

DEFINITION OF NORMAL BEHAVIOUR

1. The usual
2. Not sick
3. Operating as intended
4. Conforming to a cultural norm and
5. The best.

DEFINITION OF ABNORMAL BEHAVIOUR

Clinical psychologists diagnose and treat mental disorders. These comprise anxiety and mood disorders like depression and obsessive-compulsive disorder, eating disorders like anorexia nervosa, and psychotic disorders like schizophrenia. In all cases, people's conduct goes beyond the acceptable norms of society and appears to be maladaptive, that is, likely to be damaging to themselves or others.

DISTINGUISHING NORMAL FROM ABNORMAL

Mental disorders are frequently difficult to diagnose, because several symptoms are part of normal conduct. For instance, several people show symptoms of depression in response to the death of a loved one, but this is an expectable reaction. The psychologist must make a judgement as to the severity of symptoms and how long they have prevailed. A disorder would only be diagnosed if an individual showed no voluntary control over their feelings or conduct. So a political prisoner who deliberately goes on hunger strike would not be diagnosed as anorexic.

BIOLOGICAL EXPLANATIONS OF MENTAL DISORDER

In their research, clinical psychologists try to establish what causes mental disorders. Some emphasise biological factors that lead to brain dysfunction. These comprise genetic predispositions to mental sickness, as with schizophrenia, but also damage to the brain caused by accidents or by toxins like alcohol. Some disorders with a biological cause can be treated with drugs. For instance, the drug clozapine is used to reduce the symptoms of schizophrenia by inhibiting excessive production of dopamine and other transmitters in the brain.

THE VALUE OF 'TALKING CURES'

Not all mental disorders have plain biological causes, and researchers must also consider the personal history of people in the search for causes and treatments. There are several different kinds of so-called "talking cures", but all therapies have the aim of overcoming maladaptive ways of thinking and behaving. It has been found that about 75% of people improve when given some form of therapy.

CLASSIFICATION

There are seven elements - any of which would be indicative of potentially abnormal conduct:

- Psychological suffering
- Maladaptiveness of conduct patterns
- Irrationality and incomprehensibility
- Unpredictability and loss of control
- Vividness and unconventionality
- Observer discomfort
- Violation of moral and ideal standards

1. Abnormality as defined above is a social judgement.
2. Encourages idea that the person is flawed, rather than their conduct.
3. Elements of conduct highly dependent on context.

Symptom classification scheme based on

- Clinical interview
- Psychological testing
- Observation
- Physiological examination

Diagnostic and Statistical Manual of Mental Disorders

(DSM-V)

- Axes I and II Classification of abnormal behaviour
- Axis III Physiological disorders relevant to psychological ones
- Axis IV Type and severity of psycho-social stress
- Axis V Clinical judgement of patient's highest level of adaptive functioning during the previous year, i.e. Cumulative picture of patient's current state, taking into account nature of symptoms, environmental circumstances, context and personal history.

Problems Associated with the Use of the DSM

- Individual differences in what is regarded as 'abnormal' and society's norms will differ over the years.
- Observers/clinicians will differ in assessment of any given behaviour, and the behaviours will differ in terms of the symptoms which present.
- Discrete 'states' of listed features fosters false impression of discontinuity between normal and abnormal.
- Loss of information relevant to uniqueness of person and their problem
- Classification which may stigmatize individual and encourage inflexible view of psychotic condition.

Benefits of DSM

- Symptom classification provides key to cause and potential treatment

- Label releases patient from conviction that they are flawed and that the problem is incurable.

1. Cultural Differences
   - How people express disturbance and what they do about it
   - Personal inadequacy vs. family dishonour
   - Treatment
   - Helpseeking
   - Role of social group/family

   Failure to recognize cultural differences may lead to
   - Bias in clinical judgement
   - Bias in test and assessment procedures
   - Bias in research
2. Sex Differences
   - Bias in diagnostic system e.g., inclusion of Late Luteal Phase Dysphoric Disorder
   - Bias in clinician's use of labels
   - Bias in methods of evaluation
   - Bias in sampling
3. Causal factors which have been considered in attempts to explain abnormal behaviour

1. Biological Causes
   - Neurotransmitter imbalance/Hormonal imbalance
   - Genetic inheritance
   - Influence of genotype on environment
   - Chromosomal abnormalities
   - Constitutional liabilities
   - Gross brain damage
   - Physical deprivation/disruption
2. Psychosocial Causes
   - Schemas and self-schemas
   - Inadequate parenting
   - Early deprivation or trauma
   - Pathogenic family structures
   - Maladaptive peer relationships

3. Sociocultural Causes
   - Sociocultural inheritance
   - Low socioeconomic status
   - Prejudice and discrimination
   - Economic/employment problems
   - Social change and uncertainty

CURRENT MODELS OF ABNORMAL BEHAVIOUR

There are quite a few different ways in which it is possible to define 'abnormal' as opposed to our ideas of what is 'normal'. One way is the statistical methodology which is based on the premise that abnormal behaviour is statistically rare. For instance anxiety can be assessed utilizing Spielberger's State-Trait Anxiety Inventory. The mean score for trait anxiety is 40 and people who achieve over 55 are seen as statistically rare as only 1 in 50 score that high.

Thus those with high scores are seen as deviant from the greater bulk of the population. The statistical methodology helps to address what is meant by normal in a statistical context, but it still does not help us define the term. There are several people who have high levels of anxiety, but would still not be categorised as clinically abnormal - it is also equally true that people with very low scores on the anxiety scale are also statistically abnormal!

Social Deviance is emphasised by some psychologists as a measure of abnormal conduct. This methodology would see people who act in a socially deviant way that makes other people uncomfortable should be considered abnormal. Nevertheless there are problems inherent in this methodology. For example German citizens who objected to and spoke out against Nazi atrocities were seen as being socially deviant. It is also true to say that what is considered deviant varies from culture to culture. Kwakiutl Indians burn valuable blankets in order to cast shame on their enemies, conduct that would seem decidedly odd in Western culture.

So far both the approaches discussed only tell us a little about what we mean by 'abnormal'. Abnormality is a complex concept that is difficult to define precisely. Abnormality can take several different forms and there is no single feature that can help us distinguish abnormality from normality. Rosenhan and Seligman (1989) propose seven main features of abnormality that appear in abnormal conduct as opposed to normal conduct. The more of these features that are possessed by the individual, the more likely they are to be regarded as abnormal.

Rosenhan and Seligman's seven Features

- Suffering: Most abnormal people (such as those suffering with anxiety disorders) report that they are suffering. Nevertheless normal people can suffer at times in their lives and some abnormal people, such as those with personality disorders, treat others badly but don't appear to suffer themselves
- Maladaptiveness: Maladaptive behaviour is behaviour that prevents a person from achieving main life goals; from having fulfilling relationships with others or working effectively (for example an agrophobic will not venture out of the house because of fear).
- Vividness and unconventionality: Vivid and unconventional conduct is relatively unusual. It is conduct that differs substantially from the way in which you would expect normal people to act in similar situations. Nevertheless there are several people who act in this way that are not deemed to be abnormal.
- Unpredictability and loss of control: With most people, you normally predict what they will do in known situations. In contrast, abnormal conduct is frequently highly unpredictable and uncontrolled and inappropriate for the situation.
- Irrationality and incomprehensibility: One of the characteristics of abnormal conduct is that there appears to be no good reason why the person should choose to act in that way.
- Observer discomfort: Our social conduct is governed by a number of unspoken rules about conduct, such as the way we maintain eye contact or personal space. When others break these rules we experience discomfort. But this does not necessarily indicate abnormal conduct, for example different cultures may well have different social rules about conduct.
- Violation of moral and ideal standards: When moral standards are violated, this conduct may be judged to be abnormal
- One of the problems with utilizing the seven features of abnormality is that they rely on subjective judgements and it can be quite difficult to decide which of the features are actually present in an individual's conduct. One family may try to commit an elderly relative due to eccentric behaviour which other people may find harmless.

THE DIAGNOSTIC STATISTICAL MANUAL OF MENTAL DISORDERS

(DSM-III-R) is employed by psychiatrists to help diagnose mental disorders. It tries to distinguish between social deviance or nonconformity and mental disorder or abnormality stating: Neither deviant behaviour, e.g. political, religious or sexual, nor conflicts that are mainly between the individual and society are mental disorders unless the deviance or condition is a symptom of a dysfunction (i.e. impairment of function) in the person.

Categorisation of Mental Disorders

Most psychiatrists and clinical psychologists accept that abnormality exists and that those people who exhibit abnormal symptoms should receive a diagnosis that labels the specific abnormality. This helps determine the appropriate form of treatment. This view has had a number of critics over the years, for example Scheff (1966) argued that this form of labelling could actually create part of the symptoms.

The Diathesis-stress Approach

This approach is a general model that argues that any mental disorder happens as a joint function of a pre-disposition towards the disorder (or diathesis) and stress. Thus an individual with a high diathesis or predisposition would need less stress to react in an abnormal way.

REFERENCES

Baly, M. (1982). A leading light. Nursing Mirror, 155(19), 49–51.

Doona, M. (1984). At least well cared for . . . Linda Richards and the mentally ill. Image, 16(2), 51–56.

Gollaher, D. (1995). Voice for the mad: The life of Dorothea Dix. New York: The Free Press.

Haugland, G., Siegel, C., Hopper, K., & Alexander, M. J. (1997). Mental illness among homeless individuals in a suburban county. Psychiatric Services, 48(4), 504–509.

Lamb, H. R., & Bachrach, L. L. (2001). Some perspectives on deinstitutionalization. Psychiatric Services, 52(8), 1039–1045.

Lamb, H. R., & Weinberger, L. E. (1998). Persons with severe mental illness in jails and prisons: A review. Psychiatric Services, 49(4), 483–492.

McMillan, I. (1997). Insight into Bedlam: One hospital's history. Journal of Psychosocial Nursing, 3(6), 28–34.

Mellow, J. (1986). A personal perspective of nursing therapy. Hospital and Community Psychiatry, 37(2), 182–183.

Mohr, W. K. (2003). Johnson's psychiatric-mental health nursing: Adaptation and growth (5th ed.). Philadelphia: Lippincott Williams & Wilkins. National Institute of Mental Health (NIMH). (2002).

Ries, R. (1997). Advantages of separating the triage function from the emergency service. Psychiatric Services, 48(6), 755–756.

Rosenblatt, A. (1984). Concepts of the asylum in the care of the mentally ill. Hospital and Community Psychiatry, 35, 244–250.

2

Principles and Concepts of Mental Health Nursing

Mental health and mental sickness are difficult to define precisely. People who can carry out their roles in society and whose behaviour is appropriate and adaptive are viewed as healthy. Conversely those who fail to fulfil roles and carry out duties or whose behaviour is inappropriate are viewed as sick. The culture of any society strongly influences its values and beliefs, and this in turn affects how that society defines health and sickness. What one society may view as acceptable and appropriate, another society may see as maladaptive or inappropriate.

DEFINITION: MENTAL HEALTH NURSING

Mental Health Nursing encompasses autonomous and collaborative care of people of all ages, families, groups and communities, sick or well and in all settings. Nursing comprises the promotion of health, prevention of sickness, and the care of sick, disabled and dying people. Advocacy, promotion of a safe environment, research, participation in shaping health policy and in patient and health systems management, and education are also key nursing roles.

Mental health nursing encompasses an identification and treatment of those problems that occur as a result of human reactions to an actual or potential menace posed to an individual's mental health. This branch of nursing has developed into a specialized field of practice, employing the use of various theories about human behaviour and the learned skill of therapeutic intervention. Mental health care providers have met numerous challenges in their effort to furnish a vision of wellness for those with mental sickness and to increase public awareness of its existence. Historically, the journey to furnish this humane and therapeutic methodology to those with mental alterations has been a difficult one.

CLASSIFICATION OF MENTAL DISORDERS

The classification of mental disorders, also known as psychiatric nosology or taxonomy, is a key aspect of psychiatry and other mental health professions and a significant issue for consumers and providers of mental health services. There are currently two widely established systems for classifying mental sickness - Chapter V of the International Classification of Diseases (ICD-10) produced by the World Health Organization (WHO) and the Diagnostic and Statistical Manual of Mental Disorders (DSM-IV) produced by the American Psychiatric Association (APA). Both list classes of disorders thought to be distinct types, and have deliberately converged their codes in recent revisions so that the manuals are frequently broadly comparable, though important differences remain. Other classification schemes may be in use more locally, for instance the Chinese Classification of Mental Disorders. Other manuals are used by those of alternative theoretical persuasions, such as the Psychodynamic Diagnostic Manual. In general there is an important scientific debate about the relative merits of a categorical system or a dimensional system (also known as a continuum or spectrum system), as well as important controversy about the function of science and values in classification schemes and the professional, legal and social uses to which they are put.

INTERNATIONAL CLASSIFICATION OF DISEASES

The International Classification of Diseases (ICD) is an international standard diagnostic classification for a wide variety of health conditions. Chapter V focuses on "mental and behavioural disorders" and consists of 10 main groups:

- F0: Organic, together with symptomatic, mental disorders
- F1: Mental and behavioural disorders because of use of psychoactive substances
- F2: Schizophrenia, schizotypal and delusional disorders
- F3: Mood [affective] disorders
- F4: Neurotic, stress-related and somatoform disorders
- F5: Behavioural syndromes linked with physiological disturbances and physical factors
- F6: Disorders of personality and behaviour in adult individuals
- F7: Mental retardation
- F8: Disorders of psychological growth

- F9: Behavioural and emotional disorders with onset normally taking place in childhood and adolescence
- Unspecified mental disorders

Within each group there are more specific subcategories. The ICD comprises personality disorders on the same domain as other mental disorders, unlike the DSM. The ICD-10 states that mental disorder is "not an exact term", though is in general used ".to imply the existence of a clinically recognisable set of symptoms or behaviours linked in most cases with distress and with interference with personal functions."

PERSONALITY DEFENCE MECHANISMS

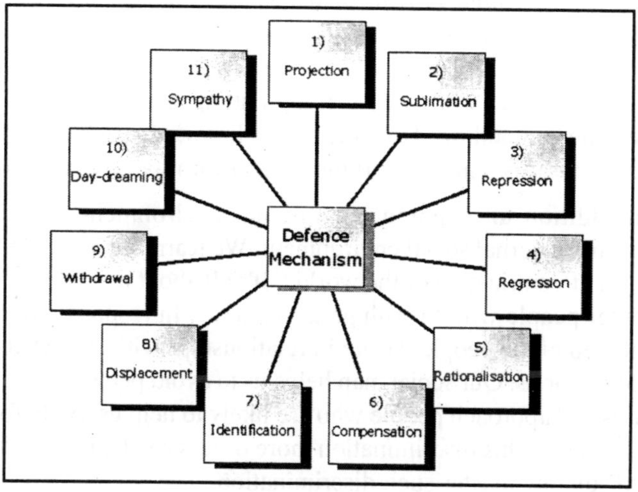

Fig. Personality Defence Mechanisms

Personality defences (coping techniques, defence mechanisms) are significant things in that they strongly influence the ease with which people are able to form and maintain healthy relationships and reject unhealthy relationships. Developing organically in response to frustrating, difficult and painful situations and experiences, they function as the human equivalent of a computer firewall, helping to defend against hurtful and abusive relationships, while hopefully also permitting healthy and nurturing relationships to pass. Discriminating when to be defensive and when not to be defensive is key for health.

MAPPING THE WORLD AND THE SELF

Becoming defensive is all about learning to identify and avoid painful and dangerous situations. We are born mostly open and undefended. We learn to avoid painful and dangerous situations by learning to map or represent (in our heads, not on paper) the world and where the dangerous, painful things exist in the world. We start doing this even as very young children and continue it with ever increasing sophistication as we mature. As our representation of the world becomes more sophisticated, our capability to control, tolerate or avoid pain also becomes likewise sophisticated.

The first pains we become aware of are internal - having to do with instinctual drives such as hunger, elimination and emotion. These drives create worries in our infant bodies that over time we learn to represent and react to. For instance, we instinctually cry when we are hungry but probably can not initially distinguish the pain of hunger from other pains. Over time we learn to recognize and represent hunger pains as a distinct sort of painful signal that can be avoided by eating. More time goes by and we learn to request food, thereby cutting hunger pains off before they become compelling. This sort of self-knowledge and control is easy for adults, but it is a major learning project for infants and toddlers.

In addition to mapping our internal environment, we also start mapping our external social environment. We learn, for example, that our initial infant-centric map of the world ("It's all about me") doesn't predict what other people will do with great accuracy. In response, we develop a social map of the people we are in relationships with and what they are likely to do for us. Our social map helps us to avoid people who are likely to hurt us and approach people who are likely to help us. As before, most adults can make this discrimination more or less easily, but children take years to suitably master such discrimination.

The level to which representation or mapping of the self and the social world takes place is always in relationship with an individual's developmental level. Infants and young children (who are not very developed, physically or mentally) have representations of the self and of others that are more primitive, while older children and adults tend to have more sophisticated self and other representations. An individual's developmental level is influenced both by biology and by experience. Children act in childlike ways both because they are inexperienced, and because their brains are literally immature and not fully physically developed. The biological facets of children's brain growth work themselves out by the teen years, and thereafter (assuming everything else has gone well), further growth and maturity is mostly a function of experience and personality. Not everyone is able to benefit from experience, nevertheless. Most everyone has probably met someone chronologically adult who functions to one level or another in an immature, child-like and primitive way.

All people are motivated to avoid (or at least control) pain (physical and psychological both), and they do this by developing representations of themselves and their world that help them to predict when pain will occur. People use these personal representations of self and world to come up with a stable of strategies for avoiding pain. Such strategies (like the representations they are based on) start out primitive and flawed and tend to become more sophisticated, functional and adaptive as maturity occurs. At each stage of growth people use their representations of self and other to cope as best they can. As people age and mature more sophisticated means of coping tend to be developed and older, less sophisticated and less effective means of coping tend to be discarded. At least, this is what happens in theory. In reality, several people get stuck, fail to move past specific developmental milestones in specific fields of their lives, and to not develop more effective means of coping in those several fields. While they will have aged chronologically and may even function as adults in most facets of their lives (holding down a job, being responsible, etc.), they may also show surprisingly child-like and primitive means of coping when stressed.

Mental health professionals differ on what to call these personality defences. Psychoanalyst types (followers of Freud & company) have tended to call them 'defence mechanisms', emphasizing the more primitive and less functional means of coping people have come up with. Other writers refer to 'coping methods' and tend to emphasize the more functional, sophisticated and effective means of coping that people use.

MORE PRIMITIVE DEFENCES

The most primitive (or developmentally early) defence strategies are frequently predicated on a mistaken or inaccurate representation of social reality - which is the major reason why we call them 'primitive'. Although they may work to some extent as a means of avoiding short term pain, they also in general don't normally result in constructive outcomes and aren't much help to someone looking for ways to resolve problems. As a class, they are likely to be the defences that are present during early childhood, and which may prevail in adults who were harmed in some important way during childhood.

Dissociation is the term given to a condition where memories and attention become unnaturally disconnected. Under normal conditions, people's memory and attention are fairly integrated and continuous (meaning that an individual can move between memories without any trouble and that they are able to remember where they began and the route they took to get to a specific thought. In contrast, dissociated memories are isolated from each other with no clear association between them that leads from thought to thought. A several amount of dissociation is normal; everyone dissociates to one level or another even if it is just occasional forgetfulness. Nevertheless, some people have a talent for dissociation, and they use it as a way of coping with emotion. In extreme cases, important disorders based entirely on dissociative processes (such as what used to be called Multiple Personality Disorder, fugues, or amnesia) can occur. More generally, nevertheless, dissociation figures as a process upon which other defences form.

A case in point is Splitting, which is said to be taking place when positive and negative representations of self and other are dissociated from one another inside an individual's mind. It is frequently related to early abuse and appears to be a mechanism by which people can preserve some semblance of happiness in the face of very negative experiences. Unlike people with more integrated self and other representations who can represent people's complexity (their capability to have both good and bad facets at once), people with split representations struggle with highly polarized "black or white, but not gray" views of others and self. They may substantially devalue someone for what others would consider minor failings, or unrealistically idealize someone else, perhaps expecting that person to save them.

In Projection people come to believe that other people are experiencing the feeling that they themselves have. This doesn't happen with all feelings, but rather, with feelings that are regarded as inappropriate or otherwise unacceptable. Owning that one feels an unacceptable feeling would be painfully anxiety-provoking, and defences are all about avoiding pain, remember? Anger is often projected onto other people, for instance, as several people have a hard time acknowledging that they are angry.

Projection involves a failure to appropriately distinguish between representations of self and other, and as such, represents a bit of a break with reality. Though an individual's feeling is identified, it is inaccurately identified as originating inside a separate person, rather than being correctly identified as originating within the self. People make a very similar mistake in Reaction Formation, wherein people react strongly to their own unacknowledged desires by acting to suppress or even destroy those desires in others (all the while denying that they themselves have those desires).

Acting Out occurs when an individual who is otherwise unable to articulate their feelings, acts those feelings out in a directly impulsive manner. Performing the acted out actions serves as a pressure release and in some way calms or reassures the actor, even if the actions are incomprehensible to outside observers. Self-mutilation ('cutting'), explosive tempers and abusive actions can fall into this class.

Denial is perhaps the most famous of the classical defence mechanisms, in part because it was a significant concept as taught by Freud, but also because is has been emphasized by addiction recovery communities. In denial, an individual simply refuses to accept that something which is true is in fact true. Examples of denial are legion and differ with regard to the depth of reality distortion present. Examples of greater reality distortion comprise the alcoholic who denies she has a drinking problem, and the battered wife who can't make the connection that her life is in danger. Examples of lessor reality distortion comprise the lover who doesn't pick up on the subtle signs that his relationship is breaking apart.

IN-BETWEEN DEFENCES

'In-Between' defences also play to some extent fast and lose with social reality, but far less so than the primitive defences (or in a less destructive manner). They are not necessarily constructive in nature, but utilizing them probably won't make problems worse. Adults use these defences all the time, but they're nothing necessarily to be proud about.

The concept of Repression has a history. Originally, Freud thought of it as a sort of force holding uncomfortable thoughts beneath the surface of consciousness. Although such 'repressed' thoughts wouldn't rise into awareness, they would motivate behaviour in round-about ways. The term Suppression has a similar but more voluntary meaning; where people are never conscious of repressed thoughts, suppressed thoughts are consciously pushed out of consciousness by people who decided they simply didn't want to think about them.

More recently, the same term Repression has been used to describe a coping style designed to reduce anxiety by way of avoiding information that might provoke anxiety. An opposite conception, Sensitization, describes an anxiety coping strategy in which a nervous person seeks out more and more information, regardless of how anxiety provoking it might be, so that a more complete menace picture might be obtained.

Displacement is the classic "kicking the dog" defence. An individual is upset about something they can't control (such as a boss' bad review), and takes that upset out on something that they can control (the dog), in effect displacing their upset feeling, in the process, transforming their psychological position from one of powerless humiliation to dominant control.

In Intellectualization, people deal with painful or anxiety producing events by retreating into a cognitive analysis of the event, in so doing, creating a sort of insulating distance from the emotions surrounding the event. A very similar manoeuvre, Rationalization, occurs when people make up reasons post-hoc (after the fact) to explain away a course of action they have taken that they feel conflicted about.

Where Intellectualization and Rationalization use inventive thought to buffer painful emotion, Undoing uses compensatory behaviours to attain the same end. In Undoing, conflicted actions and motives that one may or may not be conscious of are counteracted by other 'atoning' actions that, on the whole, attempt to balance things out.

MATURE DEFENCES

The 'mature' defence strategies are based on a pretty solid and accurate understanding of social reality, and tend to be more constructive and adaptive in nature than their younger cousins. Utilizing them may work to correct underlying problems rather than just gloss them over. Although helpful, they are difficult for people stuck in more primitive defensive modes to appreciate and engage.

Sublimation occurs when people consciously redirect energies away from unacceptable impulses and put them to productive use. While Freud originally had in mind the substitution of art work for deviant sexual urges, the strategy is far more flexible than that. Sublimation is in operation, for instance, when a student grieving an important loss pours her energy into school and pulls straight A's.

A number of mature defences work by helping people to gain perspective on their problems. Humour works well to break up negativity, to inject silliness and laughter into what is otherwise serious and deathly, and to force people to look at a brighter side of their various predicaments. Humour simultaneously distracts (permitting distance from seriousness) and instructs.

Affiliation, or the drive to socialize with others so as to benefit from their company and counsel, is probably not a proper defence, but it is a perfect offensive strategy for effective coping with anxiety and pain. Being with others provides opportunities for venting, distraction, reality testing and a host of other helpful emotional supports. Self-Observation (such as through journaling) is an alternative to seeking out others that offers some of the same benefits, together with venting of feelings, distancing and increased perspective.

Assertiveness is a communication posture that exists between aggressiveness and passivity. Passive postured people allow others to invade them, while aggressive postured people invade other people. Assertive postured people defend themselves against the invasions of aggressive people, but don't themselves become aggressive and invade others - not even those who try to invade them. Assertiveness seems plain enough, but actually calls for considerable finesse, self-confidence and a healthy and accurate understanding of social dynamics to function, unlike passivity and aggressiveness which don't call for a whole lot of thought.

DEFENSIVENESS, MATURITY AND RELATIONSHIPS

In reading through this brief and incomplete survey of the spectrum of defensive coping strategies you have hopefully picked up on the way relationship skills correlate with maturity of defences. Being able to maintain reasonable relationships is a pretty essential ingredient for a happy and functional lifestyle, inasmuch as relationships are a primary means for satisfying basic human needs for affection, attachment and economic support. Defences based on more accurate understandings of social reality tend to improve people's functioning and their capability to relate to others. Vice versa, defences based on more primitive, distorted understandings of social reality tend to sabotage people's capability to distinguish good from bad relationships. Knowing this, it may strike you as ironic to note that relationships are perhaps the best means known through which people whose representation of social reality are faulty can receive correction (Such folk need to be in healthy relationships to mature, but they all too often sabotage those relationships to which they have access).

Fully functioning mature adults are flexible - they are capable of a range of defensive manoeuvres ranging from reactive pain avoidance to constructive and adaptive efforts at problem solving. They are able to meet their needs through this flexibility - the need to protect themselves, and the need to connect with others to satisfy intimate and economic needs. A significant part of a mature adult's coping flexibility has to do with their capability to know when to be which way. Because their fundamental understanding of social reality is sound, they are less likely to misjudge situations; trusting when trust is worthy and mistrusting when mistrust is appropriate. In contrast, people operating at a more primitive level tend to lack this significant equilibrium and instead fall into more rigid applications of their defences.

MALADAPTIVE BEHAVIOUR

A maladaptive behaviour is a behaviour or trait that is not adaptive - it is counterproductive to the individual. Maladaptivity is often used as an indicator of abnormality or mental dysfunction, because its assessment is relatively free from subjectivity. Nevertheless, several behaviours regarded as moral can be evidently maladaptive, such as dissent or abstinence.

The application of modern theories of learning and conditioning in the treatment of behaviour disorders. The basic assumption of this methodology is that maladaptive behaviour can be changed without insight into its underlying causes. Behavioural therapy depends on precise observations of behaviour and concentration on symptoms. It is assumed that both normal and abnormal behaviours are learned and maintained in the same way, so procedures that alter normal behaviour should also be useful in altering maladaptive behaviour. This therapy is beneficial to patients with depression, anxiety and obsessive-compulsive disorder (OCD), where patients may have 'learnt' how to be depressed, nervous or obsessive-compulsive.

ETIOLOGY: BIO-PSYCHO-SOCIAL FACTORS

Mental disorders produce a wide range of distressing symptoms. Patients may suffer from the profound gloom of depression, the terror of a panic attack, or the disturbing unreality of psychosis. By and large, psychiatric symptoms are experienced as alien and painful. Personality disorders, in contrast, may or may not cause subjective distress. Their core features are maladaptive patterns of behaviour. Some patients report painful inner experiences, but others may not even agree that they have pathology. Some behaviours lead to consequences that make people unhappy, while other behaviours, at least in the short run, are more likely to make other people unhappy.

In essence, personality disorders are characterized by inflexible, pervasive, and stable behaviours that cause important dysfunction in the life of the patient. They begin early in the life and are enduring. We can illustrate these basic attributes with two clinical vignettes, describing one patient with distress, and one with almost no distress.

The term psychosocial refers to the psychological and social factors that influence mental health. Social influences such as peer pressure, parental support, cultural and religious background, socioeconomic status, and interpersonal relationships all help to shape personality and influence psychological makeup. People with psychosocial disorders often have difficulty functioning in social situations and may have problems effectively communicating with others.

American Psychiatric Association distinguishes 16 different subtypes (or classes) of mental sickness. Though psychosocial variables arguably have some level of influence on all subtypes of mental sickness, the major classes of mental disorders thought to involve important psychosocial factors comprise:

- Substance-related disorders: Disorders related to alcohol and drug use, abuse, dependence, and withdrawal.
- Schizophrenia and other psychotic disorders: These comprise the schizoid disorders (schizophrenia, schizophreniform, and schizoaffective disorder), delusional disorder, and psychotic disorders.
- Mood disorders: Affective disorders such as depression (major, dysthymic) and bipolar disorders.
- Anxiety disorders: Disorders in which a several situation or place triggers excessive fear and/or anxiety symptoms (i.e., dizziness, racing heart), such as panic disorder, agoraphobia, social phobia, obsessive-compulsive disorder, post-traumatic stress disorder, and generalized anxiety disorders.
- Somatoform disorders: Somatoform disorders involve clinically important physical symptoms that can't be explained by a medical condition (e.g., somatization disorder, conversion disorder, pain disorder, hypochondriasis, and body dysmorphic disorder).
- Factitious disorders: Disorders in which a person creates and complains of symptoms of a non-existent sickness in order to assume the function of a patient (or sick role).
- Sexual and gender identity disorders: Disorders of sexual desire, arousal, and performance. It should be noted that the categorization of gender identity disorder as a mental sickness has been a point of some contention among mental health professionals.

- Eating disorders: Anorexia and bulimia nervosa.
- Adjustment disorders: Adjustment disorders involve an excessive emotional or behavioural reaction to a stressful event.
- Personality disorders: Maladjustments of personality, together with paranoid, schizoid, schizotypal, antisocial, borderline, histrionic, narcissistic, avoidant, dependent, and obsessive-compulsive personality disorder (not to be confused with the anxiety disorder OCD).
- Disorders normally first diagnosed in infancy childhood, or adolescence. Some learning and developmental disorders (i.e., ADHD) may be partially psychosocial in nature.

It is significant to note that the causes of mental sickness are various and not completely understood. The bulk of psychological disorders are thought to be caused by a complex combination of biological, genetic (hereditary), familial, and social factors or biopsychosocial influences. In addition, the role that each of these play can differ from person to person, so that a disorder such as depression that is caused by genetic factors in one person may be caused by a traumatic life event in another.

The symptoms of psychosocial disorders differ depending on the diagnosis in question. In addition to disorder-specific symptoms, people with psychosocial dysfunction normally have difficulty functioning normally in social situations and may have trouble forming and maintaining close interpersonal relationships.

PSYCHOPATHOLOGY OF MENTAL DISORDERS

Psychopathology is a term which refers to either the study of mental sickness or mental distress or the manifestation of behaviours and experiences which may be indicative of mental sickness or psychological impairment. Most notably, psychiatrists and clinical psychologists are especially interested in this field and may either be involved in clinical treatment of mental sickness, or research into the origin, growth and manifestations of such states, or frequently, both. More widely, several different specialties may be involved in the study of psychopathology. For instance, a neuroscientist may concentrate on brain changes related to mental sickness. Thus, someone who is referred to as a psychopathologist, may be one of any number of professions who have specialised in studying this field. Psychiatrists in specific are interested in descriptive psychopathology, which has the aim of describing the symptoms and syndromes of mental sickness.

This is both for the diagnosis of individual patients (to see whether the patient's experience fits any pre-existing classification), or for the creation of diagnostic systems (such as the Diagnostic and Statistical Manual of Mental Disorders) which define exactly which signs and symptoms should make up a diagnosis, and how experiences and behaviours should be grouped in specific diagnoses (e.g. clinical depression, schizophrenia). Psychopathology is not the same as psychopathy, which has to do with antisocial personality disorders and criminality.

BRAIN: STRUCTURE AND FUNCTION

The brain, together with the spinal cord, makes up the central nervous system. This is the 'control centre' which coordinates the body's functions.

Between the surfaces of the brain and the skull there are three layers of membrane called the meninges, which completely cover the brain and spinal cord. Between two of these layers is a space called the subarachnoid space. The subarachnoid space contains a fluid called cerebrospinal fluid (CSF).

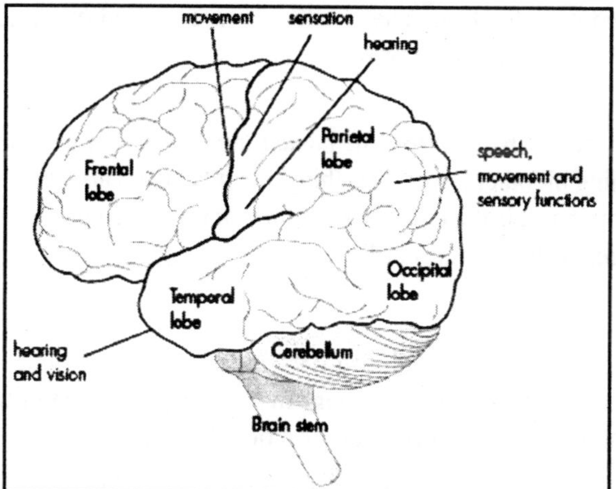

Fig. Brain Structure and Function

Like every other organ in the body, the brain is made up of cells. There are about 40 billion nerve cells, known as neurones, within the brain. Everyone is born with a similar amount. Unlike other cells, nerve cells are not able to replace themselves. In fact, as we get older there is a gradual decrease in their number.

The nerve cells communicate with each other and other parts of the body by sending messages (nerve impulses) through a system of nerve pathways or networks. The nerve cells are held in place and supported by glial cells. There are different types of glial cells, including astrocytes, oligodendrocytes and ependymal cells.

The main parts of the brain are:

- The cerebrum (the forebrain) made up of the right and left cerebral hemispheres
- The cerebellum (the hindbrain)
- The brain stem.

Cerebrum: This is the largest area of the brain and is concerned with all higher mental functions, such as thinking and memory. It is made up of two halves or hemispheres. The right cerebral hemisphere controls the left side of the body and the left cerebral hemisphere controls the right side of the body. Each cerebral hemisphere is divided into four areas, known as lobes: the frontal, parietal, temporal and occipital lobes. Each lobe controls a different range of activities.

Cerebellum: This is the back part of the brain and is concerned with balance and coordination. These activities are carried out automatically (subconsciously) by this area of the brain and are not under a person's control.

Brain stem: This controls the basic functions essential to maintaining life, including blood pressure, breathing, heart beat and also eye movements and swallowing. It is the bottom part of the brain and connects the cerebral hemispheres to the spinal cord.

LIMBIC SYSTEM

Emotion involves the entire nervous system, of course. But there are two parts of the nervous system that are especially significant: The limbic system and the autonomic nervous system.

The limbic system is a complex set of structures that lies on both sides and underneath the thalamus, just under the cerebrum. It includes the hypothalamus, the hippocampus, the amygdala, and several other nearby areas. It appears to be primarily responsible for our emotional life, and has a lot to do with the formation of memories. In this drawing, you are looking at the brain cut in half, but with the brain stem intact. The part of the limbic system shown is that which is along the left side of the thalamus (hippocampus and amygdala) and just under the front of the thalamus (hypothalamus):

Hypothalamus

The hypothalamus is a small part of the brain located just below the thalamus on both sides of the third ventricle. (The ventricles are areas within the cerebrum that are filled with cerebrospinal fluid, and connect to the fluid in the spine.) It sits just inside the two tracts of the optic nerve, and just above (and intimately connected with) the pituitary gland.

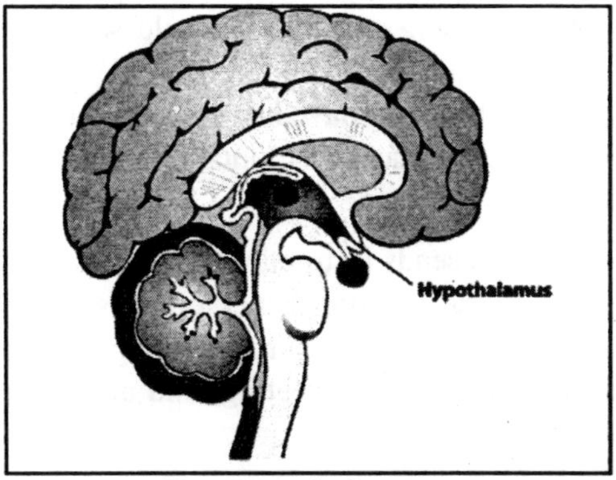

Fig. Hypothalamus

The hypothalamus is one of the busiest parts of the brain, and is mainly concerned with homeostasis. Homeostasis is the process of returning something to some "set point." It works like a thermostat: When your room gets too cold, the thermostat conveys that information to the furnace and turns it on. As your room warms up and the temperature gets beyond a certain point, it sends a signal that tells the furnace to turn off.

The hypothalamus is responsible for regulating your hunger, thirst, response to pain, levels of pleasure, sexual satisfaction, anger and aggressive behaviour, and more. It also regulates the functioning of the parasympathetic and sympathetic nervous systems, which in turn means it regulates things like pulse, blood pressure, breathing, and arousal in response to emotional circumstances.

The hypothalamus receives inputs from a number of sources. From the vagus nerve, it gets information about blood pressure and the distension of the gut (that is, how full your stomach is). From the reticular formation in the brainstem, it gets information about skin temperature. From the optic nerve, it gets information about light and darkness. From unusual neurons lining the ventricles, it gets information about the contents of the cerebrospinal fluid, including toxins that lead to vomiting. And from the other parts of the limbic system and the olfactory (smell) nerves, it gets information that helps regulate eating and sexuality. The hypothalamus also has some receptors of its own, that provide information about ion balance and temperature of the blood.

In one of the more recent discoveries, it seems that there is a protein called leptin which is released by fat cells when we overeat. The hypothalamus apparently senses the levels of leptin in the bloodstream and responds by decreasing appetite. It would seem that some people have a mutation in a gene which produces leptin, and their bodies can't tell the hypothalamus that they have had enough to eat. However, many overweight people do not have this mutation, so there is still a lot of research to do!

The hypothalamus sends instructions to the rest of the body in two ways. The first is to the autonomic nervous system. This allows the hypothalamus to have ultimate control of things like blood pressure, heartrate, breathing, digestion, sweating, and all the sympathetic and parasympathetic functions.

The other way the hypothalamus controls things is via the pituitary gland. It is neurally and chemically connected to the pituitary, which in turn pumps hormones called releasing factors into the bloodstream. As you know, the pituitary is the so-called "master gland," and these hormones are vitally important in regulating growth and metabolism.

Hippocampus

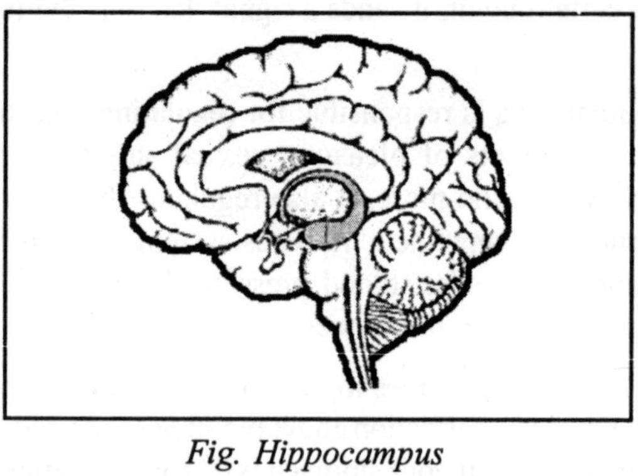

Fig. Hippocampus

The hippocampus consists of two "horns" that curve back from the amygdala. It appears to be very important in converting things that are "in your mind" at the moment (in short-term memory) into things that you will remember for the long run (long-term memory). If the hippocampus is damaged, a person cannot build new memories, and lives instead in a strange world where everything they experience just fades away, even while older memories from the time before the damage are untouched.

Amygdala

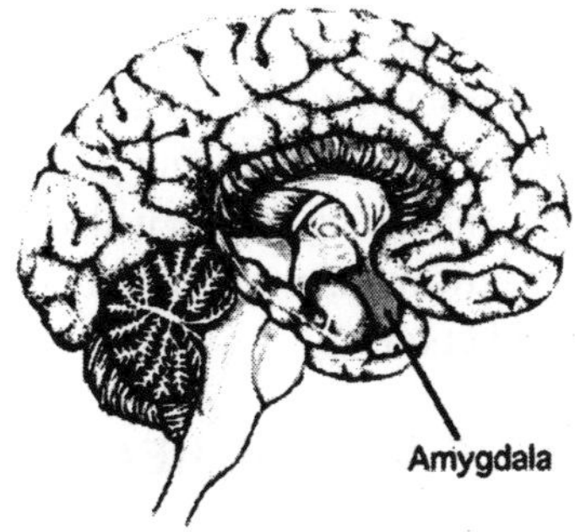

Fig. Amygdala

The amygdalas are two almond-shaped masses of neurons on either side of the thalamus at the lower end of the hippocampus. When it is stimulated electrically, animals respond with aggression. And if the amygdala is removed, animals get very tame and no longer respond to things that would have caused rage before. But there is more to it than just anger: When removed, animals also become indifferent to stimuli that would have otherwise have caused fear and even sexual responses.

Related Areas

Besides the hypothalamus, hippocampus, and amygdala, there are other areas in the structures near to the limbic system that are intimately connected to it:

Cingulate gyrus: The cingulate gyrus is the part of the cerebrum that lies closest to the limbic system, just above the corpus collosum. It provides a pathway from the thalamus to the hippocampus, seems to be responsible for focusing attention on emotionally significant events, and for associating memories to smells and to pain.

Septum: The septum, which lies in front of the thalamus, has areas that seem to be centres for orgasm.

Ventral tegmental area: The ventral tegmental area of the brain stem (just below the thalamus) consists of dopamine pathways that seem to be responsible for pleasure. People with damage here tend to have difficulty getting pleasure in life, and often turn to alcohol, drugs, sweets, and gambling.

Basal ganglia: The basal ganglia (including the caudate nucleus, the putamen, the globus pallidus, and the substantia nigra) lie over and to the sides of the limbic system, and are tightly connected with the cortex above them. They are responsible for repetitive behaviours, reward experiences, and focusing attention.

Prefrontal cortex: The prefrontal cortex, which is the part of the frontal lobe which lies in front of the motor area, is also closely linked to the limbic system. Besides apparently being involved in thinking about the future, making plans, and taking action, it also appears to be involved in the same dopamine pathways as the ventral tegmental area, and plays a part in pleasure and addiction.

PRINCIPLES OF MENTAL HEALTH NURSING

To make sense of mental health nursing practice calls for an understanding of the factors that can influence it. These comprise mental health policy, current theories about the various facets of mental health, and the attitudes, values and beliefs that guide our thinking. People's thinking changes over time and this is determined by the experiences they have had and by changes in thinking about what constitutes appropriate practice.

In mental health in the past few decades, the rate of change in thinking about practice has been important. It can be tempting to think that mental health nursing is a discrete field of practice of little value to the general nurse, but this is far from the truth.

Mental health nursing is built on several principles or beliefs about people and the care they observe:

- Every person is worthy of dignity and respect.
- Every person has the potential to change and grow.
- All people share basic human needs.
- All behaviour is meaningful and can be understood from the person's perspective.
- People have the right to partake in decisions affecting their health and treatment.
- Through the therapeutic use of self, via therapeutic relationships and communication, nurses help people adjust, change, and grow.

STANDARDS OF MENTAL HEALTH NURSING PRACTICE

Assessment: The psychiatric-mental health nurse collects patient health data.

Diagnosis: The psychiatric-mental health nurse analyzes the data in determining diagnoses.

Outcome Identification: The psychiatric-mental nurse identifies expected outcomes individualized to the patient.

Planning: The psychiatric-mental health nurse develops a plan of care that prescribes interventions identified in the plan of care.

Counselling: The psychiatric-mental health nurse employs counselling interventions to assist patients in improving or regaining their previous coping abilities, fostering mental health, and preventing mental sickness and disability.

Milieu Therapy: The psychiatric-mental health nurse provides, structures, and maintains a therapeutic environment in collaboration with the patient and other health care providers.

Self care activities: The psychiatric-mental health nurse structures interventions around the patient's activities of daily living to foster selfcare and mental and physical well-being.

Psychobiologic Interventions: The psychiatric-mental health nurse employs knowledge of psychobiologic interventions and applies clinical skills to restore the patient's health and prevent further disability.

Health Teaching: The psychiatric-mental health nurse, through health teaching, assists patients in achieving satisfying, productive, and healthy patterns of living.

Case Management: The psychiatric health nurse provides case management to coordinate complete health services and ensure continuity of care.

Health Promotion and Maintenance: The psychiatric health nurse employs strategies and interventions to promote and maintain mental health and prevent mental sickness.

Evaluation: The psychiatric health nurse assesses the patient's progress in attaining expected outcomes.

Quality of Care: The psychiatric health nurse systematically assesses the quality of care and effectiveness of psychiatric-mental health nursing practice.

Performance Appraisal: The psychiatric health nurse assesses his or her own psychiatric-mental health nursing practice in relation to professional practice standards and relevant statutes and regulations.

Education: The psychiatric health nurse acquires and maintains current knowledge in nursing practice.

Collegiality: The psychiatric health nurse contributes to the professional growth of peers, colleagues, and others.

Ethics: The psychiatric health nurse's decisions and actions on behalf of others are determined in an ethical manner.

Collaboration: The psychiatric health nurse collaborates with the patient, significant others, and health care providers in providing care.

Research: The psychiatric health nurse contributes to nursing and mental health through the use of research.

Resource Utilization: The psychiatric health nurse considers factors related to safety, effectiveness, and cost in planning and delivering patient care.

THEORETICAL MODELS AND THE ROLE OF NURSE

Following are the theoretical models of nursing in mental health nursing:

Existential Model: The existential model centres on an individual's present experiences rather than his past ones. It holds that alienation from the self causes deviant behaviour, and that people can make free choices about which behaviours to exhibit. Based on the existential model of behaviour, nursing developed the concept that the nurse works to restore the patient to a state of "full life" from a state of "self-alienation."

Psychoanalytical Model: As per the psychoanalytic model, the personality consists of the:

Id: encompassing the primitive instincts and energies underlying all psychic activity.

Ego: the conscious part of the personality, and the part that most immediately controls thought and behaviour.

Superego: the conscience.

During childhood, growth occurs in five psychosexual stages - oral, anal, phallic, latency, and genital, Deviations in behaviour result from unsuccessful task accomplishment during earlier developmental stages.

Freud also proposed that behaviour is motivated by anxiety, the cornerstone of psychopathology.

Understanding the psychosexual stages of childhood provides a model for the nurse to understand adult behaviours. Also, the nurse can promote effective parenting by teaching parents about the child's needs during each psychosexual stage.

Behavioural Model: As per the behavioural model, all behaviour - together with mental sickness - is learned. Unlike other models, which concentrate on the patient's emotions, behavioural theory focuses on the patient's actions. Behaviourist's believe that behaviour that's rewarded will prevail. Desired behaviours can be learned through rewards and negative behaviours can be eliminated through punishment. Thus, people can learn to act in socially desirable ways.

Interpersonal Model: The interpersonal model holds that human growth results from interpersonal relationships, and that behaviour is motivated by avoidance of anxiety and attainment of satisfaction.

Peplau drew on Sullivan's original theory to propose an interpersonal nursing theory, which advanced the practice of psychiatric nursing by defining it as an interpersonal process. She proposed that:

- Nurses must promote the nurse-patient relationship to build trust and foster healthy behaviour.
- Therapeutic use of self promotes healing.
- The therapeutic relationship is directed toward meeting the patient's needs.

REFERENCES

Allison, D. B., & Casey, D. E. (2001). Antipsychotic-induced weight gain: A review of the literature. Journal of Clinical Psychiatry, 62(suppl. 7), 22–31.

Beaubrun, G., & Gray, G. E. (2000). A review of herbal medicines for psychiatric disorders. Psychiatric Services, 51(9), 1130–1134.

Casey, D. E., & Zorn, S. H. (2001). The pharmacology of weight gain with antipsychotics. Journal of Clinical Psychiatry, 62(suppl. 7), 4–10.

Green, A. I., Patel, J. K., Goisman, R. M., Allison, D. B., & Blackburn, G. (2000). Weight gain from novel antipsychotic drugs: Need for action. General Hospital Psychiatry, 22, 224–235.

Keck, P. E., McElroy, S. L., & Arnold, L. M. (2001). Ziprasidone: A new atypical antipsychotic. Expert Opinions in Pharmacotherapy, 2(6), 1033–1042.

Kudzma, E. C. (1999). Culturally competent drug administration. American Journal of Nursing, 99(8), 46–52.

Lawson, W. B. (1996). The art and science of psychopharmacology of African Americans. Mt. Sinai Journal of Medicine, 63(5–6), 301–305.

Lewis, D. A. (2000). Functional neuroanatomy. In B. J. Sadock & V. A. Sadock (Eds.), Comprehensive textbook of psychiatry, Vol. 1 (7th ed., pp. 3–31). Philadelphia: Lippincott Williams & Wilkins.

3

Assessment of Mental Health Nursing

The first step in the nursing process is crucial. Assess the patient in a holistic way, integrating any relevant information about the patient's life, behaviour, and feelings. The focus of care, beginning with assessment, is toward the patient's optimal level of health and independence.

The nursing process is a six-step problem-solving methodology to nursing that also serves as an organizational model for the practice of nursing. It sets the practice of nursing in motion and serves as a monitor of quality nursing care. Nurses in all specialties practice the first step, assessment.

HISTORY TAKING

The problem oriented record or history of a patient is one of the commonest ways of recording medical information. The initial collection of data should be made as significant and complete as possible. The only restrictions should be the discomfort and expense to the patient. For the nurse practitioner it is significant to create a format that allows a health-oriented methodology. The method chosen for history taking depends on the norms of the nurse practitioner's field of practice. It is necessary that the notes allow health-care professionals to communicate effectively with each other.

History taking is a significant skill and is frequently the key to diagnosis. Keeping a logical order can help the nurse practitioner cover a lot of ground and discover extensive information. The art is to be thorough without being too interrogative and to listen to patients' reactions and encourage them with verbal and non-verbal signals to tell their story. Nurse practitioners struggling to master the art of asking difficult questions can take heed from studies in physician-patient communication.

MENTAL STATUS EXAMINATION

The mental status examination abbreviated MSE, is a significant part of the clinical assessment process in psychiatric practice. It is a structured way of observing and describing a patient's current state of mind, under the domains of appearance, attitude, behaviour, mood and affect, speech, thought process, thought content, perception, cognition, insight and judgement. There are some minor variations in the subdivision of the MSE and the sequence and names of MSE domains.

The purpose of the MSE is to obtain a complete cross-sectional description of the patient's mental state, which when combined with the biographical and historical information of the psychiatric history, allows the clinician to make an accurate diagnosis and formulation, which are required for logical treatment planning. The data are collected through a combination of direct and indirect means: unstructured observation while obtaining the biographical and social information, focused questions about current symptoms, and formalised psychological tests. The MSE is not to be confused with the mini-mental state examination (MMSE) which is a brief neuro-psychological screening test for dementia.

The mental status examination is a core skill of psychiatrists and nurses and is a key part of the initial psychiatric assessment in an out-patient or psychiatric hospital setting. It is a systematic collection of data based on observation of the patient's behaviour while the patient is in the clinician's view during the interview. The purpose is to obtain evidence of symptoms and signs of mental disorders, together with danger to self and others, that are present at the time of the interview. Further, information on the patient's insight, judgment, and capacity for abstract reasoning is used to inform decisions about treatment strategy and the choice of an appropriate treatment setting.

It is carried out in the manner of an informal enquiry, utilizing a combination of open and closed questions, supplemented by structured tests to assess cognition. The MSE can also be regarded as part of the complete physical examination performed by doctors and nurses though it may be performed in a cursory and abbreviated way in non-mental-health settings. Information is normally recorded as free-form text utilizing the standard headings, but brief MSE checklists are available for use in emergency situations, for instance by paramedics or emergency department staff. The information obtained in the MSE is used, together with the biographical and social information of the psychiatric history, to generate a diagnosis, a psychiatric formulation and a treatment plan.

A complete MSE is more complete and assesses the following ten areas of functioning:

- Appearance. The examiner notes the person's age, race, sex, civil status, and overall appearance. These features are important because poor personal hygiene or grooming may reflect a loss of interest in selfcare or physical inability to bathe or dress oneself.
- Movement and behaviour. The examiner observes the person's gait (manner of walking), posture, coordination, eye contact, facial expressions, and similar behaviours. Problems with walking or coordination may reflect a disorder of the central nervous system.
- Affect. Affect refers to an individual's outwardly observable emotional reactions. It may comprise either a lack of emotional response to an event or an overreaction.
- Mood. Mood refers to the underlying emotional "atmosphere" or tone of the person's answers.
- Speech. The examiner assesses the volume of the person's voice, the rate or speed of speech, the length of answers to questions, the appropriateness and clarity of the answers, and similar characteristics.
- Thought content. The examiner evaluates what the patient is saying for indications of hallucinations, delusions, obsessions, symptoms of dissociation, or thoughts of suicide. Dissociation refers to the splitting-off of several memories or mental processes from conscious awareness. Dissociative symptoms comprise feelings of unreality, depersonalization, and confusion about one's identity.
- Thought process. Thought process refers to the logical connections between thoughts and their relevance to the main thread of conversation. Immaterial detail, repeated words and phrases, interrupted thinking (thought blocking), and loose, illogical connections between thoughts, may be signs of a thought disorder.
- Cognition. Cognition refers to the act or condition of knowing. The evaluation evaluates the person's orientation (ability to locate himself or herself) with regard to time, place, and personal identity; long- and short-term memory; capability to perform

easy arithmetic (counting backward by threes or sevens); general intellectual level or fund of knowledge (identifying the last five Presidents, or similar questions); capability to think abstractly (explaining a proverb); capability to name specified objects and read or write complete sentences; capability to understand and perform a task (showing the examiner how to comb one's hair or throw a ball); capability to draw a easy map or copy a design or geometrical figure; capability to distinguish between right and left.

- Judgment. The examiner asks the person what he or she would do about a commonsense problem, such as running out of a prescription medication.
- Insight. Insight refers to an individual's capability to recognize a problem and understand its nature and severity.

The length of time required for a mental status examination depends on the patient's condition. It may take as little as five minutes to examine a healthy person. Patients with speech problems or intellectual impairments, dementia, or other organic brain disorders may call for fifteen or twenty minutes. The examiner may choose to spend more time on several portions of the MSE and less time on others, depending on the patient's condition and answers.

MINI MENTAL STATUS EXAMINATION

The mini-mental state examination (MMSE) or Folstein test is a brief 30-point questionnaire test that is used to assess cognition. It is generally used in medicine to screen for dementia. In the time span of about 10 minutes it samples various functions together with arithmetic, memory and orientation. It was introduced by Folstein et al in 1975, and is widely used with small modifications. This test is not the same thing as a mental status examination.

Various other tests are also used, such as the Hodkinson abbreviated mental test score (1972, geriatrics) and longer formal tests for deeper analysis of specific deficits. The MMSE test comprises plain questions and problems in a number of areas: the time and place of the test, repeating lists of words, arithmetic, language use and comprehension, and basic motor skills.

Any score over 27 (out of 30) is effectively normal. Below this, 20-26 indicates some cognitive impairment; 10-19 moderate to intense cognitive impairment, and below 10 very intense cognitive impairment. The normal value is also corrected for degree of schooling and age. Low to very low scores correlate closely with the presence of dementia, though other mental disorders can also lead to abnormal findings on MMSE testing. The presence of purely physical problems can also interfere with interpretation if not suitably noted; for instance, a patient may be physically unable to hear or read instructions properly, or may have a motor deficit that affects writing and drawing skills.

NEUROLOGICAL EXAMINATION

The human nervous system is an intricate and complex network of fibres that impenetrates the entire body and functions in complicated and frequently mysterious ways. Sophisticated imaging and laboratory tests don't always furnish sufficient information about how the nerves are functioning – or not functioning, as the case may be. The neurological examination is a series of plain questions and tests that furnish crucial information about the nervous system. It is an inexpensive, non-invasive way to determine what might be incorrect.

The neurological examination is divided into many components, each focusing on a different part of the nervous system:

Mental status: The mental status examination is a series of detailed but plain questions designed to test cognitive capability, together with the patient's:

- State of consciousness (awareness and responsiveness to the environment and the senses);
- Appearance and general behaviour;
- Mood;
- Content of thought; and
- Intellectual resources (orientation with reference to time, place, and person; comprehension; capability to pay attention; insight; memory; judgment; abstract reasoning power; speech and language function; and intellectual capacity).

The patient may be asked to remember objects that had been listed earlier in the course of the exam; repeat sentences; resolve plain mathematical problems; copy a three-dimensional drawing; and draw a clock and place the numbers and hands appropriately. When speech and language are tested, the examiner listens to the character of the speech, the fluency (smoothness of speech), and the patient's capability to understand and carry out easy or complex commands, and to read and write.

In addition to specific questions that make up the actual mental status exam, the neurologist obtains significant information by observing the patient's general behaviour during the examination. Several neurological diseases, such as dementia, cause changes in intellectual status or emotional responsiveness, and specific personality features. These changes and features can be detected during the mental status portion of the neurological exam. The mental status exam is especially significant when the other parts of the neurological exam reveal no abnormalities. Sometimes, slight changes in memory or other intellectual resources may be the only indication that something is incorrect. Evaluating an individual's intellectual capacity can also be helpful in determining a course of treatment and making a prognosis.

Cranial nerves: The cranial nerves are a set of twelve nerves that relay messages between the brain and the head and neck and control motor and sensory functions, together with vision, smell, and movement of the tongue and vocal cords.

The cranial nerve exam involves testing the function of all twelve sets of cranial nerves. It is a necessary part of the neurological exam, and helps localize central nervous system dysfunction and aids in diagnosing systemic disease. Some of the functions that are generally tested as part of the cranial nerve exam comprise: eyelid strength and function; visual function; peripheral vision; pupillary light reflexes; eye muscle movements; strength of facial musculature; the gag reflex; tongue and lip movements; capability to smell and taste; hearing; and sensation in the face, head, and neck.

Motor system: The motor system comprises the brain and spinal cord motor pathways, and all the motor nerves and muscles throughout the body. Abnormalities in the motor system can frequently be detected by evaluating muscle strength and tone and by looking for a range of characteristic signs. The patient is normally asked to undress, so the neurologist can see the muscles and look for atrophy (shrinkage), twitching, or abnormal movements. Tests are done to assess strength in all the major muscle groups.

Evaluating Babinski response is a significant part of testing the motor system. The neurologist strokes or scratches, heel-to-toe, the outer side of the sole of the foot and in patients over the age of 2, the toes normally curl downward in response. If the toes fan upward, a brain or spinal cord injury is indicated. A number of neurological disorders can lead to Babinski response.

Sensory system: Sensation depends on impulses that occur as a result of stimulation of receptors located in the skin, muscles, tendons, and so on, and are sent along nerve fibers to the central nervous system (brain and spinal cord). The sensory exam is used to determine areas of abnormal sensation, the quality and type of sensation impairment, and the level and degree of tissue involvement.

A sensory exam involves evaluating different types of sensation, together with pain, temperature, pressure, and position. For instance, pinpricks may be used to test the patient's response to pain and compare the response in different parts or opposite sides of the body. A cold or warm object may be used to test the sensation of temperature. To test position, patients may be asked to close their eyes and determine in which direction the examiner is moving a part of their body (e.g., big toe). Patients also may be asked to identify objects with their eyes closed or identify numbers or letters traced on their body. The sensory exam should be repeated to furnish accurate results. Reactions may be affected by how alert, aware, and well-rested the patient is, so this part of the neurological exam is normally performed early in the course of testing.

Deep tendon reflexes: Reflexes are actions performed involuntarily in response to impulses sent to the central nervous system. Alterations in reflexes are frequently the first sign of neurological dysfunction. Observing reflexes is the most objective part of the neurological exam, because the reflexes are not under voluntary control and testing does not depend on the patient's cooperation, attitude, or awareness.

Hundreds of reflexes have been identified, but the neurological exam in general involves testing only the deep tendon reflexes. Deep tendon reflexes, also known as muscle stretch reflexes, are reflexes elicited in response to stimuli to tendons. Normally, when a specific area of the muscle tendon is tapped with a soft rubber hammer, the muscle fibers contract. Abnormal reactions may indicate injury to the nervous system pathways that produce the deep tendon reflex.

Coordination and the cerebellum: The cerebellum is the part of the brain that controls voluntary movement and motor coordination, together with posture. Testing coordination provides clues about conditions that affect the cerebellum.

The neurologist may ask patients to move their finger from their nose to the neurologist's finger, going back and forth from nose to finger, touching the tip of each. Patients also may be asked to tap their fingers together swiftly in a coordinated fashion or move their hands one on top of the other, back and forth, as smoothly as they can. Coordination in the lower limbs can be tested by asking patients to rub one heel up and down smoothly over the other shin.

Gait: Most of us take our capability to walk for granted. But as easy as it may seem, walking is a very intricate physiological process. How we walk-our gait-is influenced by a number of bodily mechanisms and nervous system reflexes. The body must be held erect; the limbs, head, and trunk must be held in the correct position; the person must be oriented to the position of all body parts; parts of motor control involved with moving must be integrated; and so on. Because walking depends on so several different parts of the nervous system, it can be affected by a range of neurological disorders. By observing gait, the neurologist can gather significant clues about what might be incorrect. The patient is normally asked to walk in different ways (e.g., heel-to-toe in a straight line, turning suddenly, walking on the toes, walking on the heels, running).

INVESTIGATIONS

Neurodiagnostic tests, also called neurodiagnostics, are done when a patient's sickness or condition is thought to be based in the central nervous system (brain and spinal cord). Signs of nervous system disorders comprise the following:

- Chronic headaches
- Dizziness
- Hearing and vision changes
- Numbness and tingling
- Seizures
- Strokes
- Weakness

There are two types of neurodiagnostic testing: imaging tests or scans (e.g., x-ray, CT scan, MRI scan, PET scan) and electrical impulse detection (e.g., EEG, EMG). Neurodiagnostic testing may be conducted as part of a neurological exam.

CT SCAN

The computed tomographic scan (also called a CT or CAT scan) uses an x-ray beam and a computer to generate 2 dimensional images of the body. The information is displayed in a cross-section or "slice" of body tissue. Neurological CT scans focus on the head or spine.

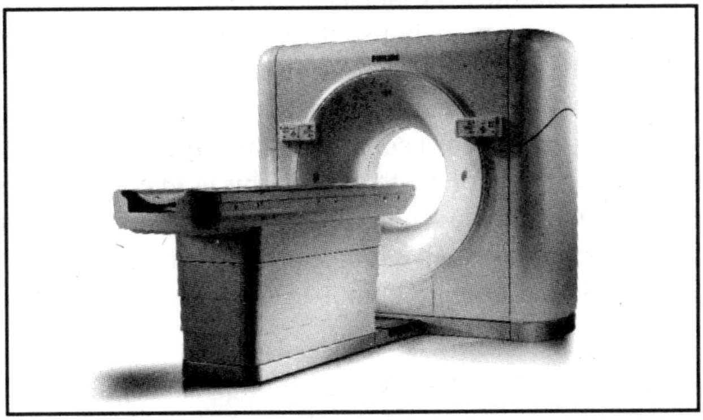

Fig. CT Scan Machine

CAT scans can help detect spinal stenosis (narrowing) or a herniated disc. They can assist in locating brain damage in patients with head injury, detect a blood clot or bleeding in patients with a stroke, detect certain brain tumours, illuminate enlarged brain ventricles (cavities) in patients with hydrocephalus, assist in planning radiation therapy for cancer of the brain, or detect bleeding in a patient with a ruptured or leaking aneurysm. CT can clearly show even the smallest bones of the body as well as surrounding muscle and blood vessels. This makes it invaluable in diagnosing and treating cranial and spinal problems.

CT scanning is fast, painless, and simple and involves little radiation exposure. If contrast material is injected, patients may experience a warm, flushed sensation or experience a metallic taste in their mouth for a few minutes. The CT scanner is a large, square machine with a donut-like hole in the centre. The patient lies on a table that can move up or down and slides into and out of the centre of the hold. The patient's body may be supported by pillows to help hold it still and in the proper position during the scanning process. Inside the machine, an x-ray tube on a rotating gantry moves around the patient's body to produce the images, making clicking and whirring sounds as the gantry moves. A CT scan usually takes from 15 minutes to 30 minutes; a CT exam of the head and brain can take between 10 and 45 minutes.

MRI SCAN

MRI and MRA(Magnetic Resonance Angiogram) are done by a machine that uses radiofrequency energy and a strong magnetic field to provide detailed images of internal organs and tissues. The image results from the different water concentration of the various tissues. No radiation exposure is involved. The conventional MRI machine consists of a closed cylindrical magnet in which the patient must lie totally still for short periods of time. MRI causes no pain, but some patients do find it uncomfortable and even claustrophobic. However, newer, more patient-friendly MRI systems are now in increasingly widespread use. Depending on the part of the body being examined, a contrast agent may be used to enhance the visibility of certain tissue or blood vessel. This is administered via a small needle connected to an intravenous line placed in vein in the arm or hand. An MRI/MRA is a non-invasive procedure and can take from 15 minutes to approximately one hour to complete, depending on the part of the body being imaged.

MRI can be used to identify and monitor tumours of the brain and spinal cord. It can also measure small metabolic changes in the active part of the brain and therefore be used to map those parts of the brain that handle critical functions such as thought, speech, movement, and sensation. It can also document changes in chronic disorders of the nervous system such as multiple sclerosis. It is also a useful diagnostic tool for identifying diseases of the blood vessels as well as stroke. It is commonly used for patients with diseases of the pituitary gland. It is also widely used to diagnose sports-related injuries and is useful in documenting brain abnormalities related to dementia or seizures. MRI can also detect tissue abnormality in patients with diseases of the eye or inner ear.

Because the MRI can give such clear pictures of soft-tissue structures in and around bones, it also is the most sensitive exam available for spinal problems. It is particularly helpful in identifying stenosis (narrowing of the spinal canal) and herniated discs. The MRI can be critical to planning surgery, radiation therapy, treatment for stroke, or other interventions to treat brain disorders. The MRA demonstrates blood vessels in the neck and brain and can help detect abnormalities.

For an MRI of the head, the patient is placed on a sliding table and a radio antenna device called a surface coil is positioned around the upper part of the head. The patient is then positioned inside the MRI gantry. The MRI exam will generally take from 15 to 45 minutes.

The functional MRI looks at how the brain is actually functioning by identify regions of increased brain activity. Increases in microscopic vessel size, chemical changes, or heat production are all signs that a particular part of the brain is processing information and giving commands to the body. For this test, the patient performs a particular task while the imaging is taking place. The metabolism in the area of the brain responsible for that task will increase, and the signal in MR image will change. By performing specific tasks that correspond to different functions, it is possible to locate the area in the brain that governs that function. This information is helpful to a surgeon so that he/she can avoid those important areas during surgery. The patient lies on a sliding table with his or her head in a brace designed to hold the head still, then is slid under or into the cylindrical magnetic unit which creates the image. As the test progresses, the patients will be asked to perform various tasks, such as tapping the thumb of one hand against each of the fingers in that hand.

PET SCAN

Positron emission tomography (PET scan or PET imagery) uses radiation from the emission of positrons (extremely small particles discharged from a radioactive substance) to create images that can help detect and evaluate cancer and the effects of cancer therapy. This test also can be used to diagnose a variety of neurological conditions, including memory disorders, tumours, and seizure disorders.

In a PET scan, a small amount of a radioactive substance is combined with a natural body compound (e.g., glucose, water, or ammonia) and is injected into the patient. Once the substance has had time to circulate through the body and accumulate in the tissues (generally 30 to 90 minutes), a PET scanner is used to detect the various levels of energy given off by the positrons and produce images. Different colours or levels of brightness indicate different levels of organ and tissue function. Cancer tissue, for example, uses more glucose than normal tissue and shows up brighter on the PET scan.

Preparation: PET scans are outpatient procedures that generally take 1 to 2 1/2 hours to perform. Patients are advised to wear loose, comfortable clothing; avoid eating for 4 hours prior to the appointment; and drink water before the appointment. Because the PET scan relies on glucose level activity, patients who have diabetes should consult a physician about how to control glucose levels during the procedure to avoid false test results.

It is important to arrive on time for PET scan appointments. The radioactive substance that is used has a short lifespan and it must be prepared immediately before the procedure to remain effective during the scan. Once the substance is injected, patients are advised to rest and avoid significant movement, so that the radioactive material can be properly localized in the tissue. Scanning usually begins after 30-90 minutes.

Procedure: The PET scanner is a large machine that is shaped like a doughnut. Inside the hole in the middle are several rings of detectors that record energy emission and send the information to computers, where the images are displayed. The patient lies on a padded examination table and is moved into the hole. The scan takes approximately 30-45 minutes. During this time, the patient must remain as still as possible.

Most people do not experience discomfort during a PET scan. However, patients who are claustrophobic or uncomfortable holding still for a long period of time may experience anxiety. The radioactive substance does not cause any physical sensations. After the procedure, patients should drink plenty of fluids to flush out the radioactive substance. There are no restrictions on activity following a PET scan.

ELECTROENCEPHALOGRAM (EEG)

An electroencephalogram (EEG or brain wave test) is a noninvasive procedure used to detect and record brain cell activity. Because normal brain waves have recognizable frequencies and amplitudes, variations or abnormalities in brain waves may suggest the following:

- Attention deficit disorders (e.g., ADHD)
- Seizure disorders (e.g., epilepsy)
- Tumours or abscesses in the brain
- Head injury
- Encephalitis and other inflammatory diseases
- Cerebral haemorrhages
- Cerebral infarct (stroke)
- Sleep disorders
- Alcohol or drug abuse
- Migraines (in some cases)
- Hallucinations
- Syncope (loss of consciousness)
- Vertigo

An EEG also is used to confirm brain death in a patient who is comatose. This neurodiagnostic test is not used to measure intelligence or diagnose mental sickness.

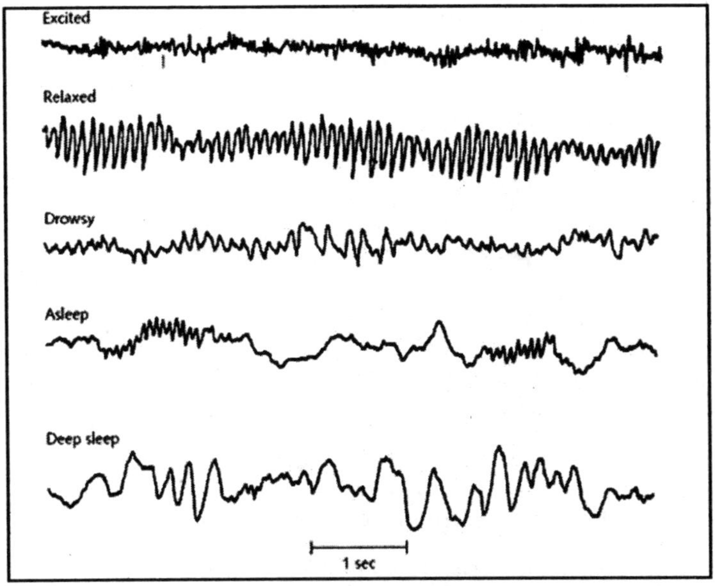

Fig. Electroencephalogram

Preparation: Patients normally are advised to wash their hair the night before the procedure, using no oils, sprays, or conditioners. Patients also should avoid caffeine for at least 8 hours prior to an EEG. If the test will be used to measure brain activity while sleeping, the patient way be asked to reduce or even eliminate their sleep time the night before. Some patients are advised to stop the use of medications before an EEG, but it is significant not to do so unless directed by a doctor.

Procedure: In an electroencephalogram, small metal disks (electrodes) are attached to the scalp to detect and record brain wave activity. These disks are attached by wires to a machine that records and converts electrical signals from the brain into wavy lines on a moving sheet of graph paper.

Before the procedure begins, an EEG technician attaches 16 to 25 disks to the scalp using a sticky paste while the patient lies still on a table or reclining chair. In some cases, the patient is asked to perform a function, such as breathing deeply and rapidly, or looking at a blinking light. In general, there is no discomfort linked with an EEG, though some patients may be bothered by the feeling of the disks.

This neurodiagnostic test normally lasts 1 to 2 hours and is performed on an out-patient basis. Nevertheless, patients who have suspected or known seizure disorders may be given a 24-hour EEG.

In this procedure, the electrodes are attached to a portable lightweight recording box that is worn over the shoulder with a strap. During the test period, the patient or a family member pushes an event button every time a seizure occurs. After 24 hours, the box is returned to the EEG centre for evaluation of the test results. In some cases, patients are admitted to a hospital for extended EEG testing.

PSYCHOLOGICAL TESTS

Psychological tests are useful in proper examining of the patient having mental disorder. Two basic types of tests are intelligence tests and personality tests. Intelligence tests are designed to assess the patient's cognitive abilities and intellectual functioning. Personality tests reflect the patient's personality in fields such as self-concept, impulse control, reality testing, and major defences. The nurse compares the patient's answers with standard answers or criteria and obtains a score or scores.

Other personality tests, called projective tests, are unstructured and are normally conducted by the interview method. The stimuli for these tests, such as pictures or Rorschach's ink blots, are standard, but patients may react with answers that are very different. The evaluator analyzes the patient's reactions and gives narrative result of testing. Both intelligence tests and personality tests are often criticized as being culturally biased. It is significant to consider the patient's culture and environment when evaluating the importance of scores or projections from any of these tests; they can furnish useful information about the patient in some circumstances but may not be suitable for all patients.

ROLE AND RESPONSIBILITIES OF NURSE

Roles of mental health nurses are as follows:

1. Obtains and accurately documents a relevant health history, with an emphasis on mental health history, for patients relevant to specialty and age.
   - Performs a complete physical and mental health assessment
   - Performs a complete psychiatric evaluation, that comprises evaluation of mental status, current and past history of violence, suicidal or self-harm behaviour, substance use, level of functioning, health behaviours, trauma, sexual behaviours, and social and developmental history

2. Analyzes the relationship between normal physiology and specific system alterations linked with mental health problems, psychiatric disorders, and treatment.
3. Identifies and analyzes factors that affect mental health such as:
   - Genetics
   - Family
   - Environment
   - Trauma
   - Psychodynamics
   - Culture & ethnicity
   - Spiritual beliefs and practices
   - Physiological processes
   - Coping skills
   - Cognition
   - Developmental stage
   - Socioeconomic status
   - Gender
   - Substance use
4. Collects data from multiple sources utilizing assessment techniques that are appropriate to the patient's language, culture, and developmental stage, together with, but not limited to, screening evaluations, psychiatric rating scales, genograms, and other standardized instruments.
5. Conducts a complete multigenerational family assessment.
6. Evaluates the impact of acute and/or chronic physical sickness, psychiatric disorders, and stressors on the family system.
7. Performs a complete assessment of mental health needs of a community.
8. Performs and accurately documents appropriate systems and symptom-focused physical examinations, with emphasis on the mental status exam and neurological exam.
9. Involves patients, significant others, and interdisciplinary team members in data collection and analysis.
10. Synthesizes, prioritizes, and documents relevant data in a retrievable form.

The following statements relate to specific nursing responsibilities:

- Nursing Assessment, together with Risk Assessment and Mental State Examination;
- Communicates with the community team to obtain collateral history;
- Gathers information from relatives/carers who accompany the patient to hospital;
- Maintenance of a constant safe environment for the patient based on the Risk Assessment;
- Complete a Missing Persons report form;
- Orientate the patient to the Ward environment and daily routine;
- Collaborate with the patient to complete a person activity proforma;
- Facilitate the daily Therapeutic Group Program;
- Ensure treatments and procedures are completed i.e. X-rays, bloods and preparation for ECT;
- Ensure patients and their carers are provided with written statements of their "Rights and Responsibilities";
- Ensure that patients are aware of, understands and is involved in their treatment plan;
- Furnish an explanation of and ensure patients understanding of rights and responsibilities;
- Ensure safe storage of the patients valuables;
- Administer prescribed medication, and PRN medication;
- Furnish ongoing monitoring and reporting of patients mental state;
- Present nursing observations and GAF score of primary patients at Ward Rounds;
- Attendance at Guardianship Board hearings for primary patients;
- Negotiate individual daily counselling sessions with primary patients to identify and problem resolve various issues;
- Liaise with the Community Mental Health Teams regarding discharge planning;
- Complete and distribute a Nursing discharge summary.

The following statements relate to broader nursing practice:

- Utilizing the nursing process to deliver complete care to patients/ patients;
- Practising within own abilities and qualifications and accepting accountability for own nursing care and service delivery, in accordance with Flinders Medical Centre standards and policies;
- The safety of patients/patients;
- The quality of patient/patient care provided to own specific caseload and/or delivered by supervised staff;
- Providing direction and supervision to less experienced Registered Nurses, Enrolled Nurses and students in the care of their patients;
- Establishing and maintaining communication that facilitates nursing teamwork and interdisciplinary collaboration;
- Functioning in accordance with common law, legislation and the profession's code of ethics;
- Participating in research and policy growth within the practice setting;
- Maintaining contemporary nursing knowledge;
- Delivering direct and complete nursing care and individual case management to patients/patients within the practice setting;
- Coordinating services together with those of other fields or agencies to individual patients/patients within the practice setting;
- Providing education, counselling and group work services orientated towards the promotion of health status improvements of patients/patients within the practice setting;
- Providing support, direction and education to newer or less experienced staff and enrolled general nurses, student nurses and student enrolled nurses;
- Accepting accountability for the employee's nursing care and service delivery, in accordance with Flinders Medical Centre standards and policies;
- Participating in action research and policy growth within the practice setting;
- Nursing staff will assume the overall management of a patient's episode of care, for instance ensuring that all appropriate

services for the patient are in place. This comprises services within the In-patient setting and may also comprise but is not limited to, liaising with the patient's family and community mental health team;

- During Ward Rounds nursing staff will outline the relevant details and history of the patient, for instance name, age, home town, diagnosis, and context of current admission. Nursing staff will summarise the decisions made in the Ward Round and will document the Nursing Care Plan as early as possible after the Ward Round;
- During discharge planning nursing staff will ensure that the local mental health team and the GP is notified of the discharge date and appropriate plans are in place to facilitate the patient's return to their community. Consideration may also need to be made to contact any existing carers.

REFERENCES

Agras, W. S. (1995). Behavior therapy. In H. I. Kaplan & B. J. Sadock (Eds.). Comprehensive textbook of psychiatry, Vol. 2 (6th ed., pp. 1877–1806). Philadelphia: J. B. Lippincott.

Aguilera, D. C. (1998). Crisis intervention: Theory and methodology (7th ed.). St. Louis: Mosby.

Caplan, G. (1964). Principles of preventive psychiatry. New York: Basic Books.

Ellis, A. (1989). Inside rational emotive therapy. San Diego: Academic Press.

Erikson, E. H. (1963). Childhood and society (2d ed.). New York: Norton.

Gabbard, G. O. (2000). Theories of personality and psychopathology: Psychoanalysis. In B. J. Sadock & V. A. Sadock (Eds.), Comprehensive textbook of psychiatry, Vol. 2 (7th ed., pp. 563–607). Philadelphia: Lippincott Williams & Wilkins.

Hemingway, S., Ashmore, R. & Askoorum, G. (2000). Telephone intervention in mental health nursing. Nursing Times, 96(22), 33–34.

Maslow, A. H. (1954). Motivation and personality. New York: Harper & Row. National Alliance for the Mentally Ill (NAMI). (2002).

Peplau, H. (1952). Interpersonal relations in nursing. New York: G. P. Putnam's Sons.

Rogers, C. R. (1961). On becoming a person: A therapist's view of psychotherapy. Boston: Houghton Mifflin.

Skinner, B. F. (1974). About behaviorism. New York: Alfred A. Knopf, Inc.

Sullivan, H. S. (1953). The interpersonal theory of psychiatry. New York: Norton.

Yalom, I. D. (1995). The theory and practice of group psychotherapy. New York: Basic Books.

4

Therapeutic Communication

Communication is the most powerful tool a psychiatric nurse should have. It is the basis of therapeutic -nurse patient relationship. We learn to communicate at an early stage of life, so we may think it quite easy. Nevertheless, communication is a complex process and needs practice to use it effectively. Therapeutic communication techniques are methods used to encourage patients to interact in a manner that promotes their development and moves them toward their treatment goals. All the communication must be aimed at preserving the self respect of both the helper and helpee.

TYPES, TECHNIQUES & CHARACTERISTICS

- Listening: Listening is an active process of receiving information and examining reaction to the messages received. It is not simply hearing. It is necessary to reach any understanding of the patient. It is the first rule of therapeutic-nurse relationship. The patient should be talking more than the nurse during the interaction. Listening is sign of respect and is powerful reinforcer. Active listening involves all the nurse's senses. E.g. maintaining eye contact and receptive nonverbal communication which helps to convey the nurse's interest and acceptance.
- Broad Openings: Here the nurse is encouraging the patient to select topics for discussion. Patient should be welcomed to the communication with warmth and respect. Patient should feel that nurse is ready to listen. Open-ended questions result in fuller, more revealing answers.

E.g.

- What are you thinking about?
- Can you tell me more about that?

- What shall we discuss today?
- Domination of the interaction by the nurse or rejecting the reactions by the nurse results in poor therapeutic relationship.
- Questioning: The nurse skilfully asks open-ended questions during the initial admission. Interviewing skills are essential to avoid asking too several personal questions in one session. Questions should be to attain relevance and depth.
- How come you stopped taking your medication?
- Tell me how you feel now?
  - Restating: Nurse is repeating of the main thought the patient has expressed. It also indicates that the nurse is listening, validating, reinforcing or calling attention to what has been said. Normally a part of patient's statement is repeated. When restating patient shouldn't feel the nurse is reassuring, judgmental or defending.
  - Clarification: Here, the nurse makes specific questions to help clear up a specific point patient makes by attempting to put in to words vague ideas or unclear ideas of the patient. Patient's verbalizations may not be clear when overwhelmed with emotions. Nothing should be allowed to pass to the patient that nurse does not hear or understand. Failure to probe and assumed understanding result in poor communication.
  - Reflection: By reflection nurse is directing back the patient's ideas, feeling, questions or content. Reflection lets the patient know that the nurse has heard what was said and understand the content. Reflection of the feelings let the patient know that the nurse is aware of what the patient is feeling. It signifies understanding, empathy, interest and respect for the patient. Other techniques may not represent empathetic understanding.

Reflecting techniques can be used incorrectly, when stereotyping patient's response, inappropriate timing of reflections and inappropriate cultural experience and educational level of the patient.

- Focusing: Focusing helps the patient expand o a topic of importance and also helps in analysing in detail. It helps the patient talk about life experiences or problem fields and accepts the responsibility for improving them. If the goal is to change thoughts, feelings or beliefs, the patient must first identify and down them. It allows the patient discuss central issues and keeps the communication goal-directed.

- Sharing Perceptions: It involves asking the patient to verify the nurse's understanding of what the patient is thinking or feeling.
- Theme Identification: Themes are underlying issues or problems experienced by the patient that emerge repeatedly during the course of the nurse-patient relationship, like anxiety, depression.
- Silence: Here, the nurse use lack of verbal communication for a therapeutic reason. It allows the patient to think and gain insights. Silence on the part of nurse has varying effects, depending on how the patient perceives it. To a vocal patient silence on the part of nurse may be welcome, but with a depressed or withdrawn patient, the nurse's silence may convey support, understanding, and acceptance.
- Humour: Humour is basic part of our personality and has a place in therapeutic nurse-patient relationship. It is the discharge of energy through the comic enjoyment of imperfect. It may be helpful with a patient experiencing mild to moderate anxiety. Humour should be consistent with social and cultural values.
- Informing: Informing or giving information is nurse shares easy facts with the patient. This skill is use in patient education like when to take medication, essential precautions and side effects.
- Suggesting: Suggesting is the presentation of alternate ideas. As a therapeutic technique, it is useful intervention in the working phase of the relationship. Suggesting or giving advice can be non-therapeutic. Patient may take nurse's advice and still have an unsuccessful outcome, the patient returns to blame nurse.
- Confrontation: Confrontation involves anger and aggression. The therapeutic dimension is assertiveness rather than aggression. Confrontation is an attempt by the nurse to make the patient aware of incongruence in is or her feelings, attitudes, beliefs, and behaviours. It may also help in discovery of ambivalent feelings in the patient. The nurse must be ready to work with the patient through the crisis after confronting the patient. Without this commitment the confrontation lack therapeutic potential and may damage nurse-patient relationship.

- Role playing: Role playing involves acting out a specific situation. It increases patient's insight in to human relations can deepen the capability to see the situation from another person's point of view. Role playing can be used for attitude change and to promote self-awareness.

One of the specific ways in which role playing can be used to solve conflicts and increase self-awareness is through a dialogue that calls for the patient to take the part of each person or each side of the problem. If the conflict is internal, the dialogue occurs in the present tense between the conflicting selves till one part of the conflict outweighs the other. If second person is involved, the patient is told to begin the dialogue by expressing wants and resentments about the other person. Then, the patient changes chairs assume the role other person, and responds to what was said. This way patient can express feelings and opinions and gives reality base for the probable response from the other party involved in the conflict.

Therapeutic Impasses: For variety of reasons therapeutic communication can be hindered. Therapeutic impasses are blocks in the progress of nurse-patient relationship. They arise for variety of reasons, but the all crates stall in the process of nurse-patient relationship. Impasse provokes variety of emotions in both he patient and nurse ranging from anxiety and apprehension to frustration, love, or severe anger. The commonest four impasses are discussed here: resistance, transference, counter transference and boundary violations.

Resistance: Resistance is the patent's reluctance or avoidance of verbalizing or experiencing troubling facets of oneself. The term was first coined by Freud. Resistance is frequently caused by patient's unwillingness to change when the need for change is recognized. Patient normally exhibits resistance during the working phase of nurse-patient relationship, because greater part of problem-solving occurs during this phase. Resistance may be because of:

- Nurse who has moved too swiftly or too deeply into the patient's feelings in to the patient's feelings.
- Intentional or unintentional communication of lack of respect.
- Nurse who is an inappropriate role model for therapeutic behaviour.
- Secondary gain -favourable environmental, interpersonal, and situational changes occur and material advantages as a result of the sickness (secondary gain can become a powerful force

in perpetuating a sickness because it makes environment more comfortable).

Transference: Transference is an unconscious response in which the patient experiences feelings and attitudes toward the nurse that were originally linked with other important figures of his or her life.

- They may be triggered by superficial similarity, such as facial features or speech, or by personality style or trait.
- These reactions are the patient's attempt to reduce anxiety.
- The nurse may be viewed as an authority figure from the past such as parent figure, or lost loved object, such as former spouse.
- Transference reactions are damaging to the therapeutic relationship only if they are ignored and unexplained.

Two types of transference are especially problematic in nurse-patient relationship: hostile transference and dependent reaction transference:

- Hostile transference: Patient may express hostility by uncooperativeness, negativism and hostile silence. If the hostility and anger are internalized, this resistance is expressed as depression and discouragement. Patient may terminate the relationship on the grounds that there is no chance of getting well. If hostility is externalized the patient may become critical, defiant, and irritable and may express doubts about nurse's training, experience or competence. Patient may undertake to compete with the nurse by reading books on psychology and debating intellectual issues rather than working on real life problems.
- Dependent reaction transference: This resistance is characterized by patient who are submissive, subordinate, and irritating and who regard nurse as godlike figure. Patient continues to demand more of the nurse.

MANAGEMENT OF TRANSFERENCE AND RESISTANCE

Resistance and transference can be difficult problems for the nurse. The psychiatric nurse must be ready to be exposed to such powerful positive and negative emotional reactions from the patient.

- Resistance may be because of the nurse and patient have not arrived mutually acceptable goals or plans of action. The appropriate action here is to return to the goals, purposes and roles of the nurse and patient relationship.

- The analysis of the resistance or transference should be directed toward the patient gaining awareness of these motivations and learning about being completely responsible for all actions or conduct.
- The first thing nurse must listen to the patient.
- When transference or resistance is recognized clarification and reflection of feelings can be used. Clarification gives the nurse a more focussed idea of what is happening. Reflection of the content ma help patients become aware of what has been going on their own mind.

Countertransfernce: It is a therapeutic impasse made by the nurse's specific emotional response to the qualities of the patient. This is inappropriate to the content and context of therapeutic nurse-patient relationship. It is transference applied to the nurse. It is natural that nurse feels warmth toward or liking for some patients more than others. The nurse also will be genuinely angry about the actions of some patient. But in countertransfernce, the nurse's reactions are not justified by reality. Here nurse identify the patient with people from their past, and personal needs interfere with their therapeutic relationship.

Types:

- Reactions of severe love or caring.
- Reactions of severe disgust or hostility.
- Reactions of severe anxiety frequently in response to resistance by the patient.

Examples:

- Difficulty in empathizing with the patient in several problem fields
- Feeling of depression during or after a session
- Feeling or anger or impatience due to the patient's unwillingness to change
- Argument with the patient or a tendency to push before the patient is ready
- Personal or social involvement with the patient
- Dreams about or preoccupation with the patient
- Sexual or aggressive fantasies about the patient

Other forms comprise staff involve in countertransfernce when they over-react the patient's aggressive conduct, ignore available patient data that would promote understanding

Ignoring patient's conduct that does not fit the staff's diagnosis, minimising a patent's behaviour, joking about or criticizing a patient or becoming in caught up in intimidation.

The nurse must be constant look out for countertransfernce, become aware when it occurs and work with it to promote therapeutic goals. The nurse must use self-examination throughout the relationship. Following questions are helpful:

- How do I feel about the patient?
- Do I feel sorry or sympathetic for the patient?
- Am I afraid of the patient?
- Do I get extreme pressure out of seeing the patient?
- Do I want to protect, reject, or punish the patient?

Countertransfernce can be damaging to the relationship; it should be dealt as early as possible. The nurse should discover the source of the problem. When it is recognized the nurse can exercise control over it. If required help, the nurse can seek individual or group supervision. 'Problem patients' may elicit strong negative feelings such as anger, fear and helplessness in the mind of nurse.

Such patients should be dealt with patience and action should be directed to making patient responsible for his own conduct. Nurse should review patient's needs and problems and use responsive dimensions of genuineness, respect, empathetic understanding, and concreteness.

Boundary Violations: Here the nurse goes beyond the boundaries of therapeutic relationship and establishes a social, economic, or personal relationship with a patient. Boundary violation is involved whenever a nurse is doing or thinking of doing something special, different or unusual for a patient. Situations where possible boundary violations can happen:

- The patient takes the nurse to a lunch or dinner
- The nurse regularly reveals personal information to the patient
- The nurse accepts free gifts from the patient
- The nurse agrees to meet the patient for treatment outside the usual therapeutic setting without therapeutic justification

Types:

- Role boundaries-problems with role boundaries call for the insight of the nurse and the setting of firm therapeutic limits with the patient.
- Time boundaries-odd and unusual hours that have no therapeutic necessity.
- Place and space boundaries-normally in an office or a hospital unit, outside that calls for strong therapeutic rationale.
- Money boundaries-regarding fee.
- Gift and service boundaries-gift acceptance may place undue obligations to the patient.
- Clothing boundaries-dress appropriately in a therapeutic manner.
- Language boundaries-addressing the patient and nurse's choice of words in implementing care. Too familiar, sexual, off-colour or leading language are boundary violations.
- Self-disclosure boundaries-inappropriately timed self-disclosure and that lacking therapeutic value.
- Post-discharge social boundaries-post-discharge social contact raise the question of boundary violation.
- Physical contact boundaries- sexual contact.

INTERVIEW SKILL

The activity of interviewing is by no means confined to mental health nursing in specific or to nursing generally. Indeed much of the empirical study of interviewing technique and effectiveness comes from other fields.

1. Mental health nursing relies heavily on the relationship between nurse and patient and the forging of a therapeutic alliance. This in turn, calls for good communication skills on the part of the nurse.
2. Self Disclosure: Revealing personal information about one-self is a controversial technique that calls for nursing experience, insight, and sophistication on the part of the interviewer. The nurse should share personal information with a patient only if, after careful evaluation the nurse believes that this sharing would benefit the patient and improve treatment. The nurse should never disclose personal information for selfish reasons.

3. Choosing Appropriate Questions: The patient's state and the subject being evaluated determine whether to ask open-ended or closed-ended questions. Open-ended questions are vague and may be answered in several different ways.

TYPES OF RELATIONSHIP

The nurse-patient relationship is by several regarded as the core of nursing. In this paper, a synthesized theory on the dynamics of that relationship is introduced from the patient's perspective. It is described as a dynamic lived reality characterized by a sense of spiritual connection which is experienced as a bond of energy. The highest quality of this connection is the life-giving nurse-patient relationship which is greatly empowering for the patient. The prerequisites for the growth of the nurse-patient relationship are perceived nurse caring, wisdom and competence in connecting with people. The dialectic nature of this relationship is discussed as well as the six main phases in the nurse-patient relationship growth.

Nurse-patient relationship to develop the nurse must be perceived by the patient as:

- Genuinely caring for the patient as an individual and as a patient.
- Competent - having the essential skills required in the relevant field of nursing and being competent in connecting with patients.
- Having professional wisdom, which is a combination of knowledge and experience.

These three necessary facets of professional nursing care created a sense of trust in the patients which is a necessary building block for the growth of a nurse-patient relationship from the patient's perspective.

The nurse-patient relationship has a dialectic nature: From the former patients' accounts it is clear that the nurse-patient relationship is dialectic in nature, involving both closeness as well as distance - which means that developing a nurse-patient relationship involves two inter-related processes - growth of connection while maintaining a comfortable distance of respect and compassion. This is symbolized with the metaphor of a bridge.

Presence or absence of relationship formation - the wall or the bridge: There are two major metaphors in the theory that of the bridge, symbolizing the openness in communication and the connectedness experienced by the patient in a life-giving nurse-patient relationship. The other metaphor is the wall, which symbolizes the negative or no communication, detachment and lack of a nurse-patient relationship, experienced by the patient in an encounter perceived as uncaring.

This theory could, thus, be called 'the wall-bridge theory of human encounters within nursing: from the patient's perspective'. The bridge is developed through mutual trust and the growth of a nurse-patient relationship. On the other hand, perceived uncaring creates distrust, disconnection and the above-mentioned 'wall' of negative or no communication.

ETHICS AND RESPONSIBILITIES

Generally, nurses think that they know what is best for their patients, frequently imposing their own methods for care and treatment decisions. This behaviour, referred to as paternalism, may occur in the psychiatric clinical setting where patients exhibit clinical symptoms of confusion, depression, or anxiety or when patients are unable to communicate their needs because of communication disorders or mental retardation. The nurse may fail to recognize an ethical dilemma because of lack of training in ethics or lack of available resources to describe ethical issues. The nurse may be subject to liability if the breach of care results in any harm or injury to the patient.

- The nurse, in all professional relationships, practices with compassion and respect for the inherent dignity, worth, and uniqueness of every individual, unrestricted by considerations of social or economic status, personal attributes, or the nature of health problems.
- The nurse's primary commitment is to the patient, whether an individual, family, group, or community.
- The nurse promotes, advocates for, and strives to protect the health, safety, and rights of the patient.
- The nurse is responsible and accountable for individual nursing practice and determines the appropriate delegation of tasks consistent with the nurse's obligation to furnish optimal patient care.
- The nurse owes the same responsibilities to self as to others, together with the responsibility to preserve integrity and safety, to maintain competence, and to continue personal and professional development.

- The nurse participates in establishing, maintaining, and improving health care environments and conditions of employment conducive to the provision of quality health care and consistent with the values of the profession through individual and collective action.
- The nurse participates in the advancement of the profession through contributions to practice, education, administration, and knowledge growth.
- The nurse collaborates with other health professionals and the public in promoting community, national, and international efforts to meet health needs.
- The profession of nursing, as represented by associations and their members, is responsible for articulating nursing values, for maintaining the integrity of the profession and its practice, and for shaping social policy.

ELEMENTS OF NURSE PATIENT CONTRACT

In the nurse patient relationship differing values are respected. The two communicate through a dialogue, or discussion, not a monologue, affirming the patient's reality and worth and permitting the patient to more fully define ego identity.

PERSONAL QUALITIES OF THE NURSE

The key therapeutic tool the psychiatric nurse employs is oneself. Thus self analysis is the first building block in providing quality nursing care.

Awareness of the self: Effective helpers must be able to answer the question, who am I? Self awareness is a key part of the psychiatric nursing experiences. The nurse's goal is to accomplish authentic, open and personal communication. The nurse must be able to examine the personal feelings, actions and reactions. This also has been described as emotional competence. A good understanding and acceptance of the self allow the nurse to acknowledge a patients differences and uniqueness.

Campbell has identified a holistic model of self awareness that consists of four interconnected components: psychological, physical, environmental and philosophical.

The psychological components comprise knowledge of emotions, motivations, self concept and personality. Being psychologically self aware means being sensitive to the feelings and outside events that affect those feelings.

The physical component is the knowledge of personal and general physiology, as well as of the bodily sensations, body image and physical potential.

The environment component consists of the sociocultural environment, relationships with others and the knowledge of the relationship between human beings and nature.

The philosophical component is the sense of life having meaning. A personal philosophy of life and death may or may not comprise a superior being, but it does take into account responsibility to the world and the ethics of behaviour.

Increasing self awareness: No one ever completely knows the inner self, as shown in Johari window.

IPR-JOHARI WINDOW

The Johari Window, named after the first names of its inventors, Joseph Luft and Harry Ingham, is one of the most useful models describing the process of human interaction. A four paned "window," as illustrated above, divides personal awareness into four different types, as represented by its four quadrants: open, hidden, blind, and unknown. The lines dividing the four panes are like window shades, which can move as an interaction progresses. In this model, each person is represented by their own window:

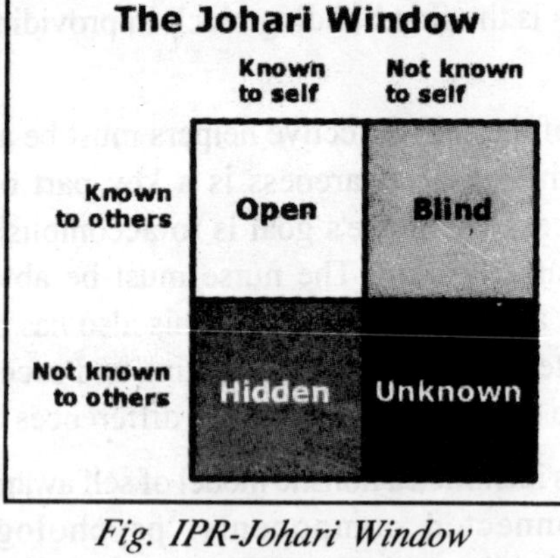

Fig. IPR-Johari Window

1. The "open" quadrant represents things that both I know about myself, and that you know about me. For instance, I know my name, and so do you, and if you have explored some of

my website, you know some of my interests. The knowledge that the window represents, can comprise not only factual information, but my feelings, motives, behaviours, wants, needs and desires. indeed, any information describing who I am. When I first meet a new person, the size of the opening of this first quadrant is not very big, because there has been little time to exchange information. As the process of getting to know one another continues, the window shades move down or to the right, placing more information into the open window, as described below.

2. The "blind" quadrant represents things that you know about me, but that I am unaware of. So, for instance, we could be eating at a restaurant, and I may have unknowingly gotten some food on my face. This information is in my blind quadrant because you can see it, but I can't. If you now tell me that I have something on my face, then the window shade moves to the right, enlarging the open quadrant's field. Now, I may also have blindspots with respect to several other much more complex things. For instance, perhaps in our ongoing conversation, you may notice that eye contact seems to be lacking. You may not say anything, because you may not want to embarrass me, or you may draw your own inferences that perhaps I am being insincere. Then the problem is, how can I get this information out in the open, because it may be affecting the level of trust that is developing between us? How can I learn more about myself? Unfortunately, there is no readily available answer. I may notice a slight hesitation on your part, and perhaps this may lead to a question. But who knows if I will pick this up, or if your answer will be on the mark.

3. The "hidden" quadrant represents things that I know about myself, that you don't know. So for instance, I have not told you, nor mentioned anywhere on my website, what one of my favourite ice cream flavours is. This information is in my "hidden" quadrant. As soon as I tell you that I love "Kwality vanilla" flavoured ice cream, I am effectively pulling the window shade down, moving the information in my hidden quadrant and enlarging the open quadrant's area. Again, there are vast amounts of information, virtually my whole life's story, that has yet to be revealed to you. As we get to know and trust each other, I will then feel more comfortable disclosing more

intimate details about myself. This process is called: "Self-disclosure."

4. The "unknown" quadrant represents things that neither I know about myself, nor you know about me. For instance, I may disclose a dream that I had, and as we both attempt to understand its significance, a new awareness may emerge, known to neither of us before the conversation took place. Being placed in new situations frequently reveal new information not formerly known to self or others. A novel situation can trigger new awareness and personal development. The process of moving formerly unknown information into the open quadrant, thus enlarging its field, has been likened to Maslow's concept of self-actualization. The process can also be viewed as a game, where the open quadrant is synonymous with the win-win situation.

The process of enlarging the open quadrant is called self-disclosure, a give and take process between nurse and the patients. Basically, as the nurse share something about herself (moving information from my hidden quadrant into the open) and if the other party is interested in getting to know me, they will reciprocate, by likewise disclosing information in their hidden quadrant. Thus, an interaction between two parties can be modelled dynamically as two active Johari windows.

We believe disclosure to be healthy, at least that's the impression one gets after reading Freud. Nevertheless, Anita Kelly recently wrote that self-disclosure of personal secrets has its dangers. We are frequently better off not telling secrets regarding our mental health problems or large-scale failures. "If you give people information about yourself, you give them power over you," she says. Be forewarned that most secrets get passed along to at least two more parties. People also misjudge how others react to secrets. Sometimes you get negative feedback.

As ones level of confidence and self esteem develops, one may actively invite others to comment on one's blind spots. A teacher may seek feedback from students on the quality of a specific lecture, with the desire of improving the presentation. Active listening skills are helpful in this endeavour. On the other hand, we all have defences, protecting the parts of ourselves that we feel vulnerable. Remember, the blind quadrant contains behaviour, feelings and motivations not accessible to the person, but which others can see. Feelings of inadequacy, incompetence, impotence, unworthiness, rejection, guilt, dependency, ambivalence for loved ones, needs to control and manipulate, are all difficult to face, and yet can be seen by others. To forcibly reveal what another wishes not to see, is "psychological rape," and can be traumatic. Fortunately, nature has provided us with a range of defence mechanisms to deal with such events, such as denial, ignoring, rationalizing, etc.

The Johari window, essentially being a model for communication, can also reveal difficulties in this field. In Johari terms, two people attempt to communicate via the open quadrants. On the simplest level, difficulties may arise because of a lack of clarity in the interaction, such as poor grammar or choice of words, unorganized thoughts, faulty logic etc. This induces the receiver to criticize you, the sender, by revealing something that was in your blind quadrant. Then, if the feedback works, you correct it immediately or perhaps on a more long term methodology take a course in reading and writing. On a deeper level, you may be in a group meeting, and while you secretly sympathize with the minority viewpoint, you voted with the majority. Nevertheless, blind to you, you actually may be communicating this information via body language, in conflict with your verbal message. On an even deeper level, you in an interaction with others, may always put on a smiling, happy face, hiding all negative feelings. By withholding negative feelings, you may be signalling to your friends to withhold also, and keep their distance. Thus, your communication style may seem bland or distant.

GOALS, PHASES, TASKS, THERAPEUTIC TECHNIQUES

Nurses should be able to answer the question, what is significant to me? Awareness helps the nurse to be honest and avoid the unethical use of patients to meet the personal needs.

CLARIFICATION OF VALUES

- Value Systems: Values are concepts that are formed as result of life experience with family, friends, culture, education, work and relaxation. Value systems furnish the model for several daily decisions and actions. By being aware of value systems, nurses can identify situations in which value systems are in conflict. Several therapeutic relationships test the nurse's values. E.g. a patient may describe a sexual behaviour that the nurse finds unacceptable; a patient may talk about the divorce where as the nurse may strongly believe that marriage contracts shouldn't be broken; or a patient may be a born again Christian but the nurse may not believe in God or religion.

- Value Clarification Process: It allows the individual to discover their values by evaluating, exploring and determining what those values are and what priority they hold in decision making process. Seven criteria are used to determine the value. These criteria should be regarded as in relation to an individual's strongest value and tested against the individuals own definition of a value.

The three criteria of choosing relay on the individual's cognitive abilities, the two criteria of prizing emphasize the emotional or affective level, and the two criteria of acting have a behavioural focus.

- The mature valuing process: It is complex. There is no guarantee that the choice made will prove to be self -actualizing. The valuing process in the mature person has the following characteristics:
  - It is fluid and flexible.
  - The valuing experience is tied to a specific time and experience.
  - Personal experience provides the value information.
- Exploration of feelings: The nurses should be open to, aware of and in control of their feelings so that they can be used to help the patient. The feelings that the nurse have serve a significant purpose. In helping others, nurses have several feelings; elation at seeing a patient improves, disappointment when a patient regresses, distress when a patient refuses the help, anger when a patient is demanding or manipulative and power when a patient express strong dependence on the nurse.
- Serving as a role model: A nurse ahs an obligation to model maladaptive and development producing behaviour. If a nurse has a chaotic personal life, it will show in the nurse's work with patients, decreasing the effectiveness of care. The effective nurse has a fulfilling and satisfying personal life that is not dominated by conflict, distress, or denial and that the nurses approach to life conveys a sense of growing, hopefulness, and adapting.
- Altruism: Altruism is concern for the welfare of others. It does not mean that an altruistic person shouldn't expect ample compensation and recognition or must practice denial or self sacrifice. A sense of altruism also can apply to changing social conditions to meet human welfare needs. One goal of all helping

professional should be to create a people -serving and development facilitating society. So the essential goal of nurse is to work to change the larger structure and process of society in ways that will promote the people health and well-being.

- Ethics and responsibility: Nurse's sense of ethics is the need to assume responsibility for behaviour. This involves knowing restrictions and strengths and being accountable for them. As a member of health team nurse has ready access to the knowledge and expertise of other people; these resources should be used appropriately.

PHASES OF THERAPEUTIC RELATIONSHIP

A vital characteristic of the nurse-patient relationship is the sharing of behaviours, thoughts and feelings. Four phases of nurse-patient relationship have been identified: pre interaction phase, introductory or orientation phase, working phase and termination phase.

PRE INTERACTION PHASE

It begins before the nurse's first contact with the patient. A common fear of nurse related to the stereotype of psychiatric patient as violent. Because this is the picture portrayed by the media several nurses are afraid of being physically hurt by the patients out burst of aggressive behaviour. Other fear is related to nurses questioning their own mental health status. Nurses may fear mental sickness and tension that exposure to psychiatric patients might cause them to lose their own needs. Other tasks of this phase comprise gathering data about the patient if information is available and planning for the first interaction with the patient.

INTRODUCTORY OR ORIENTATION PHASE

It is the introductory phase that the nurse and patient first meet. One of the nurses concerns is to find out why the patient sought help and whether it was voluntary.

Formulating Contracts: The tasks in this phase of relationship are to establish a climate of trust, understanding, acceptance and open communication and formulate a contract with the patient.

The elements of a Nurse -patient contract:

- Name of the individual
- Roles of nurse and patient
- Responsibilities of nurse and patient

- Expectations of nurse and patient
- Purpose of the relationship
- Meeting location and time
- Conditions for termination
- Confidentiality

Exploring feelings: Both the nurse and patient may experience some level of discomfort and nervousness in the introductory phase. Reasons patient have difficulty seeking help:

- It may be difficult to see or admit one's difficulties, first to oneself and then to another.
- It is not easy to trust or be open with strangers.
- Sharing personal problems with another person can threaten one's sense of independence, autonomy and self -esteem.
- Solving problems involves thinking about something that may be unpleasant, viewing life realistically, deciding on a plan of action, and then carrying out whatever it takes to bring about a change.

Other tasks of the nurse in the orientation phase of the relationship comprise the following:

- To explore the patients perceptions, thoughts, feelings and actions.
- To identify the pertinent patient problem.
- To define mutual, specific goals with the patient.

WORKING PHASE

Most of the therapeutic work is carried out during the working phase. The nurse helps the patient to master anxieties, increase independence and self -responsibility and develops constructive coping mechanisms. Actual behaviour change is the focus of this phase. Patient frequently exhibit resistance during this phase. As the relationship develops the patient begins to feel close to the nurse.

TERMINATION PHASE

Termination is one of the most difficult but most significant phases of the therapeutic nurse-patient relationship. It is the time to exchange feelings and memories and to assess mutually the patient's progress and goal attainment.

Criteria for determining patient readiness for termination:

- The patient experiences relief from the presenting problem.
- The patients functioning has improved.
- The patient has increased self-esteem and a stronger sense of identity.
- The patient employs more adaptive coping reactions.
- The patient has achieved the planned treatment outcomes.

Together the nurse and patient review the progress made in treatment and the attainment of specified goals. Feelings of rejection, sadness, loss and anger are expressed and explored. It may be helpful to prepare the patient for termination by decreasing the number of visits, incorporating others into the meetings or changing the location of the meetings. The reasons behind a change should be clarified so that the patient does not interpret it as rejection by the nurse.

Responsive dimensions: The nurse must possess several skills and qualities to establish and maintain a therapeutic relationship. Specific core conditions for facilitative interpersonal relationship can be classified into responsive dimension and action dimensions. The responsive dimensions comprise geniuses, respect, empathetic understanding and concreteness. The responsive dimensions are crucial in a therapeutic relationship establish trust and open communication. The nurse's goal is to understand the patient and to help the patient gain self understanding and insight.

Genuineness: Genuineness means that the nurse is an open, honest, sincere person who is actively involved in the relationship. Genuineness means that the nurse's response is sincere, that the nurse is not thinking and feeling one thing and saying something different. Whatever the nurse shows must be real and not merely a professional response that has been learned and repeated.

Respect: Respect also called as nonpossessive warmth or unconditional positive regard, does not depend on the patients behaviour. Caring, liking and valuing are other terms for respect. Respect can be communicated in different ways: by sitting silently with a patient who is crying, by genuine laughter with the patent over a specific event, by accepting the patients request not to share a several experience, by apologizing for the hurt unintentionally caused by a specific phase, or by being open enough to communicate anger or hurt caused by the patient.

Empathetic understanding: Empathy is the capability to enter into the life of another person and to accurately perceive his or her current feelings and their meanings. Rogers (1975) described it as "to sense the patient's private world as though it were on your own, but without losing the as though quality. There are two types of empathy. The first is basic empathy. It involves the natural, general human capacity to feel for others. The second type is trained empathy, which is taught and learned in relation to helping others. It is also called as clinical empathy or professional empathy.

Growth of empathy: Empathic understanding consists of a number of stages. If patients allow nurses to enter into their private world and attempt to communicate their perception of feelings, nurses must be receptive to this feeling; nurses must be receptive to this communication. Next nurse must understand the patient's communication by putting themselves in the place of patient. Nurses must then step back into their own rolé and communicate understanding to the patient.

Empathic reactions: First the nurse needs to furnish genuineness and unconditional positive regard for the patient. Then the understanding conveyed to the patient through empathy gives him or her personhood or identity. The patient incorporates these facets into a new changing self concept. Once self concept changes, behaviour also changes, thus producing the positive clinical outcome of therapy.

Empathetic functioning scale: Kalisch(1973)devised the nurse -patient empathetic functioning scale, which describes 5 classes of empathy.

Class 0 and 1: the nurse ignores the patient's feelings, goes off on a tangent or misinterprets what the patient's feelings. The nurse at this level may be uninterested in the patient or concentrating on the fact of what the patient says rather than on current feelings and experiences. The nurse is doing something other than listening, such as evaluating the patient, giving advice or thinking about personal problems or needs.

Class 2: a middle level of empathy shows that the nurse is making an effort to understand the patient's feelings. They are required initially to build an atmosphere of trust and openness.

Classes 3 and 4: high levels of empathy communicate "I am with you"; the nurses reactions fit perfectly with the patient's current feelings and experiences. The nurse reactions also serve to expand the patient's awareness of hidden feelings through the use of clarification and reflection. Such empathy is communicated by the language used, voice qualities and nonverbal behaviour, all of which reflect the nurses seriousness and depth of feeling.

Concreteness: It involves utilizing specific terminology rather than abstractions when discussing the patient's feelings, experiences and behaviour. It avoids vagueness and ambiguity. It has three functions: to keep the nurses reactions close to the patients feelings and experiences, to foster accuracy of understanding by the nurse, and to encourage the patient to attend to specific problem areas. In the orientation phase, concreteness should be high. It is necessary for the formulation of specific goals and plans. In the working phase, it should be at a low level to facilitate a thorough self -exploration. High levels are again desirable a t the end of the working phase, when patients are engaging in action and during the termination phase.

Action Dimensions: The action oriented conditions for facilitative interpersonal relationship are confrontation, immediacy, therapist self disclosurecatharsis and role play.

Confrontation: It is an expression by the nurse of perceived discrepancies in the patient's behaviour. The three classes of confrontation are listed in the following:

- Discrepancies between the patients expression of what she or he is and what he or she wants to be.
- Discrepancies' between the patient's verbal self expression and nonverbal behaviour.
- Discrepancies between the patient's verbal expressed experience of himself or herself and the nurses experience of him or her.

Confrontation is an attempt to by the nurse to make the patient aware of incongruence in his or her feelings, attitudes, beliefs and behaviours. It also may lead to the discovery of ambivalent feelings in the patient. It is not limited to negative facets of the patient. It comprises pointing out discrepancies involving resources and strengths that are unrecognized and unused. It calls for that the nurse collect sufficient data about the patient's history and accumulate sufficient perception and observations of verbal and nonverbal communication so that validation of reality is possible. The nurse must have developed an understanding of the patient to perceive discrepancies, inconsistencies in the word and deed, distortions and defences. The nurse must be willing and able to work through the crisis after confronting the patient. Without this commitment confrontation lacks therapeutic potential and can be harmful to both patient and nurse.

Timing in relationship before confrontation nurse should assess the following factors:

- The trust level in the relationship.
- The timing.
- The patients stress level.
- The strength of the patient's defence mechanisms.
- The patients perceived need for personal space or closeness.
- The patients level of rage and tolerance for hearing another perception.

Patients have the capacity to deny or accept nurse's observation and their response to the confrontation can serve as a measure of its success or failure. Acceptance indicates appropriate timing and patient readiness. Denial by the patient provides nurses with additional information that the patients are resisting change and are unwilling to enlarge their view of reality at this time. In the orientation phase, the nurse should use the confrontation infrequently. In the working phase of the relationship, more direct confrontation may concentrate on specific patient discrepancies. The nurse may confront the patient with areas of weakness or shortcomings or may concentrate on the discrepancies between the nurses perception of the patient and the patients self perception. This expands the patient's awareness and helps the patient move to higher levels of functioning. Confrontation is especially significant in pointing out when the patient has developed insight but has not changed the behaviour. Inexperienced nurses frequently avoid confrontation.

Immediacy: Immediacy involves focusing on the current interaction of the nurse and the patient in the relationship. It involves sensitivity to the patient's feelings and a willingness to cope with theses feelings rather than ignore them. It is not possible or appropriate for the nurse to focus continually on the immediacy of the relationship. It is most appropriate to do so when the relationship is not progressing. It is also helpful to look at the immediacy when the relationship is progressing especially well.

Nurses self disclosure: Self -disclosures are subjectively true, personal statements about the self, intentionally revealed to another person. The nurse may share experiences or feelings hat are similar to those of the patient and may emphasize both similarities and differences. It is an expression of genuineness and honesty by the nurse and is an aspect of empathy. Criteria for self disclosure comprise the following:

- To model and educate.
- To foster the therapeutic alliance.

- To validate reality.
- To encourage the patients autonomy.

The nurse should disclose in response to statements made by the patient. If the nurses disclosure is away from what the patient is experiencing, it can distract the patient from the problem or cause feelings of alienation. A patient who is experiencing intense anxiety may feel threatened by the nurses self disclosure.

Emotional catharsis: Emotional catharsis occurs when patient is encouraged to talk about things that are most bothersome. It brings fears, feelings and experiences out into the open so that they can be examined and discussed with the nurse. Forcing emotional catharsis on the patient could precipitate a panic episode because the patient's defences are attacked without sufficient alternative coping mechanisms available.

If the patient has difficulty in expressing feelings, nurses may help suggesting how they or others might feel in the patients' specific situation. Some patients react directly to the question "How did that make you feel?"

Role playing: It involves acting out a specific situation. It increases the patient's insight into human relations and can deepen the capability to see the situation from another person's point of view. Role playing consists of the following steps:

- Define the problem
- Creating a readiness for role playing
- Establishing the situation
- Casting the characters
- Briefing and warming up
- Acting
- Stopping
- Analyzing and discussing
- Evaluating

One of the specific way in which role playing can be used to solve conflicts and increase self awareness is through a dialogue that calls for the patient to take the pat of each person or each part of a problem. If the conflict is internal, the dialogue occurs in the present tense between the patients conflicting selves till one part of the conflict overweighs the other. If the conflict involves a second person, the patient is instructed to imagine that the other person is sitting in the chair across from you. The patient is told to begin the dialogue wants and resentments about the other person. Then the patient changes the chairs, assumes the function of another person and responds to what was just said. It not only helps the patient in expressing feelings and opinions but also gives a reality for the probable response from the other party involved in the conflict.

THERAPEUTIC IMPASSE AND ITS INTERVENTION

Therapeutic impasses are locks in the progress of the nurse-patient relationship. They are resistance, transference, counter transference and boundary violations.

Resistance: It is the patient's reluctance or avoidance of verbalizing or experiencing troubling facets of oneself. Resistance is frequently caused by the patient's unwillingness to change when the need for change is recognized. It normally occurs in working phase.

Transference: It is an unconscious response in which the patient experiences the feelings and attitude towards the nurse that were originally linked with other important figures in his or her life. It may be a facial feature or manner of speech or by a personality trait or style.

Counter transference: It is a therapeutic impasse created b the nurse's specific emotional response to the qualities of the patient. This response is inappropriate in therapeutic relationship.

Boundary violations: These occur when the nurse goes outside the boundaries of the therapeutic relationship and establishes a social, economic, or personal relationship with a patient.

Boundaries violations can occur in the following classes:

- Role boundaries: It is related to the psychiatric nurses role.
- Time boundaries: These relates to the time of day that the nurse implements treatment.
- Place and space boundaries: These relate to where treatment takes place. Treatment out of the office normally violates therapeutic relationship.
- Money boundaries: - These relates to the compensation for the treatment between the nurse and patient.
- Gift and service boundaries: Gift giving is a controversial issue in nursing. Gifts can be classified into the following types:

— Gifts to reciprocate for care given.
— Gifts intend to manipulate or change the quality of care given.
— Gifts given as perceived obligation by the patient.
— Gifts given to the organization to recognize excellence of care given.

- Clothing boundaries: Theses pertains to the nurses need to dress in appropriate therapeutic manner.
- Language boundaries: This boundary raises questions of when patients should be addressed by their first or last name the tone that the nurse employs when talking with the patient and the nurses choice of words in implementing care.
- Self -disclosure boundaries: Nurse self disclosure that lacks therapeutic value are suspect for boundary violation.
- Post discharge social boundaries: The post discharge social contact with a patient by the nurse always raise questions of boundary violations.
- Physical contact boundaries: All physical contact with a patient must be evaluated for possible boundary violations. Sexual contact of any kind is never therapeutic and never acceptable within the nurse patient relationship.

The nurse's effectiveness in working with the psychiatric patients is related to the knowledge base, clinical skill and self evaluation. The nurse and patient, as participants in an interpersonal relationship, are entwined in a pattern of reciprocal emotions that directly affect the therapeutic outcome.

REFERENCES

Beck, A. T. (1976). Cognitive therapy and the emotional disorders. New York: The New American Library, Inc.

Berne, E. (1964). Games people play. New York: Grove Press.

Caplan, G. (1964). Principles of preventive psychiatry. New York: Basic Books.

Crain, W. C. (1980). Theories of development: Concepts and application. Englewood Cliffs, NJ: Prentice-Hall, Inc.

Frankl, V. E. (1959). Man's search for meaning: An introduction to logotherapy. New York: The Beacon Press.

Glasser, W. (1965). Reality therapy: A new approach to psychiatry. New York: Harper & Row.

Miller, P. H. (1983). Theories of developmental psychology. San Francisco: W. H. Freeman & Co.

Millon, T. (Ed.). (1967). Theories of psychopathology. Philadelphia: W. B. Saunders.

Sugarman, L. (1986). Life-span development: Concepts, theories and interventions. London: Methuen & Co., Ltd.

Szasz, T. (1961). The myth of mental illness. New York: Hoeber-Harper.

5

Treatment Modalities and Therapies

Recent changes in health care and reimbursement have affected mental health treatment, as they have all areas of medicine, nursing, and related health fields. In-patient treatment is frequently the last, rather than the first, mode of treatment for mental sickness. Current treatment reflects the belief that it is more beneficial and certainly more cost-effective for patients to remain in the community and receive out-patient treatment whenever possible. The patient can frequently continue to work and can stay connected with family, friends, and other support systems while participating in therapy.

Out-patient therapy also takes into account that an individual's personality or behaviour patterns such as coping skills, styles of communication, and level of self-esteem, gradually develop over the course of a lifetime and can't be changed in a relatively short in-patient course of treatment. Hospital admission is indicated when the person is seriously depressed and suicidal, seriously psychotic, experiencing alcohol or drug withdrawal, or exhibiting behaviours that call for close supervision in a safe supportive environment.

The introduction of psychopharmacological treatments since the late 1940s has undoubtedly revolutionised the treatment of psychosis, affective disorders and other mental health problems. However, as in many other areas of health care, pharmacotherapy often requires long-term maintenance treatment to maintain health and prevent relapse.

This can be problematic because service users are often uncertain about taking medication, especially long term. Mental health nurses have always had an important role to play in medication management, working with service users to help them manage their treatment so that it fits in with their lifestyle and maximises their health.

PSYCHO PHARMACOLOGY

Psychopharmacology is the study of drug-induced changes in mood, sensation, thinking, and behaviour. The discipline of psychopharmacology studies a wide range of substances with various types of psychoactive properties. The professional and commercial fields of pharmacology and psychopharmacology don't mainly concentrate on psychedelic or recreational drugs, as the bulk of studies are conducted for the growth, study, and use of drugs for the modification of behaviour and the alleviation of symptoms, especially in the treatment of mental disorders (psychiatric medication). While studies are conducted on all psychoactives by both fields, psychopharmacology focuses mainly on the psychoactive and chemical interactions with the brain.

Pharmacologic treatment of patients with personality disorders focuses on the patient's symptoms rather than the specific subtype. The four symptom classes that underlie personality disorders are cognitive perceptual distortions together with psychotic symptoms; affective symptoms and mood dysregulation; aggression and behavioural dysfunction; and anxiety.

Nerve cells communicate with each other by electrical impulses. An impulse travels along the nerve axon and stimulates the release of chemical messengers known as neurotransmitters. They are released from storage vesicles in the presynaptic nerve and released into the synapse. The synapse is the gap between the presynaptic cell and the postsynaptic cell at a transmission site. The neurotransmitter travels across the synapse and binds with the appropriate receptor on the postsynaptic cell membrane. Receptors are selective cellular recognition sites for neurotransmitters, hormones and many drugs. This usually sets up an electrical impulse (an excitatory effect) in the postsynaptic nerve cell and so the message is passed on.

Sometimes neurotransmitters have an inhibitory effect and stop further transmission of the message. After transmission, the neurotransmitter usually leaves the receptor and is taken back up into the presynaptic cell (reuptake) or destroyed by enzymes such as monoamine oxidase (MAO) in the synapse. Some of the most important neurotransmitters in mental disorders are dopamine, serotonin (5-hydroxytryptamine or 5-HT), noradrenaline and gamma-aminobutyric acid (GABA). It has been hypothesised that over- or under-response within neurotransmission may be linked with some mental health problems. For example, psychosis may involve excessive dopamine neurotransmission, whilst depression and mania may involve disruption in the normal patterns of neurotransmission of noradrenaline and serotonin. This thinking about neurotransmission has led to the development of a range of pharmacological strategies to try to treat mental health problems.

For example, antipsychotic drugs stop the neurotransmitter from binding to the postsynaptic receptor site by blocking those receptors. This reduces the transmission of the message and activity of the nerves in that structure of the brain. Antidepressants stop the reuptake of noradrenaline and serotonin and regulate areas of the brain that make them.

Monoamine oxidase inhibitors (MAOIs) prevent enzymatic metabolism of noradrenaline and serotonin. Both these actions result in increasing levels available at the synapse, thus increasing the activity between nerve cells. The clinical effects of medicines used in psychiatry do not, however, confine themselves to the specific areas of the brain associated with mental health problems. Medicines will often interact with many other receptors, causing unwanted symptoms or side effects and potential drug interactions during concomitant drug therapy.

Lithium, anticonvulsant mood stabilizers, and benzodiazepines are used most frequently to treat aggression. Low-dose neuroleptics may be useful in modifying predatory aggression.

Mood dysregulation symptoms comprise emotional instability, emotional detachment, depression, and dysphoria. Emotional instability and mood swings react favourably to lithium, carbamazepine (Tegretol), valproate (Depakote), or low-dose neuroleptics such as haloperidol (Haldol).

Emotional detachment, cold and aloof emotions, and disinterest in social relations frequently react to selective serotonin reuptake inhibitors (SSRIs) or atypical antipsychotics such as risperidone (Risperdal), olanzapine (Zyprexa), and quetiapine (Seroquel). Atypical depression is frequently treated with SSRIs or monoamine oxidase inhibitor antidepressants (MAOIs) or low-dose antipsychotic medications.

Anxiety seen with personality disorders may be chronic cognitive anxiety, somatic anxiety, or intense acute anxiety. Chronic, constant anxiety responds to SSRIs and MAOIs, as does chronic somatic anxiety, or anxiety evidenced as multiple physical complaints. Episodes of acute, intense anxiety are best treated with MAOIs or low-dose antipsychotic medications.

PSYCHOLOGICAL THERAPIES

Psychological therapies are recognized by both researchers and clinicians as effective treatments for reducing the frequency and intensity of symptoms of mental illnesses. Effective psychological treatments for stress changes in behaviour and/or thoughts (sometimes called cognitions). When appropriate, behavioural and cognitive treatments are combined alone or with medication to get the best result.

THERAPEUTIC COMMUNITY

Therapeutic community is a term applied to a participative, group-based approach to long-term mental sickness, personality disorders and drug addiction. The approach is normally residential with the patients and therapists living together, is based on milieu therapy principles and comprises group psychotherapy as well as practical activities.

Therapeutic communities have and acquired some reputation for success in rehabilitation and patient satisfaction in Britain and abroad. In Britain, 'democratic analytic' therapeutic communities have tended to specialise in the treatment of moderate to intense personality disorders and complex emotional and interpersonal problems. The evolution of therapeutic communities has followed a different path with hierarchically arranged communities (or concept houses) specialising in the treatment of drug and alcohol dependence.

PSYCHOTHERAPY

Psychotherapy is an interpersonal, relational intervention used by trained psychotherapists to assist patients in problems of living. This normally comprises increasing individual sense of well-being and reducing subjective discomforting experience. Psychotherapists employ a range of techniques based on experiential relationship building, dialogue, communication and behaviour change and that are designed to improve the mental health of a patient or patient, or to improve group relationships (such as in a family). Psychotherapy may be performed by practitioners with a number of different qualifications, together with psychologists, marriage and family therapists, licensed clinical social workers, counsellors, psychiatric nurses, music therapists, and psychiatrists.

Psychotherapy Systems

There are many main broad systems of psychotherapy:

- Psychoanalysis - the first practice to be called a psychotherapy. It encourages the verbalization of all the patient's thoughts, together with free associations, fantasies, and dreams, from which the analyst formulates the nature of the unconscious conflicts which are causing the patient's symptoms and character problems.

- Cognitive Behavioural - in general seeks to by different methodologies identify and transcend maladaptive cognitions, appraisal, beliefs and reactions with the aim of influencing destructive negative emotions and problematic dysfunctional behaviours.
- Psychodynamic - is a form of depth psychology, the primary focus of which is to reveal the unconscious content of a patient's psyche in an effort to alleviate psychic worry. Though it has its roots in psychoanalysis, psychodynamic therapy tends to be briefer and less intensive than traditional psychoanalysis.
- Existential - is based on the existential belief that human beings are alone in the world. This aloneness leads to feelings of meaninglessness which can be overcome only by creating one's own values and meanings.
- Humanistic - emerged in reaction to both behaviourism and psychoanalysis and is thus known as the Third Force in the growth of psychology. It is explicitly related with the human context of the growth of the individual with an emphasis on subjective meaning, a rejection of determinism, and a concern for positive development rather than pathology. It posits an inherent human capacity to maximise potential, 'the self-actualing tendency'. The task of Humanistic therapy is to create a relational environment where this tendency might flourish.
- Brief therapy - is an umbrella term for a range of approaches to psychotherapy. It differs from other schools of therapy in that it emphasizes (1) a concentrate on a specific problem and (2) direct intervention. It is solution-based rather than problem-oriented. It is less related with how a problem arose than with the current factors sustaining it and preventing change.
- Systemic Therapy - seeks to address people not at a person level, as is frequently the focus of other forms of therapy, but as people in relationship, dealing with the interactions of groups, their patterns and dynamics (comprises family therapy & marriage counselling).
- Transpersonal Therapy - Addresses the patient in the context of a spiritual understanding of consciousness.

- Body Psychotherapy or Body-oriented Psychotherapy - addresses the whole of the person, together with their body, manifestations of symptoms in the body of the patient, body language, proprioception, emotional expression, proxemics, psychosomatics etc.

There are dozens of approaches, which continue to be developed around the wide variety of theoretical backgrounds. Several practitioners use many approaches in their work and alter their approach based on patient need.

COGNITIVE THERAPY

The cognitive therapy, which focuses on immediate thought processing- how an individual perceives or interprets his or her experience and determines how he or she feels and behaves. For instance, if an individual interprets a situation as dangerous, he or she experiences anxiety and tries to escape. Basic emotions of sadness, elation, anxiety, and anger are reactions to perceptions of loss, gain, danger, and wrongdoing by others. Aaron Beck is credited with pioneering cognitive theory in individuals with depression.

SUPPORTIVE THERAPY

Supportive therapy is the psychotherapeutic approach employed with the bulk of mentally sick people. However, most mental health professional training programs dedicate little time and effort to the teaching and learning of supportive therapy, and several mental health professionals are unable to distinctly and concisely articulate the nature or process of supportive work. Though supportive therapy incorporates several specific techniques from a wide variety of psychotherapy schools, it can be conceptualized as consisting of a more limited number of underlying strategies.

BEHAVIOURAL THERAPIES

Behavioural therapies assume that the behaviour is the problem and that there are no unconscious conflicts or underlying problems of self-esteem. Instead, psychological disorders are behaviours that have been learned - sometimes under extreme or unusual circumstances. If disordered behaviour is learned, then it can be unlearned or extinguished. "Classical conditioning" and "Operant conditioning" theories each offer variations of behavioural therapies.

Classical Conditioning Therapies

Systematic Desensitization: This therapy has been especially effective for treating phobias. It is based on the idea that a person can't be relaxed and nervous at the same time. First, the situations that trigger anxiety are identified and rank ordered based on how much anxiety each situation triggers. Second, the patient is taught relaxation techniques. Next, the patient imagines the least anxiety provoking situation and practices the relaxation techniques. Many trials of relaxing while imagining the anxiety situation may be needed till the situation triggers a relaxation response instead of an anxiety response. This process is repeated with the next situation on the hierarchy, then the next, then the next. Eventually, the patient will practice relaxation techniques in the real situations till there are no more anxiety reactions in those situations.

Aversive Conditioning: This therapy has been used most with undesirable compulsive behaviours, such as alcoholism or child molesting. It is also based on the idea that a fear response can't occur at the same time as a pleasurable or arousal response. This stimulus that has provoked a positive response is paired with an aversive stimulus. For instance, alcoholic drinks are laced with another drug that induces vomiting. Quite a few trials of drinking and vomiting should extinguish the undesirable behaviour. Unfortunately, aversive conditioning has the same problems linked with utilizing punishment as a learning tool.

Operant Conditioning Therapies

Token Economies: A system of rewards or points is created to reward positive or desirable behaviours. Rewards or points are lost when the patient performs undesirable behaviours. Token economies work best when they are used in institutional settings or group-homes where there can be frequent monitoring of behaviour and frequent rewards. As the patient gets used to the token economy, time intervals between rewards can be increased. Eventually, points or rewards also need to be replaced with naturally occurring positive or negative consequences.

RELAXATION THERAPIES

In this form of therapy the patient is helped to solve stresses that can contribute to the specific disorder. Breathing re-training and other skills are taught in which the patient is actively involved in developing skills that are useful for a lifetime. Can take time to attain results and treatment benefits are limited to active use of the techniques.

Adlerian Therapy: It is a growth model. It stresses a positive view of human nature and that we are in control of our own fate and not a victim to it. We start at an early age in creating our own distinctive style of life and that style stays relatively constant through the remained of our life. That we are motivated by our setting of goals, how we cope with the tasks we face in life, and our social interest. The therapist will gather as much family history as they can. They will use this data to help set goals for the patient and to get an idea of the patients' past performance. This will help make several the goal is not to low or high, and that the patient has the means to reach it. The goal of Adlerian Therapy is to challenge and encourage the patients' premises and goals. To encourage goals that are useful socially and to help them feel equal. These goals maybe from any component of life together with, parenting skills, marital skills, ending substance-abuse, and most anything else. The therapist will concentrate on and examine the patients' lifestyle and the therapist will try to form a mutual respect and trust for each other. They will then mutually set goals and the therapist will provided encouragement to the patient in reaching their goals. The therapist may also assign homework, setup contracts between them and the patient, and make suggestions on how the patient can reach their goals.

Existential Therapy: It focuses on freedom of choice in shaping one's own life. Teaches one is responsible to shape his/her own life and a need for self-determination and self-awareness. The uniqueness of each individual forms his/her own distinctive personality, starting from infancy. Existential therapy focuses on the present and on the future. The therapist try's to help the patient see they are free and to see the possibilities for their future. They will challenge the patient to recognize that he/she themselves were responsible for the events in their life. This type of therapy is well suited in helping the patient to make good choices or in dealing with life.Yoga: Yoga therapy technique corrects the problem from the most fundamental level. The corrections are sought from the innermost layer of our existence (Anandamaya kosa or the soul or the will - the master of the system). A total correction of the bodily disturbances is brought about by correcting the disturbances at the emotional, psychological and the vital energy levels. The integrated approach employs quite a few techniques with a distinctive aim of reaching a state of total silence or calmness of mind or deep relaxation and rest.

Meditation: Meditation is an activity that calms the mind and keeps it centred on the present. In the meditative state, the mind is not cluttered with thoughts or memories of the past, nor is it related with future events. Meditation, which has been practiced for thousands of years, is an effective means of treating stress and managing pain. There are hundreds of meditation techniques, most of which fall into one of two classes: concentrative and mindfulness. During concentrative meditation, attention is centred on a single sound, an object or one's breath, to bring about a calm, tranquil mind. During mindfulness meditation, the mind becomes aware of but does not react to the wide variety of sensations, feelings, and images tied in with a current activity. Much research has been done on trasnscendental meditation (TM). TM brings about a state of deep relaxation in which the body is totally at rest, but the mind is highly alert. Meditation relies on the body's capability to switch to an alpha (resting) or theta (relaxing) brain-wave state, during which the brain's rhythm slows appreciably, and endorphins, the body's natural painkillers, are released. Studies have shown that during meditation, metabolism is lowered, resulting in a slower heart rate, decreased blood pressure, and slower breathing. Bio feedback: Biofeedback is a therapy, in which people are trained to improve their health by utilizing signals from their own bodies. In the late 1960s research showed that several involuntary activities like brain activity, blood pressure, heart rate can be altered by tuning into our body. This was termed as Biofeedback. Simply put biofeedback is the technique of looking into the signals from our body, for instance measuring one's weight or temperature are easy methods of biofeedback, as both devices feedback information about the body. Biofeedback is used in a range of situations. It is in general used by physical therapists to help stroke victims regain movement in paralyzed muscles. Psychologists use it to help tense and nervous patients learn to relax.

ALTERNATIVE SYSTEM OF MEDICINE

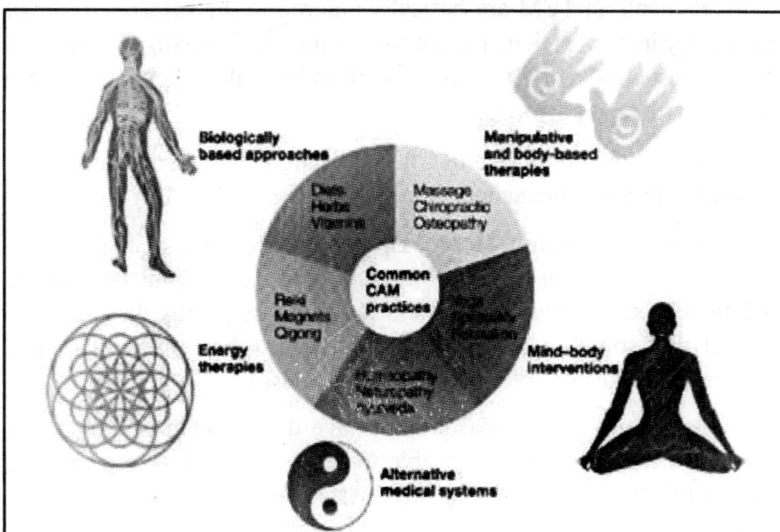

Fig. Alternative System of Medicine

Alternative system of medicine involve complete systems of theory and practice that have developed independently from or parallel to allopathic (traditional) medicine. Several are traditional systems of medicine that are exercised by individual cultures throughout the world. Major Eastern whole medical systems comprise traditional Chinese medicine (TCM) and Ayurvedic medicine, one of India's traditional systems of medicine. Major Western whole medical systems comprise homeopathy and naturopathy. Other systems have been developed by Native American, African, Middle Eastern, Tibetan, and Central and South American cultures.

TRADITIONAL CHINESE MEDICINE

TCM is a complete system of healing that dates back to 200 B.C. in written form. Korea, Japan, and Vietnam have all developed their own unique versions of traditional medicine based on practices originating in China. In the TCM view, the body is a delicate equilibrium of two opposing and inseparable forces: yin and yang. Yin represents the cold, slow, or passive principle, while yang represents the hot, excited, or active principle. Among the major assumptions in TCM are that health is achieved by maintaining the body in a "balanced state" and that disease is because of an internal imbalance of yin and yang. This imbalance leads to blockage in the flow of Qi (or vital energy) and of blood along pathways known as meridians. TCM practitioners basically use herbs, acupuncture, and massage to help unblock Qi and blood in patients in an attempt to bring the body back into harmony and wellness.

Treatments in TCM are basically tailored to the subtle patterns of disharmony in each patient and are based on an individualized diagnosis. The diagnostic tools differ from those of traditional medicine. There are three main therapeutic modalities:

Moxibustion: Moxibustion is the application of heat from the burning of the herb moxa at the acupuncture point.

Massage and manipulation: Though TCM proposes that natural products catalogued in Chinese Materia Medica or acupuncture can be used alone to treat virtually any sickness, quite frequently they are used together and sometimes in combination with other modalities (e.g., massage, moxibustion, diet changes, or exercise).

Acupuncture: Preclinical studies have documented acupuncture's effects, but they have not been able to fully explain how acupuncture works within the model of the Western system of medicine. It is proposed that acupuncture produces its effects by the conduction of electromagnetic signals at a greater-than-normal rate, thus aiding the activity of pain-killing biochemicals, such as endorphins and immune system cells at specific sites in the body. In addition, studies have shown that acupuncture may alter brain chemistry by changing the release of neurotransmitters and neurohormones and affecting the parts of the central nervous system related to sensation and involuntary body functions, such as immune reactions and processes whereby an individual's blood pressure, blood flow, and body temperature are regulated.

AYURVEDIC MEDICINE

Ayurveda, which literally means "the science of life," is a natural healing system developed in India. Ayurvedic texts claim that the sages who developed India's original systems of meditation and yoga developed the foundations of this medical system. It is a complete system of medicine that places equal emphasis on the body, mind, and spirit, and strives to restore the innate harmony of the individual.

Some of the primary Ayurvedic treatments comprise diet, exercise, meditation, herbs, massage, exposure to sunlight, and controlled breathing. In India, Ayurvedic treatments have been developed for various diseases (e.g., diabetes, cardiovascular conditions, and neurological disorders). Nevertheless, a survey of the Indian medical literature indicates that the quality of the published clinical trials in general falls short of contemporary methodological standards with regard to criteria for randomization, sample size, and ample controls.

NATUROPATHY

Naturopathy is a system of healing, originating from Europe, that views disease as a manifestation of alterations in the processes by which the body naturally heals itself. It emphasizes health restoration as well as disease treatment. The term "naturopathy" literally translates as "nature disease." There are six principles that form the basis of naturopathic practice:

- The healing power of nature
- Identification and treatment of the cause of disease
- The concept of "first do no harm"
- The physician as teacher
- Treatment of the whole person
- Prevention

The core modalities supporting these principles comprise diet modification and nutritional supplements, herbal medicine, acupuncture and Chinese medicine, hydrotherapy, massage and joint manipulation, and lifestyle counselling. Treatment protocols combine what the practitioner deems to be the most suitable therapies for the individual patient.

HOMEOPATHY

Homeopathy is a complete system of medical theory and practice. Its founder, German physician Samuel Christian Hahnemann (1755-1843), hypothesized that one can select therapies on the basis of how closely symptoms produced by a remedy match the symptoms of the patient's disease. He called this the "principle of similars.

" Hahnemann proceeded to give repeated doses of several common remedies to healthy volunteers and carefully record the symptoms they produced. This procedure is called a "proving" or, in modern homeopathy, a "human pathogenic trial." As a result of this experience, Hahnemann developed his treatments for sick patients by matching the symptoms produced by a drug to symptoms in sick patients.

Hahnemann emphasized from the beginning carefully examining all facets of an individual's health status, together with emotional and mental states, and tiny idiosyncratic characteristics.

Because homeopathy is administered in minute or potentially nonexistent material dosages, there is an a priori skepticism in the scientific community about its efficacy. Nonetheless, the medical literature provides evidence of ongoing research in the discipline.

OCCUPATIONAL THERAPY

Occupational Therapy incorporates meaningful and meaningful occupation to enable people with restrictions or impairments to partake in everyday life. Occupational therapists work with people, families, groups and populations to facilitate health and well-being through engagement or re-engagement in occupation.

Occupational therapists are becoming increasingly involved in addressing the impact of social and environmental factors that contribute to exclusion and occupational deprivation.

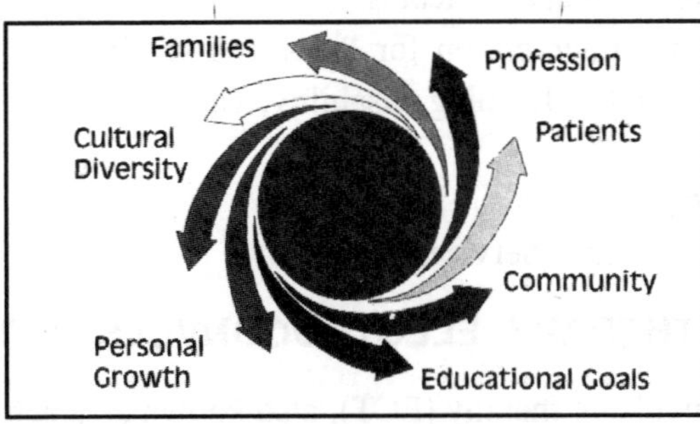

Fig. Occupational Therapy

The World Federation of Occupational Therapists defines occupational therapy as a profession related with promoting health and well-being through occupation. The primary goal of occupational therapy is to enable people to partake in the actions of everyday life. Occupational therapists attain this outcome by allowing people to do things that will improve their capability to partake or by modifying the environment, or the activity to better support participation.

Another way of thinking about the ideas contained in these definitions could be: occupational therapy is about understanding the importance of an activity to an individual, being able to analyze the physical, mental and social components of the activity and then adapting the activity, the environment and/or the person to enable them to resume the activity. Putting differently, occupational therapists would ask, "Why does this person have difficulties managing his or her daily activities (or occupations), and what can we adjust to make it possible for him or her to manage better and how will this then impact his or her health and well-being?"

- Mental health in-patient units
  - Adolescent, adult and older people's acute mental health wards
  - Adult and older people's rehabilitation wards
  - Prisons/secure units (Forensic psychiatry)
  - Psychiatric intensive care unit
  - Specialist units for Eating Disorders, Learning disabilities
- Community based mental health teams
  - Child and adolescent mental health teams
  - Adult and older people's community mental health teams
  - Rehabilitation and recovery and Assertive Outreach community teams

— Primary care services in GP practices
— Home treatment teams
— Early Intervention for Psychosis services
— Specialist learning disability, eating disorder community services
— Day services
— Vocational Services

PHYSICAL THERAPY: ELECTROCONVULSIVE THERAPY

Electroconvulsive therapy (ECT), also known as electroshock, is a well established, albeit controversial psychiatric treatment in which seizures are electrically induced in anaesthetized patients for therapeutic effect. Today, ECT is most frequently used as a treatment for intense major depression which has not responded to other treatment, and is also used in the treatment of mania (frequently in bipolar disorder), catatonia, schizophrenia and other disorders. It was first introduced in the 1930s and acquired widespread use as a form of treatment in the 1940s and 1950s; today, an estimated 1 million people worldwide receive ECT every year, normally in a course of 6-12 treatments administered 2 or 3 times a week.

Electroconvulsive therapy can differ in its application in three ways; electrode placement, length of time that the stimulus is given, and the property of the stimulus. The variance of these three forms of application have important differences in both adverse side effects and positive outcomes. In a study, ECT was shown clinically to be the most efficient treatment for intense depression, and to result in improved quality of life in both short- and long-term. After treatment, drug therapy can be continued, and some patients receive continuation/maintenance ECT.

ECT may become the treatment of first choice for depression if a patient with intense depression or psychotic symptoms is at increased danger of committing suicide and has not responded to other treatments. Though antidepressant medications are effective in several cases, they may take two to six weeks to begin to work. Some patients with mania and schizophrenia may not be able to tolerate the side effects of the antipsychotic medications used to treat these disorders. In addition, some patients may be unable to take their prescribed medications. For these people, ECT is a significant option. ECT is also indicated when patients need a treatment that brings about rapid improvement because they are refusing to eat or drink, or presenting some other danger to themselves.

ECT is also recommended for several subgroups of patients diagnosed with depression. Several elderly patients, for instance, react better to ECT than to antidepressant medications. Pregnant women are another subgroup that may benefit from ECT. Because ECT does not harm a foetus as some medications might, pregnant women suffering from intense depression can safely choose ECT for relief of their depressive symptoms.

GERIATRIC CONSIDERATIONS

Older adults have special physical, emotional, and social needs. Understanding this, the geriatric psychiatrist takes a complete approach to diagnosis and treatment, together with listening and responding to the concerns of the older adult, helping families, and when essential, working with other health care professionals to develop effective approaches to treatment. Co-existing medical illnesses, medications, family issues, social concerns, and environmental issues are integrated into a complete program of care. Older adults with a variety of concerns see a geriatric psychiatrist. These concerns comprise difficulty coping with change, stress, death, depression, memory problems, family history of dementia, anxiety, or agitation linked with dementia or poor sleep. Sometimes emotional problems occur for the first time in older adults who suffer with chronic pain, Parkinson's disease, heart disease, diabetes, stroke, or other medical disorders.

The geriatric psychiatrist offers valuable help to older adults who are coping with changes in health and function. Because the geriatric psychiatrist also understands the family's role in caring for the patient, the physician educates the family about the nature of the sickness and how they can best cope, and may comprise referral to other appropriate service.

ROLE OF NURSE IN MENTAL HEALTH THERAPIES

Nurse participates in providing these therapies on a daily basis. In health care setting the nurse serves on or led task groups that create policy, describe procedures and plan client care. They are also involved in a variety of other activities aimed at the institutional efforts of serving the clients. Nurses are encouraged to use the steps of the nursing process as a framework. Nurses working in this field should continuously strive for expanding their knowledge and use of nursing process for the effective approach. Nursing interventions may be classified into the following classes:

PSYCHIATRIC MEDICATION

Psychiatric medication is a generally used intervention and several psychiatric mental health nurses are involved in the administration of medicines, both in oral (e.g., tablet or liquid) form or by intramuscular injection. Nurses will monitor for side effects and response to these medical treatments by utilizing assessments. Nurses will also offer information on medication so that, where possible, the person in care can make an informed choice, utilizing the best evidence available.

ELECTROCONVULSIVE THERAPY

Psychiatric mental health nurses are also involved in the administration of the treatment of electroconvulsive therapy and assist with the preparation and recovery from the treatment, which involves an anaesthesia. This treatment is only used in a tiny proportion of cases and only after all other possible treatments have been exhausted

PHYSICAL CARE

Along with other nurses, psychiatric mental health nurses will intervene in areas of physical need to ensure that people have acceptable levels of personal hygiene, nutrition, sleep etc as well as tending to any concomitant physical ailments.

PSYCHOSOCIAL INTERVENTIONS

Psychosocial interventions are increasingly delivered by nurses in mental health settings and comprise psychotherapy interventions such as cognitive behavioural therapy, family therapy and less generally other interventions such as milieu therapy or psychodynamic approaches. These intervention can be applied to broad range of problems together with psychosis, depression and anxiety. Nurses will work with people over a period of time and use psychological methods to teach the person psychological techniques that they can then use to assist recovery and help manage any future crisis in their mental health. In practice, these interventions will be used frequently, in conjunction with psychiatric medications.

Psychosocial interventions are based on evidence based practice and thus the techniques tend to follow set guidelines based upon what has been demonstrated to be effective by nursing research. There has been some criticism that evidence based practice is focused mainly on quantitative research and should reflect also a more qualitative research approach that seeks to understand the meaning of people's experience.

SPIRITUAL INTERVENTIONS

The basis of this approach is to look at mental sickness or distress from the perspective of a spiritual crisis. Spiritual interventions concentrate on developing a sense of meaning, purpose and hope for the person in their current life experience. Spiritual interventions involve listening to the person's story and facilitating the person to connect to God, a greater power or greater whole, perhaps by utilizing meditation or prayer. This may be a religious or non-religious experience depending on the individual's own spirituality.

Spiritual interventions, along with psychosocial interventions, emphasize the importance of engagement, nevertheless, spiritual interventions focus more on caring and 'being with' the person during their time of crisis, rather than intervening and trying and 'fix' the problem. Spiritual interventions tend to be based on qualitative research and share some similarities with the humanistic approach to psychotherapy.

Psychiatric mental health nurses work in a variety of hospital and community settings.

- People in general call for an admission to hospital, voluntarily or involuntarily if they are experiencing a crisis that means they are dangerous to themselves or others in some immediate way. Nevertheless, people may gain admission for a concentrated period of therapy or for respite. In spite of changes in mental health policy in several countries that have closed psychiatric hospitals, several nurses continue work in hospitals although patient length of stay has decreased significantly.
- Community nurses in mental health work with people in their own homes (care in the community) and will frequently emphasize work on mental health promotion. Psychiatric mental health nurses also work in rehabilitation settings where people are recovering from a crisis episode and the where the aim is social inclusion and a return to living independently in society.
- Psychiatric mental health nurses also work in forensic psychiatry with people who are detained as they have committed a crime or are especially dangerous.
- People in the older age group who are more prone to dementia tend to be cared for in separate places than younger adults and there are also specialist services for the care of adolescents

with mental health problems. Some times there have been efforts to integrate psychiatric units across the age spectrum.

REFERENCES

Caton, C., & Gralnick, A. (1987). A review of issues surrounding length of psychiatric hospitalization. Hospital and Community Psychiatry, 38, 858–863.

Collins, A. M., & Diego, L. (2000). Mental health promotion and protection. Journal of Psychosocial Nursing, 38(1), 27–32.

Dickey, B., Gonzalez, O., Latimer, E., Powers, K., Schutt, R., & Goldfinger, S. (1996). Use of mental health services by formerly homeless adults residing in group and independent housing. Psychiatric Services, 47(2), 152–158.

Dilonardo, J. D., Connely, C. E., Gurel, L., Kendrick, K., & Deutsch, S. I. (1998). Scheduled intermittent hospitalization for psychiatric patients. Psychiatric Services, 49(4), 504–509.

Finkelman, A. W. (2000). Self-management for the psychiatric patient at home. Home Care Provider, 6, 95–103.

Haugland, G., Siegel, C., Hopper, K., and Alexander, M. J. (1997). Mental illness among homeless individuals in a suburban county. Psychiatric Services, 48(4), 504–509.

Gantt, A. B., Cohen, N. L., & Saintz, A. (1999). Impediments to the discharge planning effort for psychiatric inpatients. Social Work in Health Care, 29(1), 1–14.

Gibson, D. M. (1999). Reduced hospitalizations and reintegration of persons with mental illness into community living: A holistic approach. Journal of Psychosocial Nursing, 37(11), 20–25.

6

Management of Psychotic Disorders

Psychotic disorders are intense mental disorders that cause abnormal thinking and perceptions. People with psychoses lose touch with reality. Two of the main symptoms are delusions and hallucinations. Delusions are false beliefs, such as thinking that someone is plotting against you or that the TV is sending you secret messages.

Hallucinations are false perceptions, such as hearing, seeing or feeling something that is not there. Schizophrenia is one type of psychotic disorder. There are different types of psychotic disorders, such as:

- Schizophrenia: People with this sickness have changes in behaviour and other symptoms – such as delusions and hallucinations – that last longer than six months, normally with a decline in work, school and social functioning.
- Schizoaffective disorder: People with this sickness have symptoms of both schizophrenia and a mood disorder, such as depression or bipolar disorder.
- Schizophreniform disorder: People with this sickness have symptoms of schizophrenia, but the symptoms last more than one month but less than six months.
- Brief psychotic disorder: People with this sickness have sudden, short periods of psychotic behaviour, frequently in response to a very stressful event, such as a death in the family. Recovery is frequently quick – normally less than a month.
- Delusional disorder: People with this sickness have delusions involving real-life situations that could be true, such as being followed, being conspired against or having a disease. These delusions prevail for at least one month.

- Shared psychotic disorder: This sickness occurs when an individual develops delusions in the context of a relationship with another person who already has his or her own delusion(s).
- Substance-induced psychotic disorder: This condition is caused by the use of or withdrawal from some substances, such as alcohol and crack cocaine, that may cause hallucinations, delusions or confused speech.
- Psychotic disorder because of a medical condition: Hallucinations, delusions or other symptoms may be the result of another sickness that affects brain function, such as a head injury or brain tumour.
- Paraphrenia: This is a type of schizophrenia that starts late in life and occurs in the elderly population.

Other possible symptoms of psychotic illnesses comprise:

- Disorganized or incoherent speech.
- Confused thinking.
- Strange, possibly dangerous behaviour.
- Slowed or unusual movements.
- Loss of interest in personal hygiene.
- Loss of interest in activities.
- Problems at school or work and with relationships.
- Cold, detached manner with the inability to express emotion.
- Mood swings or other mood symptoms, such as depression or mania.

CLASSIFICATION: ICD

The ICD is the international standard diagnostic classification for all general epidemiological, several health management purposes and clinical use. These comprise the analysis of the general health situation of population groups and monitoring of the incidence and prevalence of diseases and other health problems in relation to other variables such as the characteristics and circumstances of the people affected, reimbursement, resource allocation, quality and guidelines.

It is used to classify diseases and other health problems recorded on several types of health and vital records together with death certificates and health records. In addition to allowing the storage and retrieval of diagnostic information for clinical, epidemiological and quality purposes, these records also furnish the basis for the compilation of national mortality and morbidity statistics by WHO Member States.

The ICD-10-classification for mental disorders consists of 10 main groups:

F0 Organic, including symptomatic, mental disorders

F1 Mental and behavioural disorders due to use of psychoactive substances

F2 Schizophrenia, schizotypal and delusional disorders

F3 Mood [affective] disorders

F4 Neurotic, stress-related and somatoform disorders

F5 Behavioural syndromes associated with physiological disturbances and physical factors

F6 Disorders of personality and behaviour in adult persons

F7 Mental retardation

F8 Disorders of psychological development

F9 Behavioural and emotional disorders with onset usually occurring in childhood and adolescence

In addition, there is a group of "unspecified mental disorders".

F2 group is dedicated to Psychotic disorders. The classification according to ICD-10 is:

F20: F29: Schizophrenia, schizotypal and delusional disorders

F20: Schizophrenia

F20.0 Paranoid schizophrenia
F20.1 Hebephrenic schizophrenia
F20.2 Catatonic schizophrenia
F20.3 Undifferentiated schizophrenia
F20.4 Post-schizophrenic depression
F20.5 Residual schizophrenia
F20.6 Simple schizophrenia
F20.8 Other schizophrenia
F20.9 Schizophrenia, unspecified

A fifth character may be used to classify course:

.x0 Continuous

.x1 Episodic with progressive deficit

.x2 Episodic with stable deficit

.x3 Episodic remittent

.x4 Incomplete remission

.x5 Complete remission

.x8 Other

.x9 Course uncertain, period of observation too short

F21: Schizotypal disorder

F22: Persistent delusional disorders

F22.0 Delusional disorder

F22.8 Other persistent delusional disorders

F22.9 Persistent delusional disorder, unspecified

F23: Acute and transient psychotic disorders

F23.0 Acute polymorphic psychotic disorder without symptoms of schizophrenia

F23.1 Acute polymorphic psychotic disorder with symptoms of schizophrenia

F23.2 Acute schizophrenia-like psychotic disorder

F23.3 Other acute predominantly delusional psychotic disorder

F23.8 Other acute and transient psychotic disorders

F23.9 Acute and transient psychotic disorder, unspecified

A fifth character may be used to identify the present or absence of associated acute stress:

.x0 Without associated acute stress

.x1 With associated acute stress

F24: Induced delusional disorder

F25: Schizoaffective disorders

F25.0 Schizoaffective disorder, manic type

F25.1 Schizoaffective disorder, depressive type

F25.2 Schizoaffective disorder, mixed type

F25.8 Other schizoaffective disorders

F25.9 Schizoaffective disorder, unspecified

A fifth character may be used to classify the following subtypes:

.x0 Concurrent affective and schizophrenic symptoms only

.x1 Concurrent affective and schizophrenic symptoms, plus persistence of the schizophrenic symptoms beyond the duration of the affective symptoms

F28: Other nonorganic psychotic disorders

F29: Unspecified nonorganic psychosis *(Source: ICD-10)*

SCHIZOPHRENIA

Schizophrenia causes distorted and bizarre thoughts, perceptions, emotions, movements, and behaviour. It cannot be defined as a single illness; rather, schizophrenia is thought of as a syndrome or disease process with many different varieties and symptoms, much like the varieties of cancer. For decades, the public vastly misunderstood schizophrenia, fearing it as dangerous and uncontrollable and causing wild disturbances and violent outbursts.

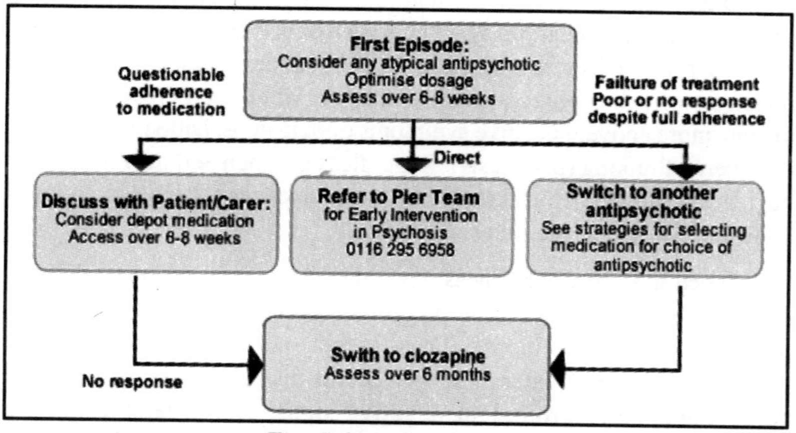

Fig. Schizophrenia Care

Many people believed that those with schizophrenia needed to be locked away from society and institutionalized. Only recently has the mental health industry come to learn and educate the community at large that schizophrenia has many different symptoms and presentations and is an illness that medication can control. Thanks to the increased effectiveness of newer atypical antipsychotic drugs and advances in community based treatment, many clients with schizophrenia live successfully in the community. Clients whose illness is medically supervised and whose treatment is maintained often continue to live and sometimes work in the community with family and outside support. Schizophrenia usually is diagnosed in late adolescence or early adulthood.

Rarely does it manifest in childhood. The peak incidence of onset is 15 to 25 years of age for men and 25 to 35 years of age for women. The prevalence of schizophrenia is estimated at about 1% of the total population. The incidence and the lifetime prevalence are roughly the same throughout the world.

The symptoms of schizophrenia are divided into two major categories: positive or hard symptoms/signs, which include delusions, hallucinations, and grossly disorganized thinking, speech, and behaviour, and negative or soft symptoms/signs such as flat affect, lack of volition, and social withdrawal or discomfort. Medication can control the positive symptoms, but frequently the negative symptoms persist after positive symptoms have abated. The persistence of these negative symptoms over time presents a major barrier to recovery and improved functioning in the client's daily life.

Onset may be abrupt or insidious, but most clients slowly and gradually develop signs and symptoms such as social withdrawal, unusual behaviour, loss of interest in school or work, and neglected hygiene. The diagnosis of schizophrenia usually is made when the person begins to display more actively positive symptoms of delusions, hallucinations, and disordered thinking (psychosis). Regardless of when and how the illness begins and the type of schizophrenia, consequences for most clients and their families are substantial and enduring.

When and how the illness develops seems to affect the outcome. Age of onset appears to be an important factor in how well the client fares. Those who develop the illness earlier show worse outcomes than those who develop it later. Younger clients display a poorer premorbid adjustment, more prominent negative signs, and greater cognitive impairment than do older clients. Those who experience a gradual onset of the disease (about 50%) tend to have both a poorer immediate and long-term course than those who experience an acute and sudden onset. Approximately 30% of clients with schizophrenia relapse within 1 year of an acute episode; this figure doubles by the end of the second year.

Related Disorders

Other disorders are related to but distinguished from schizophrenia in terms of presenting symptoms and the duration or magnitude of impairment. The DSMIV- TR (APA, 2000) categorizes these disorders as:

Schizophreniform disorder: The client exhibits the symptoms of schizophrenia but for less than the 6 months necessary to meet the diagnostic criteria for schizophrenia. Social or occupational functioning may or may not be impaired.

Schizoaffective disorder: The client exhibits the symptoms of psychosis and, at the same time, all the features of a mood disorder, either depression or mania.

Delusional disorder: The client has one or more nonbizarre delusions-that is, the focus of the delusion is believable. Psychosocial functioning is not markedly impaired, and behaviour is not obviously odd or bizarre.

Brief psychotic disorder: The client experiences the sudden onset of at least one psychotic symptom, such as delusions, hallucinations, or disorganized speech or behaviour, which lasts from 1 day to 1 month. The episode may or may not have an identifiable stressor or may follow childbirth.

Shared psychotic disorder (folie à deux): Two people share a similar delusion. The person with this diagnosis develops this delusion in the context of a close relationship with someone who has psychotic delusions.

Two other diagnoses, schizoid personality disorder and schizotypal personality disorder, are not psychotic disorders and should not be confused with schizophrenia even though the names sound similar.

Etiology

The exact cause of psychotic disorders is not known, but researchers believe that many factors may play a role. Some psychotic disorders tend to run in families, suggesting that the tendency, or likelihood, to develop the disorder may be inherited. Environmental factors may also play a role in their development, including stress, drug abuse and major life changes.

In addition, people with certain psychotic disorders may have an imbalance of certain chemicals in the brain. They may be either very sensitive to or produce too much of a chemical called dopamine. Dopamine is a neurotransmitter, a substance that helps nerve cells in the brain send messages to each other. An imbalance of dopamine affects the way the brain reacts to certain stimuli, such as sounds, smells and sights and can lead to hallucinations and delusions.

One of the reasons for the ongoing difficulty in classifying schizophrenic disorders is incomplete understanding of their causes. As of 2001, it is thought that these disorders are the end result of a combination of genetic, neurobiological, and environmental causes. A leading neurobiological hypothesis emphasizes the connection between the disease and excessive levels of dopamine, a chemical that transmits signals in the brain (neurotransmitter). The genetic factor in schizophrenia has been underscored by recent findings that first-degree biological relatives of schizophrenics are 10 times more likely to develop the disorder than are members of the general population.

Prior to recent findings of abnormalities in the brain structure of schizophrenic persons, several generations of psychotherapists advanced a number of psychoanalytic and sociological theories about the origins of schizophrenia. These theories ranged from hypotheses about a person's problems with anxiety or aggression to theories about stress reactions or interactions with disturbed parents.

Psychosocial factors are now thought to influence the expression or severity of schizophrenia, rather than directly cause it. Another hypothesis suggests that schizophrenia may be caused by a virus that attacks the hippocampus, a part of the brain that processes sense perceptions. Damage to the hippocampus would account for a schizophrenic person's vulnerability to sensory overload. As of mid-2001, researchers are testing antiviral medications on schizophrenics.

Symptoms

People with a possible diagnosis of schizophrenia are evaluated on the basis of a set or constellation of symptoms. There is no single symptom that is unique to schizophrenia. In 1959, the German psychiatrist Kurt Schneider proposed a list of so-called first-rank symptoms, which he regarded as diagnostic of the disorder. These symptoms include:

- Delusions
- Somatic hallucinations
- Hallucinations
- Hearing voices commenting on a person's behaviour
- Thought insertion or thought withdrawal

Somatic hallucinations refer to sensations or perceptions concerning body organs that have no known medical cause or reason, such as the notion that one's brain is radioactive. Thought insertion and/or withdrawal refer to delusions that an outside force (for example, the FBI, the CIA, Martians, etc.) has the power to put thoughts into one's mind or remove them.

Positive Symptoms

The positive symptoms of schizophrenia are those that represent an excessive or distorted version of normal functions. Positive symptoms include Schneider's first-rank symptoms as well as disorganized thought processes (reflected mainly in speech) and disorganized or catatonic behaviour. Disorganized thought processes are marked by such characteristics as looseness of association, in which a person rambles from topic to topic in a disconnected way; tangentiality, which means that an individual gives unrelated answers to questions; and flights of ideas or "word salad," in which a person's speech is so incoherent that it makes no grammatical or linguistic sense. Disorganized behaviour means that a person has difficulty with any type of purposeful or goal-oriented behaviour, including personal self-care or preparing meals. Other forms of disorganized behaviour may include dressing in odd or inappropriate ways, sexual self-stimulation in public, or agitated shouting or cursing.

Negative Symptoms

The DSM-IV definition of schizophrenia includes three so-called negative symptoms. They are called negative because they represent the lack or absence of behaviours. The negative symptoms that are considered diagnostic of schizophrenia are a lack of emotional response (affective flattening), poverty of speech, and absence of volition or will. In general, the negative symptoms are more difficult for doctors to evaluate than the positive symptoms.

Diagnosis

A doctor must make a diagnosis of schizophrenia on the basis of a standardized list of outwardly observable symptoms, not on the basis of internal psychological processes. There are no specific laboratory tests that can be used to diagnose schizophrenia. Researchers have, however, discovered that persons with schizophrenia have certain abnormalities in the structure and functioning of the brain compared to normal test subjects. These discoveries have been made with the help of imaging techniques such as computed tomography scans (CT scans).

When a psychiatrist assesses an individual for schizophrenia, the doctor will begin by excluding physical conditions that can cause abnormal thinking and some other behaviours associated with schizophrenia. These conditions include organic brain disorders (including traumatic injuries of the brain), temporal lobe epilepsy, Wilson's disease, Huntington's chorea, and encephalitis. The doctor will also need to rule out substance abuse disorders, especially amphetamine use.

After ruling out organic disorders, a clinician will consider other psychiatric conditions that may include psychotic symptoms or symptoms resembling psychosis. These disorders include mood disorders with psychotic features; delusional disorder; dissociative disorder not otherwise specified (DDNOS) or multiple personality disorder; schizotypal, schizoid, or paranoid personality disorders; and atypical reactive disorders. In the past, many individuals were incorrectly diagnosed as being schizophrenic. Some people who were diagnosed prior to the changes in categorization introduced by DSM-IV should have their diagnoses, and treatment, reevaluated. In children, a doctor must distinguish between psychotic symptoms and a vivid fantasy life, and also identify learning problems or disorders. After other conditions have been ruled out, a person must meet a set of criteria specified by DSM-IV:

- Characteristic symptoms. To make a diagnosis of schizophrenia, a person must exhibit two (or more) of the following symptoms during a one-month period: delusions; hallucinations; disorganized speech; disorganized or catatonic behaviour; negative symptoms.
- Decline in social, interpersonal, or occupational functioning, including self-care.
- Duration. The disturbed behaviour must last for at least six months.

NURSING ASSESSMENT

HISTORY

The nurse first elicits information about the patient's previous history with schizophrenia to establish baseline data. He or she asks questions about how the patient functioned before the crisis developed such as "How do you normally spend your time?" and "Can you describe what you do each day?" The nurse evaluates the age of onset of schizophrenia, knowing that poorer outcomes are linked with an earlier age of onset. Learning the patient's previous history of hospital admissions and response to hospitalization also is significant.

The nurse also evaluates the patient for previous suicide attempts. Ten percent of all people with schizophrenia eventually commit suicide. The nurse might ask, "Have you ever attempted suicide?" or "Have you ever heard voices telling you to hurt yourself?" Similarly, it is significant to elicit information about any history of violence or aggression because a history of aggressive behaviour is a strong predictor of future aggression.

The nurse might ask "What do you do when you are angry, frustrated, upset, or scared?"

The nurse evaluates if the patient has been utilizing current support systems by asking the patient or significant others the following questions:

- Has the patient kept in contact with family or friends?
- Has the patient been to scheduled groups or therapy appointments?
- Does the patient seem to run out of money between paychecks?
- Have the patient's living arrangements changed recently?

Finally the nurse evaluates the patient's perception of his or her current situation-that is, what the patient believes to be significant present events or stressors. The nurse can gather such information by asking,

"What do you see as the primary problem now?" or

"What do you need help managing now?"

ASSESSMENT

Three kinds of assessment in nursing exist for mental sickness patients: complete, focused, and screening assessments.

Comprehensive: A comprehensive assessment comprises data related to the patient's biologic, psychological, cultural, spiritual, and social needs. This type of assessment is in general completed in collaboration with other health care professionals such as a doctor, psychologist, neurologist, and social worker. A physical examination is performed to rule out any physiologic causes of disorders such as anxiety, depression, or dementia. Several psychiatric facilities call for a comprehensive assessment, together with medical clearance, before or within 24 hours of admission to avoid medical emergencies in the psychiatric setting.

Focused: A focused assessment comprises the collection of specific data regarding a specific problem as determined by the patient, a family member, or a crisis situation. For instance, in the event of a suicide attempt, the nurse would assess the patient's mood, affect, and behaviour. Data regarding the attempted suicide and any previous attempts of self-destructive behaviour would also be collected.

Screening: A screening assessment comprises the use of assessment or rating scales such as the Brief Psychiatric Rating Scale (BPRS), Drug Attitude Inventory (DAI-10), or the Hamilton Rating Scale for Depression (HRSD) to assess data regarding a specific problem. For instance, a screening assessment utilizing the Abnormal Involuntary Movement Scale could be done for a patient taking neuroleptic medication to stabilize clinical symptoms of schizophrenia to assess the patient's movement disorder.

During any assessment, the psychiatric mental health nurse employs a psychosocial nursing history and assessment tool to obtain factual information, observe patient appearance and behaviour, and assess the patient's mental or cognitive status.

TREATMENT MODALITIES

Treatment modalities for psychoses comprise psychopharmacology, individual psychotherapy, group therapy, family therapy, milieu therapy, psychoeducation, psychiatric rehabilitation, and self help groups.

PSYCHOPHARMACOLOGY

Typical (older) antipsychotics comprise haldol, thorazine, prolixin, trilafon, mellaril, navane, moban and stelazine. They block dopamine at mesolimbic pathways in the temporal lobes. Atypical (newer) antipsychotics comprise zyprexa, risperdol, abilify, and clozaril. In addition to blocking excess dopamine, they also block serotinin at mesocortical pathways in the frontal lobe. This makes atypical antipsychotic good with controlling both positive and negative symptoms. Patients taking Clozaril need frequent and regular blood checks because the medication can cause fatal agranulocytosis. Haldol and prolixin decanoate (given by injection every two weeks) are good for patients who are non-adherent with their medications. Encourage patients not to stop taking their medications simply because symptoms have subsided. Watch out for side effects of antipsychotics, e.g. extrapyramidal symptoms (EPS) such as dystonia, akathysia, tardive dyskenesia, neuroleptic malignant syndrome, and pseudoparkinsonism. Dystonias are spasms, stiffness and contractions of muscles especially of the face and neck. They can be painful and frightening to patient especially if airways are compromised. Benadryl or cogentin are normally given to treat dystonias. Reassure the patient. Furnish a quiet non-stimulating environment. Akathisia is restlessness, restless leg syndrome, and inability to sit still. It may make patient very nervous. Benadryl, cogentin, clonidine, propanolol, diazepam or lorazepam can be given. Dose of the antipsychotic might be reduced. Tardive Dyskinesia is a late occurring irreversible side-effect of antipsychotics. It manifests by abnormal involuntary movement e.g. tongue-thrusting, writhing of wrists, lip pursing, lip smacking, facial grimacing, and grunting. Teach patient to recognize and report early warning signs. Administer the Abnormal Involuntary Movement Scale (AIMS) every 6 months for early detection. Reduce antipsychotics or change from typical to atypical. Neuroleptic Malignant Syndrome (NMS) is a clinical emergency resulting from antipsychotics. It involves altered consciousness; unstable blood pressure, breathing and pulse rates; fever; lead pipe rigidity; diaphoresis; tremors; and drooling. Withhold the antipsychotic immediately and notify the prescriber. Care for the patient's breathing, fever, anxiety, and hydration. Dantrolene or Bromocryptine may be prescribed. NMS is fatal in 15-20% cases.

Pseudoparkinsonism involves muscle rigidity, slow movement, shuffling gate, tremors, masklike face, hypersalivation and drooling. Notify the prescriber of the antipsychotic. The dose may be reduced. Artane or cogenting may be ordered. Other side effects of antipsychotics are sedation, drowsiness, orthostatic hypotension, increased appetite, agranulocytosis (from clozaril), hyperglycemia, allergy, rash, and photosensitivity.

PSYCHOSOCIAL TREATMENT

In addition to pharmacologic treatment, many other modes of treatment can help the person with schizophrenia. Individual and group therapy, family therapy, family education, and social skills training can be instituted for clients in both inpatient and community settings. Individual and group therapy sessions are often supportive in nature, giving the client an opportunity for social contact and meaningful relationships with other people. Groups that focus on topics of concern such as medication management, use of community supports, and family concerns also have been beneficial to clients with schizophrenia.

Clients with schizophrenia can improve their social competence with social skills training, which translates into more effective functioning in the community. Bustillo describe three forms of social skills training: the basic model; the social problem-solving model; and the cognitive remediation model. The basic model involves breaking complex social behaviour into simpler steps, practicing through role-playing, and applying the concepts in the community or real-world setting. The social problem-solving model focuses on improving impairments in information processing that are assumed to cause deficits in social skills. This includes medication and symptom management, recreation, basic conversation, and self-care. The cognitive remediation model focuses on improving underlying cognitive impairments by emphasizing such things as paying attention and planning. Improvements in these basic cognitive functions enhance learning in the other two models as well.

Family education and therapy are known to diminish the negative effects of schizophrenia and reduce the relapse rate. While inclusion of the family is a factor that improves outcomes for the client, family involvement often is neglected by health care professionals. Families often have a difficult time coping with the complexities and ramifications of the client's illness. This creates stress among family members that is not beneficial for the client or family members. Family education helps to make family members part of the treatment team. In addition, family members can benefit from a supportive environment that helps them cope with the many difficulties presented when a loved one has schizophrenia.

These concerns include continuing as a caregiver for the child who is now an adult; worrying about who will care for the client when the parents are gone; dealing with the social stigma of mental illness; and possibly facing financial problems, marital discord, and social isolation. Such support is available through the NAMI and local support groups. The client's health care provider can make referrals to meet specific family needs.

GERIATRIC CONSIDERATIONS

Following are the geriatric considerations for the psychotic disorder patients:

Abnormal suspiciousness: Most elderly individuals who exhibit abnormal suspiciousness don't have contact with mental health practitioners. Nevertheless, they frequently have medical disorders and are seen by a primary care doctor or a geriatrician. These patients may have vague complaints of external forces controlling their lives. Some times, these beliefs become focal, frequently directed at their children; e.g., they believe their children have deserted them or have plotted to obtain control of their finances or property. Perception of a loss of control, coupled with an inability to assess the social milieu, favours the growth of abnormal suspiciousness.

Doctors may also encounter suspiciousness linked with dementia and attention deficits. Institutionalized patients with dementia are frequently suspicious of family and staff members; psychosis because of dementia is, nevertheless, uncommon. Their accusations are normally disjointed, unfocused, and unaccompanied by sustained emotional distress. Common complaints concern objects being stolen, medicines being swapped, and attendants misbehaving. Symptoms derive from the patient's inability to organize environmental stimuli and comprehend the frequently confusing activities of the institution. It is unknown whether an underlying paranoid personality contributes to excessive paranoid behaviour in individuals with dementia. Nevertheless, doctors must keep in mind that elderly patients, especially those with dementia, at times are mistreated in long-term care facilities and in hospitals and that suspiciousness may be grounded in fact.

Transitional paranoid reactions: These reactions normally occur in women who live alone; they believe that someone is plotting against them. Social isolation and perceptional difficulties contribute to these reactions. The focus of hallucinations and delusional thinking normally moves gradually from outside the home to inside it, e.g., from complaints of noises in the basement and attic to reports of physical abuse or molestation. Hence, a transition can be observed from external threats to violations of property and person.

Paraphrenia: Paraphrenia is not universally accepted as a distinct syndrome. Individuals who distinguish the syndrome emphasize that it is primary rather than secondary to an affective sickness or to an organic mental disorder. In addition, the gross disturbances of affect, volition, and function characterizing schizophrenia are not prominent. However, paranoid delusions and hallucinations almost always occur. Paraphrenia may be chronic, but deterioration to the degree observed in schizophrenia or Alzheimer's disease is not characteristic. The boundaries blur not only between paraphrenia and classic paranoid schizophrenia but also between the transitional paranoid state and paraphrenia.

Patients with paraphrenia frequently report plots against them, focusing on family members. In contrast with mild suspiciousness, these plots are pertinacious, extreme, and intricate. Normally, cognitive impairment is not present. Though the patient is physically independent (i.e., diet and hygiene are rarely compromised), social functioning and cooperation with staff members are greatly impaired. Such individuals rarely speak for long without referring to the symptoms of concern.

Patients with paraphrenia normally are female, live alone, and have evidence of difficult social interactions earlier in life. In contrast with schizophrenia, these patients are friendly and trusting, especially when they are interviewed in their homes and are not threatened with the diagnosis of a mental disorder. Patients with paraphrenia tend to have a hearing impairment, but the relationship between paraphrenia and hearing impairment is not nearly as strong as some authorities contend.

Early-onset schizophrenia: The symptoms comprise two or more of the following, each present for most of the time for at least 1 month: delusion, hallucination, disorganized speech, grossly disorganized or catatonic behaviour, and negative symptoms (e.g., flattening of affect). Overall, the symptoms must be present for at least 6 months and significantly interfere with social and occupational functioning.

Basically, the symptoms become less acute, yet social functioning continues to deteriorate gradually over time. Acute paranoid thinking may accompany an episode of major depression or acute mania. Treating the mood disorder normally eliminates the paranoid thinking in these patients and thus rules out the diagnosis of schizophrenia.

Elderly individuals who have been treated for schizophrenia for years are likely to have adverse effects of antipsychotic drugs (e.g., tardive dyskinesia).

Psychotic disorders because of neurologic, toxic-metabolic, or systemic disorders: These comprise suspiciousness and agitation because of drug intoxication, physical sickness, and postoperative psychosis (e.g., psychosis occurring among patients in intensive care units). Visual hallucinations occur more frequently (as in delirium), yet the psychosis may be organized and intricate (unlike delirium). These disorders are normally transient and solve with treatment of the underlying cause or spontaneously. In the midst of the disorder, nevertheless, acute management is essential.

FOLLOW-UP AND HOME CARE AND REHABILITATION

Home care is a critical concern for an increasing number of patients with both chronic and acute diseases. New technologies, pharmaceutical advances, changing reimbursement policies, and the continuing desire of patients and their families to remain in their homes have combined to drastically change the treatment of acute and chronic sickness. Patients with chronic sickness are living longer, and patients with acute sickness are discharged from hospitals earlier, increasing the need for complex and frequently less costly care in the home.

This has resulted in a paradigm shift in medical care delivery from hospital-based care back to home-based care. In an increasing number of situations, home care can be regarded as the "first option," preferred over hospitals, emergency departments, or nursing homes whenever care needs can safely be met at home.

Psychiatric rehabilitation involves providing services to people with intense and pertinacious mental sickness to help them to live in the community. These programs are frequently called community support services or community support programs. Psychiatric rehabilitation focuses on the patient's strengths, not just on his or her sickness. The patient actively participates in program planning. The programs are designed to help the patient manage the sickness and symptoms, gain access to needed services, and live successfully in the

community. These programs assist patients with activities of daily living such as transportation, shopping, food preparation, money management, and hygiene. Social support and interpersonal relationships are recognized as a primary need for successful community living. Psychiatric rehabilitation programs furnish opportunities for socialization such as drop-in centres and places where patients can go to be with others in a safe, supportive environment.

REFERENCES

Lamb, H. R., & Weinberger, L. E. (1998). Persons with severe mental illness in jails and prisons: A review. Psychiatric Services, 49(4), 483–492.

Mallik, K., Reeves, R. J., & Dellario, D. J. (1998). Barriers to community integration for people with severe and persistent psychiatric disabilities. Psychiatric Rehabilitation Journal, 22(2), 175–180.

McGihon, N. N. (1999). Psychiatric nursing for the 21st century: The PACED model. Journal of Psychosocial Nursing, 37(10), 22–27.

Pittman, D. C., Parson, R., & Peterson, R. W. (1990). Easing the way: A multifaceted approach to day treatment. Journal of Psychosocial Nursing, 28(11), 6–11.

Swearingen, L. (1987). Transitional day treatment: An individualized goal-oriented approach. Archives of Psychiatric Nursing, I(2), 104–110.

Ware, N. C. (1999). Evolving consumer households. Psychiatric Rehabilitation Journal, 23(1), 3–10.

Ware, N. C., & Goldfinger, S. (1997). Poverty and rehabilitation in severe psychiatric disorders. Psychiatric Rehabilitation Journal, 21(1), 3–9.

7

Management of Mood Disorders

A mood disorder is a mental sickness characterized mainly by mood swings or an abnormally high or low mood. Most mood disorders are defined and diagnosed by the occurrence of one or more mood episodes, or periods of abnormal happiness or sadness. Such episodes are not mood disorders in themselves.

Mood disorders comprise major depression, dysthymia and bipolar disorder, among others. Major depression and dysthymia involve periods of sadness and lack of pleasure or interest in normal activities as well as fatigue. Bipolar disorder comprises episodes of both depression and mania, which is an elevated mood of (euphoria), combined with increased self-esteem, racing thoughts and reckless behaviour or impulsive activity. If intense, episodes of high and low mood can involve psychotic symptoms, such as hallucinations and delusions.

The causes of mood disorders are not completely understood. Nevertheless, a chemical imbalance in the brain seems to play a major role in their growth. Brain chemicals called neurotransmitters convey messages between the nerves. Abnormalities in the regulation of these neurotransmitters are believed to cause alterations in mood. Mood disorders also appear to be linked to genetics. People who have relatives with a history of a mood disorder have a greater danger of developing a mood disorder.

The diagnosis of a mood disorder involves a physical examination by a doctor and a mental health evaluation by a doctor or a mental health professional. Mood episodes or mood disorders can be triggered or imitated by other illnesses, substance abuse or side effects of medications, so a doctor must rule out these potential causes first. The mental health evaluation comprises a complete history of symptoms, together with when they started, how long they have lasted and how intense they are.

It is also noted whether the patient has experienced these symptoms before and, if so, whether and how they were treated.

Depressive mood disorders are basically treated with antidepressants. Mood stabilizing drugs, especially lithium, are the primary medications for bipolar disorder. Patients with mood disorders may also benefit from different types of therapy, together with psychotherapy and cognitive behaviour therapy (CBT), in addition to medications. Electroconvulsive therapy (ECT) may be used in intense cases or in cases where medications are not effective or are not safe to use (e.g., pregnancy).

BIPOLAR AFFECTIVE DISORDER

Bipolar disorder is a mood disorder in which feelings, thoughts, behaviours, and perceptions are altered in the context of episodes of mania and depression. Formerly known as manic depression, bipolar disorder was once thought to occur rarely in youth. Nevertheless, approximately 20% of adults with bipolar disorder had symptoms beginning in adolescence. The Diagnostic and Statistical Manual of Mental Disorders, Fourth Edition Text Revision (DSM-IV TR), does not distinguish adult onset from childhood or adolescent onset of symptoms of bipolar disorder. Indeed, the diagnostic criterion for bipolar disorder is the same regardless of the patient's age at the onset of symptoms. In spite of clinically significant differences in the way mood disorders, especially behavioural differences, may manifest in a child or an adolescent, no diagnostic accommodation has been made on the basis of age.

The DSM-IV TR employs universal symptoms to define the diagnostic criteria for mood episodes, together with major depressive and manic episodes. One true manic episode, with or without psychotic features, is the essential and sufficient criterion for type I bipolar disorder. A depressive episode is insufficient for this diagnosis, even in the presence of a strong family history of bipolar disorder. Type II bipolar disorder is diagnosed on the basis of at least 1 hypomanic episode. Thus, bipolar disorders are viewed as having a spectrum of symptoms that range from mild hypomania to the most extreme mania, which may comprise life-threatening behaviours, dysphoria, and psychotic features.

MANIA DEPRESSION

Hallmark symptoms of mania comprise an abnormal, frequently expansive, and elevated mood lasting for at least 1 week. Mania may also comprise a decreased need for sleep, racing thoughts or a sense that thoughts are out of control, rapid and frequently pressured speech, increased goal-directed activities or projects, hypersexuality, reckless behaviours and risk taking, and delusions of grandeur. Delusions linked with mania often centre around an expansive sense of self that goes well beyond narcissism, e.g., believing oneself to have special (e.g., supernatural) powers or to be the chosen leader of the world or universe.

For some, the elevated and elated mood may transform into a state of dysphoria during which agitated and irritable behaviours may develop. Cognitive impairment in mania may manifest as episodes of confusion with a flight of ideas and disorganization of thought. In addition, increased risk taking may involve physical, emotional, or financial endangerment.

Moreover, poor insight into one's disorder or behaviours and poor judgment accompany mania. Thus, the person's financial accounts or significant relationships may be in such disarray as to lead to adverse outcomes, together with loss of significant friends and family support or connections, serious financial setbacks, job losses, legal problems, and homelessness.

As per the DSM-IV TR, criteria for a manic episode are as follows:

- The individual has a distinct period of abnormally and pertinaciously elevated, expansive, or irritable mood lasting at least 1 week (or any duration if hospitalization is essential).
- During the period of mood disturbance, 3 or more of the following symptoms persisted (4 if the mood is only irritable) and have been present to a important degree:

— Inflated self-esteem to levels of grandiosity

— Decreased need for sleep

— More talkative than usual, frequently with pressured speech with a sense of a need to keep talking

— Flight of ideas or subjective feeling that thoughts are racing

— Distractibility

— Increased goal-directed activity or psychomotor agitation

— Excessive involvement in pleasurable activity that has a high potential for painful consequences (e.g., hypersexuality, excessive spending, impetuous traveling)

The symptoms don't meet the criteria for a mixed episode.

The mood disturbance is sufficiently intense to cause marked social impairment in occupational functioning, social activities, or relationships with others. Hospitalization may be essential to prevent harm to self or others or if psychotic features are present.

The symptoms are not because of the direct physiologic effects of a substance or a general medical condition.

Hypomania is to some extent similar to mania, but it is less intense and less debilitating than true mania. As such, hypomania is defined as an elevated mood during which (1) no hospitalization has ever been essential, and (2) no state of delusional or other psychotic thinking ever coincided with the elevated mood. Hypomanic and manic states must cause impairment of normal functioning to be regarded as pathologic states.

An abnormal behavioural episode may be designated a bipolar disorder after the frequency and type of abnormal mood are considered. Thus, an episode may be reported as a bipolar disorder with a single manic episode, with recurrent manic episodes, or by the mood state of the most recent episode (e.g., depressed, mixed, hypomanic, manic). Descriptors such as with psychosis or without psychosis are used to further clarify and reflect the severity of the state of the disorder.

Mood disturbances in children and adolescents are frequently more difficult to recognize and diagnose than those in adults. Some of the difficulty arises in recognizing atypical symptoms, together with irritability, tantrums, physical aggression, and other behavioural problems, such as expressions of mood disruptions. Perhaps this difficulty is best demonstrated in symptom recognition and proper, but controversial, diagnosis of bipolar disorder in youths. The classic symptoms of mania, together with racing thoughts, pressured speech, hypersexuality, and grandiosity, more frequently match the presentation of bipolar disorder in late adolescence. In childhood- or prepubertal-onset bipolar disorder, such a classic cluster of symptoms is uncommon. Nonetheless, as early as 1921, Kraepelin reported that 38% of his 900 patients who had manic episodes had symptom onset when younger than 20 years, and 0.4% had onset of symptoms when younger than 10 years.

In spite of Kraepelin's early observation and description of childhood-onset and adolescent-onset bipolar disorders, the controversy about diagnosing bipolar disorder in young individuals persists. This is partially driven by the requirement of discrete episodes of disturbed mood to diagnose bipolar disorder. Unlike what is noted in adults, well-defined and discrete episodes of abnormal mood are frequently missing in children and adolescents with this disorder. In specific, as per the DSM-IV TR criteria, at least 1 discrete episode of mania or hypomania is essential to diagnose bipolar disorder type I or II.

Clinicians frequently use the diagnosis of bipolar disorder not otherwise specified (NOS) in children and adolescents with a chronically mixed or vacillating mood state. Children with this diagnosis may have clinically important impairment although they don't meeting specific criteria for bipolar disorder type I or II.

Because no distinction is made for symptoms of adult-, adolescent-, or childhood-onset bipolar disorder, clinicians are challenged to distinguish abnormal mood symptoms in adolescents and children from normal developmental behaviours, oppositional or defiant behaviours, inattention or hyperactivity, and conduct problems. Childhood-onset bipolar disorder often has an insidious onset with affective storms frequently linked with the presentation of mental sickness.

DYSTHYMIA

Dysthymia is a mood disorder that falls within the depression spectrum. It is considered a chronic depression, but with less severity than major depressive disorder. This disorder tends to be a chronic, long-lasting illness. Dysthymia is a type of low-grade depression. Harvard Health Publications states that, "the Greek word dysthymia means 'bad state of mind' or 'ill humor'. As one of the two chief forms of clinical depression, it usually has fewer or less serious symptoms than major depression but lasts longer."

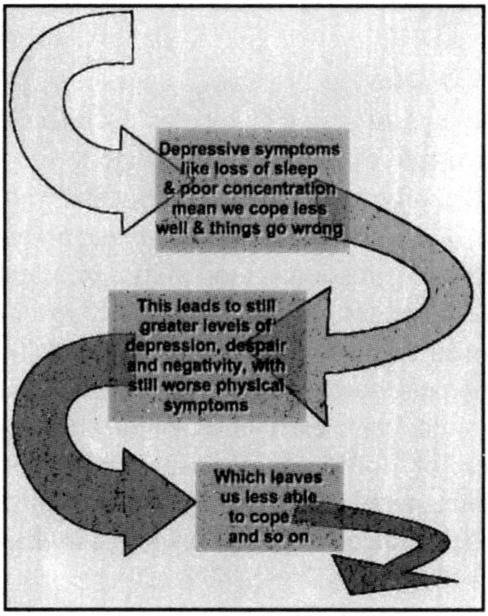

Fig. Dysthymia

Harvard Health Publications says, "at least three-quarters of patients with dysthymia also have a chronic physical illness or another psychiatric disorder such as one of the anxiety disorders, drug addiction, or alcoholism". The Primary Care Journal says that dysthymia "affects approximately 3% of the population and is associated with significant functional impairment". Harvard health Publications says: "The rate of depression in the families of people with dysthymia is as high as 50% for the early-onset form of the disorder." "Most people with dysthymia can't tell for sure when they first became depressed".

CAUSES OF BIPOLAR DISORDER

- Genetic and familial factors have profound influence in the propagation of bipolar disorder.
  - Chang and colleagues (2000) reported that children who have at least 1 biologic parent with bipolar I or bipolar II disorder have increased psychopathology. The specific finding was that 28% of the children examined had attention deficit/hyperactivity disorder (ADHD). This rate is far above the prevalence of 3-5% in the general population of school-aged children. Also, 15% of the children had a bipolar disorder or cyclothymia. Approximately 90% of children who have bipolar disorders had comorbid ADHD. Moreover, both bipolar disorder and ADHD were more likely to be diagnosed in boys than in girls.
  - Early age of onset of bipolar disorder is predictive of a higher rate of mood disorder among first-degree relatives of the proband. Also, adolescents who have onset of true mania with childhood-linked psychotic symptoms, such as aggression, mood shifts, or attention difficulties, have a greater genetic risk (family loading) for bipolar I disorder than adolescents with more adult-related psychotic symptoms, such as grandiosity. Other distinctive features of youths with early-onset bipolar disorder comprise (1) poor or ineffective response to lithium therapy (administered as Eskalith) and (2) an linked increased danger of alcohol-related disorders in the family members of the probands.
  - Twin studies of bipolar disorder showed a 14% concordance rate in dizygotic twins and a 65%

concordance rate (range, 33-90%) in monozygotic twins. The risk for the offspring of a couple in which 1 parent has bipolar disorder was estimated to be 30-35%. For an offspring of a couple in which both parents have bipolar disorder, the risk was approximately 70-75%.

- Faraone et al further delineated the differences among children with mania, adolescents with childhood-onset mania, and adolescents with adolescence-onset mania.

- Socioeconomic status (SES) was statistically lower in families of children with mania and adolescents with childhood-onset mania than in others.
- Increased energy was twice as common in childhood mania than in other forms, euphoria was most common in adolescents with childhood-onset mania, and irritability was least common in adolescents with adolescent-onset mania.
- On statistical analysis, adolescents with adolescent-onset mania abused psychoactive drugs and had more impaired parent-child relationships than people in the other 2 groups with mania.
- ADHD was more common in children and adolescents with childhood-onset mania than in patients with adolescent-onset mania. This finding led the authors to theorize that ADHD may be a marker for juvenile-onset mania.
  - Data from this and other studies suggest that a subtype of bipolar disorder may exist. This subtype may have a high familial transmission rate, and affected people present with childhood-onset of mania symptoms suggestive of ADHD.
  - Faraone et al propose that early-onset mania may be the same as the comorbid state of ADHD and bipolar disorder, which has a high rate of familial transmission. The question exists regarding whether youths who are later given the diagnosis of bipolar disorder may have a prodromal phase in early life that appears to be ADHD or another behavioural disturbance or whether several simply have bipolar disorder and comorbid ADHD.
- Cognitive and neurodevelopmental factors also seem to be involved in the growth of bipolar disorder.
  - A case-cohort study of adolescents with affective disorders revealed that neurodevelopmental delays are

overrepresented in early-onset bipolar disorders. These delays occur in language, social, and motor growth approximately 10-18 years before affective symptoms appear.

— Adolescents who had early developmental antecedents were at high danger of developing psychotic symptoms. In addition, intelligence quotient (IQ) scores were significantly lower in patients with early-onset bipolar disorder than in patients with unipolar depression.

— Finally, a statistically important difference in the mean verbal IQ and mean performance IQ was found only in patients with bipolar disorder. The reason for this discrepancy is unclear but should be the subject of further investigation.

— Overall, patients with intense bipolar disorder had a mean IQ lower than that of patients with mild-to-moderate forms of the disorder.

- Finally, environmental factors also contribute to the growth of bipolar disorder. These may be behavioural, educational, family-related, toxic, or substance abuse induced.
- Diagnoses of mental health problems increase the danger of suicide in adolescents compared with their healthy peers.

— Adolescent patients in whom bipolar disorder is diagnosed are at higher danger of suicide than adolescents with other behavioural illnesses. Family conflict and substance abuse exponentially increase this risk.

— Another risk factor for suicide in youths is legal problems. One study showed that 24% of adolescents who attempted suicide had faced legal charges or consequences in the past 12 months.

- Incarcerated youths also have an inordinately high number of mental illnesses. Some are facing legal consequences as a direct result of behaviours that arise from uncontrolled or untreated mental disorders. The manic state of bipolar disorder can be especially problematic for adolescents because the disinhibited risk-taking behaviours driven by the disorder can easily lead to legal problems, such as public disorderly conduct, theft, drug seeking or use, and an agitated and irritable mood that results in verbal and physical altercations.

Biologic and Biochemical Factors

- Sleep disturbances frequently assist in defining abnormal mood states of bipolar disorder in either the manic or depressed state.
  - — A profoundly decreased need for sleep in the absence of a sense of fatigue is a strong indicator of a manic state.
  - — An uncomfortable reduction of sleep is a pattern of an atypical depression episode in which more sleep is wanted but can't be achieved. Conversely, a typical depression episode may be indicated by hypersomnolence, an excessive but irresistible need for sleep.
  - — The biology that drives these anomalies of sleep in mood disturbances is not fully appreciated. Some suggest that neurochemical and neurobiologic shifts cause these episodic sleep disturbances in conjunction with other shifts that occur in the evolution of manic or depressed states.
- Bipolar disorder and other mood disorders are increasingly understood in the context of neurochemical imbalances in the brain.
  - — Though the circuits of the brain that modulate mood, cognition, and behaviour are not well defined, the database of neuroimaging studies that facilitate increased appreciation of possible modulating pathways that connect many brain regions to work in unison to regulate thoughts, feelings, and behaviours is regularly growing.
  - — An association of neurotransmitters acts upon various brain regions and circuits to modify and regulate brain activity.
  - — One proposal suggests that many neurotransmitters acting in unison but with dynamic equilibrium act as modulators of mood states. In specific, serotonin, dopamine, and norepinephrine appear to modify mood, cognition, and sense of pleasure or displeasure.
  - — Pharmacotherapy for the regulation of bipolar mood swings is thought to be based on the use of medications that facilitate the regulation of these and perhaps other neurochemicals to restore a normal mood and cognition state.

DIAGNOSIS OF BIPOLAR DISORDER

No laboratory study can be used to confirm the diagnosis of bipolar disorder. Thus, gathering the history of present and past disturbances of mood, behaviour, and thought is critical to properly diagnose a psychiatric condition such as bipolar disorder. Unlike other areas of medicine in which the clinician frequently relies on laboratory or imaging studies to identify or characterize a disorder, mental health professionals rely almost exclusively on descriptive symptom clusters to diagnose mental disorders. As a consequence, the history is an necessary part of the patient examination.

- The appropriate first step in evaluating an individual for a psychiatric disorder is to ensure that no other medical condition is causing the mood or thought disturbance. Thus, evaluation of the patient is best began by obtaining their oral history of current and past medical and behavioural symptoms and treatments. To further clarify the problem, gathering additional information from family and friends always is urged for an individual experiencing an altered mood or behavioural state.
- After interviewing the patient, perform a physical examination. Gather information from family, friends, and perhaps other doctors to whom the patient is known. The problem might be classified as being mainly caused by a physical health problem or by a mental health problem.
  - While obtaining the history, the doctor must explore the possibilities that substance abuse or dependence, trauma to the brain in the present or past, and/or seizure disorders may be contributing to or causing the current symptoms of sickness.
  - CNS insults, such as encephalopathy or medication-induced mood changes (ie, steroid-induced mania), must also be considered. Delirium is one of the most significant medical conditions to exclude early in individuals presenting with altered mental states or acute disturbances of mood and conduct.
  - Perhaps more relevant to youth is the evaluation of substance abuse patterns because acute drug intoxication states may mimic bipolar disorder.
- If the physical examination does not reveal a medical condition contributing to the patient's mental state, a thorough mental health evaluation is appropriate. Through observation and interviewing, mental health professionals may learn of mood, behavioural, cognitive, or judgment and reasoning abnormalities.

- The mental status examination (MSE) is the necessary component of a mental health evaluation. This examination goes beyond the mini-mental status examination (e.g., Folstein Mini-Mental State Examination to screen for dementia) frequently used in emergency departments. Rather, the MSE is used to assess the general appearance and demeanor, speech, movement, and interpersonal relatedness of the patient with the examiner and others.
  - Mood and cognitive abilities (e.g., orientation to circumstance; attentiveness; immediate-, short-, and long-term modes of memory) are assessed in the MSE.
  - Some of the most significant components of the MSE are those addressing issues of safety of people and members of a community. Thus, suicidal and homicidal issues are explored.
  - Similarly, screens for the more subtle forms of psychosis, such as paranoid or delusional states, in addition to screens for overt psychosis, such as observing the patient responding to unseen others or other non-reality-based internal stimuli, are explored.
  - Finally, insight into the patient's mental and physical states, the current circumstances of medical or mental healthcare, and the patient's capability to use age-appropriate judgments are assessed and integrated into the evaluation of the global mental state of the patient at that moment.
- Because bipolar disorder may cause a transient but marked impairment of judgment, insight, and recall, quite a few sources of information are crucial to understand a specific patient. Thus, family members, friends, teachers, caregivers, or other doctors or mental healthcare workers may be interviewed to clarify the full clinical picture.
- Nonetheless, the patient's subjective experience is necessary in the evaluation and treatment processes, and the establishment of a therapeutic alliance and trust early in the assessment is vital to obtaining an accurate and useful history from the patient.
- Knowledge of the family's psychiatric history is another necessary part of the patient's history because bipolar disorder has genetic transmission and familial patterns. A genogram may be developed to further describe a specific patient's risk bipolar

disorder based on familial and genetic attributes in the family system.

Physical

- Physical examination must comprise general neurologic examination, together with examination of the cranial nerves, muscular bulk, and tone and deep tendon reflexes.
- Cardiovascular, pulmonary, and abdominal examinations are also necessary because abnormal pulmonary function or poor vascular perfusion of the brain may cause abnormal mood, behaviour, or cognition.
- Both physical and laboratory thyroid examination should be performed due to the potential mood alteration in hypothyroid and hyperthyroid states.
- If these examinations don't reveal a medical condition contributory to the current mental state, a mental health evaluation should be performed.

NURSING ASSESSMENT OF DEPRESSION

Nursing assessment of depression as the first step of the nursing process involves systematic, thorough consideration of the patient's safety and mental status, together with mood, affect, thought processes, and intellectual processes. It also necessitates careful review of physiologic and psychomotor activities, as well as behavioural and social activities. Suicidality is the priority safety issue and a primary concern for patients suffering from depression, but a patient with agitated depression may threaten not only to harm self but also others. When evaluating an individual's suicidality, the nurse should remember factors that increase risk for suicide, together with expression of current thoughts or plans about suicide, past history of suicidal attempts or behaviours, formulation of a plan, availability of means for completing suicide, interpersonal conflicts, failure at personal endeavours, and substance abuse.

The assessment of depression in elders may call for a slightly different approach because older adults tend to express their symptoms of depression by anxiety and somatic complaints that can mask the depth of ongoing depression. They may be at increased risk for depression and suicide because they frequently experience multiple losses (spouse, friends, job), co-morbid medical conditions, cognitive decline, and socioeconomic changes (retirement, limited and fixed income). In older adults, frequently it is difficult to determine whether cognitive symptoms (disorientation, apathy, difficulty concentrating, memory loss) are better accounted for by dementia or by a major depressive episode. A thorough medical evaluation and an evaluation of the onset of the disturbance, temporal sequencing or depressive and cognitive symptoms, course of sickness, and treatment response are helpful in making this determination.

Mental status examination is a significant tool to assess depression. The exam must be complete and thorough, and reperformed at intervals based on the patient's acuity of depressive symptom manifestation, together with safety issues. Quite a few components should be noted when the nurse performs a mental status examination for the depressed patient.

First, appearance and general behaviour assessment comprises age, grooming, clothing, posture, hygiene, and stature. Then overall behavioural presentation during the interview must be evaluated. The patient with depression may neglect personal hygiene with poor grooming, a disheveled appearance, and a dejected facial expression, and may show no interest in engaging the interviewer.

Second, assessment of mood and affect normally can be done by direct verbalization by the patient and also through observation of the patient's behaviour because mood and affect manifest themselves mainly as disturbances in the patient's emotional tone and expression in response to external and internal stimuli. Putting differently, mood can be assessed by evaluating the content of the patient's verbal communication, tone of voice, facial expression, posture, and gestures. In depression, affect normally is constricted but appropriate to content.

Third, thought content and process assessment comprises the ideas, vocabulary, and actual subject matter about which the patient speaks; content, degree of logic, and clarity of thought determine whether the patient's thoughts are coherent as process. The depressed patient frequently has to cope with issues of loss and abandonment, worthlessness, guilt, suicidality, and hopelessness. The patient may exhibit confusion, poor concentration and attention span, and thought blocking (DSM-IVTR).

Fourth, intellectual process assessment involves the patient's judgment and decision-making abilities. Depression can cause disturbed judgment, possibly related to anergia (lack of energy) and withdrawal. Insight is frequently limited in the patient with major depression because he or she can't assess the situation objectively. Assessment of the individual's physiologic integrity and function is significant because the depressed patient frequently exhibits poor appetite or excessive appetite, insomnia or hypersomnia, sexual dysfunction, gastrointestinal disturbance, and neglect in selfcare.

TREATMENT MODALITIES OF PATIENTS WITH MOOD DISORDERS

DEPRESSIVE DISORDER AND PSYCHOSOCIAL TREATMENTS

Psychosocial treatment is frequently effective in combating the symptoms of an episode if an individual has Depressive Disorder. Nevertheless, it must be understood that medication and the prescription of drugs might also be a requirement in several situations. As a subset of psychosocial therapy, counselling and family therapy methods are also useful in recovery. Family therapy is especially significant when it comes to the cases where children or adolescents have been affected with Depression.

Psychotherapy is a requirement in several cases because medical science has not yet advanced to a level where every mood disorder or mental ailment could be cured by a pill. Science has not fully identified the neurological or chemical basis of why several people have feelings of love, courage, or compassion just as science has not identified why some people feel depressed, angry or lose control of their emotional state. Nevertheless, therapy for patients suffering from a mood disorder is essential and is frequently.

The primary aim of psychosocial therapy is to furnish aid to the patient in understanding the disease, relieve symptoms and to try and alter behaviour patterns in combination with efforts from the patient. After undergoing successful psychosocial therapy, a patient is able to communicate more effectively with others and can continue to improve till the disease becomes completely manageable. A large portion of the therapy provided to the patient looks at ways in which the patient can improve their outlook of the world as well as their own person. Because such methods seek to renew the cognitive behaviour of the individual they are regarded as to be a part of Cognitive Behaviour Therapy.

The success of CBT for depressed patients who are undergoing psychosocial treatments is limited because there is a high rate of relapse into an episode of depression once the therapy is stopped. This distinctly suggests that the patient should have a social support group or an understanding family which continues to assist and monitor the patient. Psychosocial therapy coming in the shaper of interpersonal therapy centres can be quite helpful here because such centres help a person deal with personal grief, drastic changes in life and other difficulties for patients with mood disorders.

Depending on the requirements of individual cases, psychosocial therapies for patients with Clinical Depression comprise elements from CBT, interpersonal supportive therapy, as well as social group/family support. The delivery of such therapies can be given in both in-patient and out-patient settings, depending on medical recommendations based on the psychosocial assessments of the patient. Modern research also suggests that patients with milder forms of depression can battle their mood disorder with self help sessions as well as therapy. A patient suffering from Clinical Depression may think that no one cares for them or that the people around him don't understand the state he is in. Psychosocial treatment in such cases is tremendously beneficial since it distinctly shows that there are people who do care and are willing to sacrifice a lot to ensure that the patient gets better.

There might be a misconception about the depressed person that he is lazy and can easily snap out of his present state. Nurses and social workers have to do their part in psychosocial therapy to educate and inform the people around the patient that a mood disorder calls for medical aid as much as any other disease. Emotional support from the friends of the patient must continue to come with understanding, patience, love and supportive guidance. A depressed person needs to be listened to whenever he is willing to communicate and his feelings shouldn't be belittled. For instance, remarks about suicide or thoughts/plans about committing suicide are red flags for both nurses and the people around the individual which should be reported to the doctor/therapist handling the case.

If possible, the depressed person should be taken for short walks in natural environment, taken to see a movie, or engaged in some activity which helps them take their mind off the disease. This must not be enforced on them, but rather they should be gently persuaded towards it. Goals and milestones setup for an individual with mood disorders can be monitored to see how much progress they have made and how they can help in improving their condition. Nevertheless, a failure to meet goals can depress the person further; thus, small goals should be set and met before larger ones can be given. Finally, engagement in social groups, religious activities, sports and hobbies can also help an individual suffering from depression.

BIPOLAR DISORDER AND PSYCHOSOCIAL TREATMENTS

According to the case of Depressive Disorder, treatment with medicine alone is not always an effective method to control Bipolar Disorder. Generally accepted psychosocial therapies like interpersonal therapy, family oriented therapy and cognitive behaviour therapy are thus essential for the treatment of Bipolar Disorder.

It was formerly thought that patients with Bipolar Disorder couldn't benefit as much as patients with Depression since bouts of mania would greatly interfere with the therapy process. The newest research on the subject considers other factors like family support, CBT and monitoring of the patient as elements of psychosocial therapy which can act as effective counters to the impulsive behaviour or uncooperative mood of an individual suffering from BD. Additionally, it was found that patients (especially children) could continue learning, engage in active discussion, and make self-assessments if provided sufficient guidance from family members.

With Bipolar Disorder, family therapy becomes especially significant because, along with the individual, the whole family may suffer the effects of the disease since the social relationships of the patients are affected negatively. The function of the social worker or the nurse in such situations is to furnish aid, education and guidance as much as possible. Nurses and social workers are frequently recruited by physicians to furnish several aid in the course of such psychotherapies for monitoring progression in out-patient or in-patient settings. The cognitive therapy for Bipolar Disorder teaches the patient to recognize when they are going through one of their depressive or manic phases and how they can control their thoughts to control their behaviour.

The process of education about the disease for the patient, as well as the family of the patient, helps them recognize patterns of behaviour which can be adjusted over time. Additionally, the family members need to be watchful of any signs of relapse or fresh symptoms which show that the help being given is not sufficient. In such situations, additional therapy could be recommended, or a change in medication might be ordered by the physicians to ensure that the fresh symptoms don't develop into a full episode. Moreover, psychosocial therapy is frequently more cost effective than medical or surgical procedures for combating mood disorders.

Both Clinical Depression and the Bipolar Disorder can be helped with psychosocial treatments which comprise the following:

- Helping the patient as well as the family of the patient understand the disorder, its causes and symptoms.
- Monitoring the changes in the mood of the patient, the feelings of the patient and sleep patterns.
- Teaching the patient and related parties how to deal with the stress of the disease and reduce the effect of other stressors which can make the condition worse.
- Helping the patient manage his/her relationships to avoid/reduce the difficulties linked with decisions made or actions taken during a depressive or manic episode.
- Permitting patients to share experiences and offer helping hands in situations where group therapy is prescribed
- Offering an alternative to the patients for whom the side effects of pharmacological treatments are difficult to manage or for those who can't have pharmacological treatment at all.

REDUCING THE STIGMA

A significant role played by nurses and social workers in psychosocial therapy, as well as the treatment of other mental illnesses, is trying to reduce the social stigma linked with mood disorders. The main method with which the stigma can be reduced is through the creation of a therapeutic alliance.

GERIATRIC CONSIDERATIONS

Among patients who are seen in the psychiatric emergency department, geriatric patients-defined as patients aged 65 years and older-are statistically underrepresented. Geriatric individuals account for only 5 to 6 percent of all psychiatric emergency service visitors-although they account for about 12 percent of the population at large and represent the fastest growing segment of the population.

In addition to differences in demographic characteristics-such as the gender imbalance (more females than males) or the preponderance of patients with a fixed income-other special considerations exist for geriatric patients in the psychiatric emergency service. First is the high rate of comorbid medical and neurological problems, which can be chronic or acute. Behavioural disturbances can result from major medical problems, such as stroke, and from relatively minor problems, such as urinary tract infection. The increased danger of medical problems carries with it a danger of adverse drug reactions from the simultaneous use of multiple medications. The psychiatric consultant must be vigilant in screening for medical and neurological problems or be confident that the other doctors in the emergency department have already addressed them.

Geriatric patients are also at danger of pharmacological emergencies-medical emergencies that are related to psychiatric medications. Possible problems comprise agranulocytosis secondary to antipsychotics, hypotension or cardiac conduction disturbances that are caused by the use of antipsychotics or antidepressants, neuroleptic malignant syndrome, lithium toxicity, anticholinergic delirium, and acute dystonia.

Another critical factor in evaluating geriatric patients in the psychiatric emergency service is the danger of suicide, which is much higher among geriatric patients than younger patients. The suicide rate for white men aged 80 to 84 years is six times that of the general adult population. Clinicians in the psychiatric emergency service need to calibrate their index of concern about the danger of completed suicide for elderly psychiatric emergency service patients who present with depression, alcohol abuse, or other risk factors for suicide.

Due to these and other special considerations that apply to the geriatric patient, we suggest several maxims that may prove useful in guiding the clinician's work. They are formulated as ten "do's" and "do not's" for the psychiatric emergency service clinician, constituting a list that can't claim to be complete. These are:

Establish the situational context: It is no accident that more patients from nursing homes are referred to the emergency psychiatric service on Friday nights than on any other night of the week. Normally, Friday evening is when staffing levels and programming decline for the weekend, which leads to an increased likelihood that nursing home residents will become symptomatic and that staff members will worry about their capacity to handle residents' problem behaviours. Only 5 percent of individuals who are aged 65 years and older live in nursing homes; nevertheless, the prevalence of psychiatric disorders in these settings is at least 80 percent. Resources to take care of patients with psychiatric sickness-together with training and supervising caregivers as well as having access to psychiatric consultation-may be lacking. The same resource shortages could be true for caregivers in the home.

Communicate with third parties, taking the presenting complaint of the referral source seriously: In the evaluation of children, the involvement of parents, teachers, and other people is taken for granted-if only for legal reasons. Nevertheless, in the evaluation of an older person, family members' or caregivers' input is frequently invaluable in determining a pattern of behavioural change-such as threatening or assaultive behaviours toward caregivers or roommates-that easily escapes a one-point observation.

Obtaining consent and calling family members, primary care physicians, visiting nurses, adult protective workers, and other parties should be part of the protocol for evaluating geriatric patients. Most elderly patients don't come to the psychiatric emergency service on their own but are brought in by family members or others. Elderly patients may minimize or outright deny significant issues, such as environmental problems-together with changes in the home environment-and psychiatric symptoms.

Determine the accompanying psychopathology: Rarely will an older person develop new psychiatric symptoms without precipitants. For example, a new onset of psychotic symptoms demands an evaluation of cognitive functions to determine whether underlying dementia or delirium exists. Attention to the milieu interne and milieu externe is critical. An infectious disease, a transient ischemic episode, a change of cardiovascular medication, the loss of a pet, or the death of a roommate in the nursing home can trigger a psychiatric crisis. As with younger patients, it is appropriate to screen for affective and anxiety symptoms-such as changes in sleep, appetite, energy, and mood-as well as psychotic symptoms-such as auditory hallucinations and paranoid ideation.

Assess cognitive functioning: The Folstein Mini-Mental State Examination is a brief objective screen for cognitive impairment. Although behavioural problems, not memory problems, lead to admission to the psychiatric emergency service, a cognitive evaluation is mandatory for each geriatric patient. The presenting complaint of the referral source should be taken seriously. Nursing home staff members are all too swiftly accused of "dumping" patients. Nevertheless, nursing home staff members can't rationally be expected to manage an agitated patient with dementia who threatens to assault staff or his roommate. Combativeness among elderly people with dementia is dangerous and calls for a high level of staff monitoring as well as access to psychopharmacological medication, seclusion rooms, and restraints, which are available only in a hospital setting.

Suspect extrinsic substances: Elderly patients receive a disproportionate number of prescribed medications. Polypharmacy is probably the most common reason for delirium in the elderly patient, and a review of all medications in the patient's nursing home chart or in the home medicine cabinet is essential. Older individuals have a reduced tolerance for the central nervous system effects of prescribed medications and of alcohol and street drugs. Although substance abuse seems to be less common among elderly individuals, intoxication and withdrawal should be regarded as in the differential diagnosis for patients who present in a psychiatric emergency service, irrespective of their age. Also, a breath analysis and urine drug screens should be obtained if substance abuse is suspected.

Screen carefully for suicidal ideation and behaviour: Among geriatric patients, compared with other age groups, suicidal action is highly correlated with lethal outcomes. Mood disorders are common among older psychiatric patients, and the presenting affect, even in a manic state, is more frequently dysphoric compared with that of younger patients. Other risk factors for suicide, such as being unmarried and having a chronic medical sickness, are also common in this population.

Consider the situation that awaits the patient after discharge from the psychiatric emergency service: Questions to be considered comprise: Did this patient's home situation contribute to admission to the psychiatric emergency service? If so, has the home situation changed? Evaluators should try to put themselves in the patient's and caregiver's shoes. For example, the case should be handled as it would if it involved a family member. The presence of an outreach team can dramatically alter the disposition options.

Consider the possibility of elder abuse: The patient may be the carrier of symptoms for a dysfunctional social unit. The elderly person with "failure to thrive" or with multiple falls shouldn't be too swiftly seen as depressed. Memory impairment or intimidation can disguise recent abuse by the spouse, adult children or grandchildren, and others. The patient should be interviewed separately from the caregivers after the initial part of the interview and screened for abuse.

Get a second opinion when in doubt: Older patients may not be routinely seen in the psychiatric emergency service. So that a significant aspect of a geropsychiatric assessment will not be missed, a consultation with a colleague may be helpful. An internist or family practitioner with experience in geriatrics may be especially helpful in dealing with medical and psychosocial problems.

Document the dispositional decision and its rationale, and communicate it to the referral source: An attempt should be made to give the patient's caregivers and primary care doctor a copy of any notes relating to the dispositional decision and its rationale. The failure to communicate across institutional or disciplinary boundaries creates specific problems for older individuals who are served by a variety of systems or agencies.

The assessment of geriatric patients in the psychiatric emergency service can be more time intensive due to the necessity of investigating multiple domains-medical conditions; medications, whether prescribed or not; substances of abuse; and psychiatric symptoms. In addition, the patient may not be a reliable historian due to cognitive impairment or acute behavioural disturbance. Good outcomes depend on careful, complete assessments. Frequently, psychiatrists will need to work with other health care professionals, together with internists, family practitioners, social workers, and nurse specialists. This team approach promotes good communication and aids in establishing a complete biopsychosocial database. This approach can also decrease the individual clinician's burden of performing a time-intensive assessment. The patient also benefits from a team of professionals who may be able to furnish increased resources after the psychiatric emergency has been solved but ongoing treatment needs to be continued on an out-patient or institutional basis.

A bulk of older patients are not demented, frail, depressed, or suicidal. But all these conditions are more prevalent among older adults. In addition, all these conditions can be predisposing factors for psychiatric emergencies. Chronic medical conditions, social problems, and depression all contribute to the markedly elevated danger of suicide among older patients. A careful assessment of a geriatric patient should lead to a safe disposition and be the first step in a well-designed treatment plan.

FOLLOW UP AND HOME CARE REHABILITATION

Outcome identification for the patient with major depression focuses on the patient's needs such as safety and security, physical health, acceptance, belonging, positive self-concept, and empowerment. In addition to those for the patient with depression, outcomes for the manic patient will concentrate on opportunities to channel energy and to accurately perceive reality.

Planning interventions for patients with mood disorders can be done with a feeling of optimism and satisfaction, because most mood disorders are time-limited or can be stabilized with medication and other therapies that enable the patient to attain a healthier state of functioning. For instance, patients exhibiting clinical symptoms of a mood disorder secondary to a stressful life event frequently experience a time-limited mood disorder that responds positively to therapeutic interventions. Conversely, patients with the diagnosis of BPD frequently do well when taking medication but are at risk for an exacerbation of clinical symptoms if they discontinue taking prescribed medication.

Be alert to a personal vulnerability to depressive disorders. Working with such patients may cause one to react to the atmosphere of depression, and in turn, experience symptoms of depression. When planning care for patients with the diagnosis of depression or BPD, strive to attain and maintain the following personal attitudes:

- Acceptance: Patients with depression are not always able to express their feelings and may exhibit peculiar behaviour or low self-esteem. Patients with manic behaviour may be manipulative and demanding.
- Honesty: Patients with low self-esteem are less able to tolerate disappointment.
- Empathy: Any attempts to cheer up a patient with depression or to minimize negative, painful feelings will be viewed as an inability to understand the patient's feelings or problems. Doing so may lead to further withdrawal, isolation, or depression.
- Patience: Patients with depression may be unable to make decisions as easy as what to eat for breakfast or what clothing to wear. Patients who exhibit manic behaviour may elicit feelings of irritation, frustration, or anger on the part of the caregiver.

Patients with depression may attempt self-inflicted harm or suffer injury because of intense depression, lack of interest, psychomotor retardation, the inability to concentrate, or the inability to defend themselves against aggressive individuals. Be aware of the potential for self-destructive behaviour. Such an action may occur as the patient's psychomotor retardation lessens, the capability to concentrate returns, and the person is able to formulate a plan of action. Instituting protective care is necessary.

Protective care may be essential for the patient with mania as well as for the patient with depression. Individuals who exhibit manic behaviour may injure themselves because of excessive motor activity, inability to concentrate, distractibility, or poor judgment. Their destructive tendencies, frequently because of poor impulse control, may comprise self-inflicting behaviour and accidental injury. They may provoke self-defensive actions unintentionally from others who fear injury. If the patient is experiencing psychotic symptoms, the potential for homicidal behaviour could exist.

Planning care may call for a multidisciplinary team approach to address additional risk factors such as a medical condition that may or may not contribute to the patient's clinical symptoms; dual diagnosis such as the presence or history of alcohol or substance abuse; history of treatment-resistant depression; lack of social support; or a stressful life event such as the death of a spouse or divorce. A thorough knowledge base about psychotropic medication and a proficiency in administration; firm foundational understanding about the current use of somatic therapies; and the capability to furnish patient and family education are key elements of planning care.

Implementation: Implementing appropriate nursing interventions can occur in a variety of settings. Basically, hospitalization is recommended for patients who are seriously depressed, exhibit suicidal ideation, or call for medical care secondary to depression. Patients displaying symptoms of acute manic behaviour call for hospitalization as well. Providing a safe environment is of the utmost importance.

Assistance in Meeting Basic Needs: The severity of the patient's symptoms directly influences the degree of importance for physical care. The more intense the depression or mania is, the more significant physical care becomes because the patient loses interest in selfcare and may have difficulty making decisions. Aid with bathing, grooming, personal hygiene, and selection of appropriate attire to wear may be essential.

Dietary needs also call for close monitoring. The patient with depression may exhibit lack of appetite or anorexia, whereas the patient with mania may be too hyperactive to eat. Nutritional supplements, dietary snacks, or finger foods may be essential. Also monitor intake and output daily till the patient is able to take the responsibility of meeting nutritional needs.

Assess the patient's periods of rest and activity. The patient with depression may sleep continuously in an attempt to avoid the problems and anxieties of reality. Dysthymic depression is characterized by increased feelings of depression as the day progresses. Such patients in general "feel better in the morning" and are more productive at that time. As the day progresses, clinical symptoms of depression become more pronounced. Patients tend to withdraw and lose interest in their environment and selfcare. Patients with major depressive disorder or psychotic depression fall asleep early, awaken early, and feel better as the day progresses. The patient with mania may experience sleep deprivation because of hyperactivity. A patient exhibiting manic behaviour generally stays awake for a few days and then succumbs to physical exhaustion.

For the patient with a short attention span or one who is unable to concentrate, engage the patient in easy activities, such as a card game or a short walk. These activities are most efficient because the patient's self-esteem is enhanced when the tasks are completed. Also consider the patient's energy level for activities. The more energy the task calls for, the less energy the patient will have to engage in hostile, aggressive behaviour.

Displaying acceptance can be challenging when a patient exhibits hyperactivity, anger, hostility, or demanding, manipulative behaviour. Limit-setting may be essential as the patient attempts to express feelings and emotional needs.

Interpersonal, family, group, cognitive, or behavioural psychotherapy may be tailored to each patient depending on that person's specific conditions and coping capacities. The approach chosen is influenced by patient preference, stage and severity of sickness, concurrent life situations, and psychological traits. The frequency of the therapy chosen depends on the need to monitor medication compliance and suicide risk; severity of the sickness; the patient's own support network; and the nature of the psychotherapeutic goals.

Patients with mania should show some response to medication, such as decreased agitation and restlessness and an increased attention span, before therapy sessions begin. Patients with depression don't benefit from therapy if they exhibit psychomotor retardation.

In addition, occupational and recreational therapy may be used to channel the activity level of patients exhibiting manic behaviour or psychomotor agitation. Patients with depression may exhibit growth in self-esteem as they partake in these therapies.

Patient Education: Patient education, an ongoing process, begins as soon as the patient exhibits the capability to concentrate and process information. Education focuses on teaching patients to recognize the onset or recurrence of clinical symptoms of depression or mania; understand the dynamics of mood disorders; recognize the adverse effects of prescribed medication; and understand the consequences of medication noncompliance and the importance of establishing a support system. Caution patients who exhibit manic behaviour to not assume too several responsibilities or overextend themselves. Instruct patients with depression to contact a support person if feelings of depression return or increase in intensity.

Evaluation: The patient's response to interventions is evaluated based on the attainment of desired outcomes. The nurse compares the patient's clinical symptoms as initially seen when entering treatment with symptoms exhibited following completion of a plan of care. Input by family members and members of the treatment team is significant.

A significant aspect of evaluation involves determining the solution of clinical symptoms. Not all clinical symptoms improve at the same time. Residual symptoms (the phase of a sickness that occurs after the remission of the initial clinical symptoms) have been identified in some patients on antidepressant therapy. These symptoms comprise anergia (sluggishness or listlessness), apathy (indifference), asthenia (profound fatigue with loss of motivation and short-term memory problems), excessive daytime somnolence, fatigue, and hypersomnia.

REFERENCES

Carper, B. (1978). Fundamental patterns of knowing in nursing. Advances in Nursing Science, 13–23.

Deering, C. G. (1999). To speak or not to speak? Selfdisclosure with patients. American Journal of Nursing, 99(1), 34–39.

Hancock, C. (1998). How to decide about self-disclosure. Nursing, 98(3), 12–13.

Hewitt, J. (2002). A critical review of the arguments debating the role of the nurse advocate. Journal of Advanced Nursing, 37(5), 439–445.

Kohnke, M. F. (1982). Advocacy: What is it? Nursing and Health Care, 3(6), 314–318.

Mohr, W. K., & Horton-Deutsch, S. (2001). Malfeasance and regaining nursing's moral voice and integrity. Nursing Ethics, 8(1), 19–35.

Munhall, P. (1993). Unknowing: Toward another pattern of knowing in nursing. Nursing Outlook, 41(3), 125–128.

Peplau, H. E. (1952). Interpersonal relations in nursing. New York: J. P. Putnam's Sons.

Peternilji-Taylor, C. (1998). Forbidden love: Sexual exploitation in the forensic milieu. Journal of Psychosocial Nursing, 36(6), 17–23.

8

Management of Neurotic Disorders

Neurotic disorder is a term that refers to any mental imbalance that causes distress, but, unlike a psychosis or some personality disorders, does not prevent or affect rational thought. It is especially linked with the discipline of psychoanalysis. As a sickness, neurosis represents a variety of psychiatric conditions in which emotional distress or unconscious conflict is expressed through various physical, physiological, and mental disturbances, which may comprise physical symptoms (e.g., hysteria). The definitive symptom is anxieties. Neurotic tendencies are common and may manifest themselves as depression, acute or chronic anxiety, obsessive-compulsive tendencies, phobias, and even personality disorders, such as borderline personality disorder or obsessive-compulsive personality disorder. It has perhaps been most simply defined as a "poor capability to adjust to one's environment, an inability to change one's life patterns, and the inability to develop a richer, more complex, more satisfying personality." Neurosis shouldn't be mistaken for psychosis, which refers to loss of touch with reality.

The term connotes an actual disorder or disease, but under its general definition, neurosis is a normal human experience, part of the human condition. Most people are affected by neurosis in some form. A psychological problem develops when neuroses begin to interfere with, but not significantly impair, normal functioning, and thus cause the individual anxiety. Often, the coping mechanisms enlisted to help "ward off" the anxiety only exacerbate the situation, causing more distress. It has even been defined in terms of this coping strategy, as a "symbolic behaviour in defence against excessive psychobiologic pain which is self-perpetuating because symbolic satisfactions can't fulfil real needs."

As per psychoanalytic theory, neuroses may be rooted in ego defence mechanisms, but the two concepts are not synonymous. Defence mechanisms are a normal way of developing and maintaining a consistent sense of self (i.e., an ego), while only those thought and behaviour patterns that produce difficulties in living should be termed neuroses.

ANXIETY DISORDER

Anxiety is a vague feeling of dread or apprehension; it is a response to external or internal stimuli that can have behavioural, emotional, cognitive, and physical symptoms. Anxiety is distinguished from fear, which is feeling afraid or threatened by a distinctly identifiable, external stimulus that represents danger to the person. Anxiety is unavoidable in life and can serve several positive functions such as motivating the person to take action to resolve a problem or to solve a crisis. It is regarded as normal when it is appropriate to the situation and dissipates when the situation has been solved.

Anxiety disorders comprise a group of conditions that share a key feature of excessive anxiety with ensuing behavioural, emotional, and physiologic reactions. Clients suffering from anxiety disorders can demonstrate unusual behaviours such as panic without reason, unwarranted fear of objects or life conditions, uncontrollable repetitive actions, reexperiencing of traumatic events, or unexplainable or overwhelming tension. They experience significant distress over time, and the disorder significantly impairs their daily routine, social life, and occupational functioning.

PHOBIAS

A phobia is an illogical, severe, pertinacious fear of a specific object or a social situation that causes extreme distress and interferes with normal functioning. Phobias normally don't result from past, negative experiences. In fact, the person may never have had contact with the object of the phobia. People with phobias understand that their fear is unusual and irrational and may even joke about how "silly" it is. However, they feel powerless to stop it. People with phobias develop anticipatory anxiety even when thinking about possibly encountering the dreaded phobic object or situation. They engage in avoidance behaviour that frequently seriously limits their lives. Such avoidance behaviour normally does not relieve the anticipatory anxiety for long.

There are three classes of phobias:

- Agoraphobia (discussed earlier)
- Specific phobia, which is an irrational fear of an object or situation

- Social phobia, which is anxiety provoked by several social or performance situations

Several people express "phobias" about snakes, spiders, rats, or similar objects. These fears are very specific, easy to avoid, and cause no anxiety or tension. The diagnosis of a phobic disorder is made only when the phobic behaviour significantly interferes with the person's life by creating marked distress or difficulty in interpersonal or occupational functioning.

Specific phobias are subdivided into the following classes:

- Natural environmental phobias: fear of storms, water, heights, or other natural phenomena.
- Blood-injection phobias: fear of seeing one's own or others' blood, traumatic injury, or an invasive medical procedure such as an injection. Situational phobias: fear of being in a specific situation such as a bridge, tunnel, elevator, small room, hospital, or airplane.
- Animal phobia: fear of animals or insects (normally a specific type). Frequently this fear develops in childhood and can continue through adulthood in both men and women. Cats and dogs are the most common phobic objects.
- Other types of specific phobias: for instance, fear of getting lost while driving if not able to make all right (and no left) turns to get to one's destination.

In social phobia, also known as social anxiety disorder, the person becomes seriously nervous to the point of panic or incapacitation when confronting situations involving people. Examples comprise making a speech, attending a social engagement alone, interacting with the opposite sex or with strangers, and making complaints. The fear is rooted in low self-esteem and concern about others' judgments. The person fears looking socially inept, appearing nervous, or doing something embarrassing such as burping or spilling food. Other social phobias comprise fear of eating in public, utilizing public bathrooms, writing in public, or becoming the centre of attention. An individual may have one or quite a few social phobias; the latter is known as generalized social phobia.

DISSOCIATION AND CONVERSION DISORDER

Conversion disorder is a condition where patients present with neurological symptoms such as numbness, paralysis, or fits, but where no neurological explanation can be found. It is thought that these problems arise in response to difficulties in the patient's life, and conversion is regarded as a psychiatric disorder in the International Statistical Classification of Diseases and Related Health Problems (ICD-10) and Diagnostic and Statistical Manual of Mental Disorders 4th edition (DSM-IV). Formerly known as 'hysteria', the disorder has arguably been known for millennia, although it came to greatest prominence at the end of the 19th century, when the neurologist Jean-Martin Charcot, and psychiatrists Pierre Janet and Sigmund Freud made it the focus of their study. The term 'conversion' has its origins in Freud's doctrine that anxiety is 'converted' into physical symptoms. Although formerly thought to have vanished from the west in the 20th century, new research has suggested it is as common as ever.

DSM-IV-TR(2000) specifies six criteria for the diagnosis of conversion disorder. They are:

- The patient has one or more symptoms or deficits affecting the senses or voluntary movement that suggest a neurological or general medical disorder.
- The onset or worsening of the symptoms was preceded by conflicts or stressors in the patient's life.
- The symptom is not faked or produced intentionally.
- The symptom can't be fully explained as the result of a general medical disorder, substance intake, or a behaviour related to the patient's culture.
- The symptom is intense enough to interfere with the patient's schooling, employment, or social relationships, or is serious enough to call for a medical evaluation.
- The symptom is not limited to pain or sexual dysfunction, does not occur only in the context of somatization disorder, and is not better accounted for by another mental disorder.

OBSESSIVE COMPULSIVE DISORDER

Obsessive-compulsive disorder (OCD) is a chronic mental disorder most common generally characterized by intrusive, repetitive thoughts resulting in compulsive behaviours and mental acts that the person feels driven to perform, as per rules that must be applied rigidly, aimed at preventing some imagined dreaded event. In intense cases, it affects an individual's capability to function in every day activities. The disorder is frequently debilitating to the sufferer's quality of life. Also, the psychological self-awareness of the irrationality of the disorder can be painful. For people with intense OCD, it may take quite a few hours a day to carry out the compulsive acts.

Experts believe OCD is related to levels of a normal chemical in the brain called serotonin. When the proper flow of serotonin is blocked, the brain's "alarm system" overreacts. Danger messages are mistakenly triggered. Instead of the brain filtering out these unnecessary thoughts, the brain dwells on them-and the person repeatedly experiences unrealistic fears and doubts.

The phrase "obsessive-compulsive" has become part of the English lexicon, and is frequently used in an informal or caricatured manner to describe someone who is meticulous, perfectionistic, absorbed in a cause, or otherwise fixated on something or someone. Though these signs are frequently present in OCD, an individual who exhibits them does not necessarily have OCD, and may instead have obsessive-compulsive personality disorder (OCPD) or some other condition.

SOMATOFORM DISORDERS

The somatoform disorders are a group of mental disturbances placed in a common class on the basis of their external symptoms. These disorders are characterized by physical complaints that appear to be medical in origin but that can't be explained in terms of a physical disease, the results of substance abuse, or by another mental disorder. In order to meet the criteria for a somatoform disorder, the physical symptoms must be serious enough to interfere with the patient's employment or relationships, and must be symptoms that are not under the patient's voluntary control.

It is helpful to understand that the present classification of these disorders reflects recent historical changes in the practice of medicine and psychiatry. When psychiatry first became a separate branch of medicine at the end of the nineteenth century, the term hysteria was generally used to describe mental disorders characterized by altered states of consciousness (for instance, sleepwalking or trance states) or physical symptoms (for instance, a "paralyzed" arm or leg with no neurologic cause) that couldn't be fully explained by a medical disease. The term dissociation was used for the psychological mechanism that allows the mind to split off uncomfortable feelings, memories, or ideas so that they are lost to conscious recall. Sigmund Freud and other pioneering psychoanalysts thought that the hysterical patient's symptoms resulted from dissociated thoughts or memories reemerging through bodily functions or trance states. Prior to the categorization all mental disorders that were regarded as to be forms of hysteria were grouped together on the basis of this theory about their cause. Since 1980, nevertheless, the somatoform disorders and the so-called dissociative disorders have been placed in separate classes on the basis of their chief symptoms. Generally, the somatoform disorders are characterized by disturbances in the patient's physical sensations or capability to move the limbs or walk, while the dissociative disorders are marked by disturbances in the patient's sense of identity or memory.

POST TRAUMATIC STRESS DISORDER

Posttraumatic stress disorder (PTSD) is an emotional sickness that develops as a result of a terribly frightening, life-threatening, or otherwise highly unsafe experience. PTSD sufferers re-experience the traumatic event or events in some way, tend to avoid places, people, or other things that remind them of the event (avoidance), and are exquisitely sensitive to normal life experiences (hyperarousal). Though this condition has likely existed since human beings have endured trauma, PTSD has only been recognized as a formal diagnosis since 1980. Nevertheless, it was called by different names as early as the American Civil War, when combat veterans were referred to as suffering from "soldier's heart." In World War I, symptoms that were in general consistent with PTSD were referred to as "combat fatigue." Soldiers who developed such symptoms in World War II were said to be suffering from "gross stress reaction," and several who fought in Vietnam who had symptoms of what is now called PTSD were assessed as having "post-Vietnam syndrome." PTSD has also been called "battle fatigue" and "shell shock." Complex posttraumatic stress disorder (C-PTSD) normally results from prolonged exposure to a traumatic event or series thereof and is characterized by long-lasting problems with several facets of emotional and social functioning.

Approximately 7%-8% of people will likely develop PTSD in their lifetime, with the lifetime occurrence (prevalence) in combat veterans and rape victims ranging from 10% to as high as 30%. Some of that difference is thought to be because of higher rates of dissociation soon before and after the traumatic event (peritraumatic); a tendency for people from minority ethnic groups to blame themselves, have less social support, and an increased perception of racism for those ethnic groups; as well as differences between how ethnic groups may express distress. Other significant facts about PTSD comprise the estimate of 5 million people who suffer from PTSD at any one time and the fact that women are twice as likely to develop PTSD as men.

Almost half of people who use out-patient mental-health services have been found to suffer from PTSD. As evidenced by the occurrence of stress in several people in the United States in the days following the 2001 terrorist attacks, not being physically present at a traumatic event does not guarantee that one can't suffer from traumatic stress that can lead to the growth of PTSD.

PTSD statistics in children and teens reveal that up to more than 40% have endured at least one traumatic event, resulting in the growth of PTSD in up to 15% of girls and 6% of boys. On average, 3%-6% of high school students and as several as 30%-60% of children who have survived specific disasters have PTSD. Up to 100% of children who have seen a parent killed or endured sexual assault or abuse tend to develop PTSD, and more than one-third of youths who are exposed to community violence will suffer from the disorder.

ETIOLOGY

Genetic Theories

Anxiety may have an inherited component, because first-degree relatives of clients with increased anxiety have higher rates of developing anxiety. Heritability refers to the proportion of a disorder that can be attributed to genetic factors:

- High heritabilities are greater than 0.6 and indicate that genetic influences dominate.
- Moderate heritabilities are 0.3 to 0.5 and suggest a more even influence of genetic and nongenetic factors.
- Heritabilities less than 0.3 mean that genetics are negligible as a primary cause of the disorder.

Panic disorder and social and specific phobias including agoraphobia have moderate heritability. General anxiety disorder and OCD tend to be more common in families, but they have not been studied in-depth to determine heritability. At this point, current research indicates a clear genetic susceptibility to or vulnerability for anxiety disorders; however, additional factors are necessary for these disorders to actually develop.

Neurochemical Theories

Gamma-amino butyric acid (GABA) is the amino acid neurotransmitter believed to be dysfunctional in anxiety disorders. GABA, an inhibitory neurotransmitter, functions as the body's natural anti-anxiety agent by reducing cell excitability, thus decreasing the rate of neuronal firing. It is available in one-third of the nerve synapses especially those in the limbic system and the locus ceruleus, the area where the neurotransmitter norepinephrine that excites cellular function is produced. Because GABA reduces anxiety and norepinephrine increases it, researchers believe that a problem with the regulation of these neurotransmitters occurs in anxiety disorders. Serotonin (5-HT), the indolamine neurotransmitter usually implicated in psychosis and mood disorders, has many subtypes. 5-HT1a plays a role in anxiety as well as in affecting aggression and mood. Serotonin is believed to play a distinct role in OCD, panic disorder, and generalized anxiety disorder. An excess of norepinephrine is suspected in panic disorder, generalized anxiety disorder, and posttraumatic stress disorder.

Intrapsychic/Psychoanalytic Theories

Freud saw a person's innate anxiety as the stimulus for behaviour. He described defence mechanisms as the human's attempt to control awareness of and to reduce anxiety. Defence mechanisms are cognitive distortions that a person uses unconsciously to maintain a sense of being in control of a situation, to lessen discomfort, and to deal with stress. Because defence mechanisms arise from the unconscious, the person is unaware of using them. Some people overuse defence mechanisms, which stops them from learning a variety of appropriate methods to resolve anxiety-producing situations. The dependence on one or two defence mechanisms also can inhibit emotional growth, lead to poor problemsolving skills, and create difficulty with relationships.

Interpersonal Theory

Harry Stack Sullivan viewed anxiety as being generated from problems in interpersonal relationships. Caregivers can communicate anxiety to infants or children through inadequate nurturing, agitation when holding or handling the child, and distorted messages. Such communicated anxiety can result in dysfunction such as failure to achieve age-appropriate developmental tasks. In adults, anxiety arises from the person's need to conform to the norms and values of his or her cultural group. The higher the level of anxiety, the lower the ability to communicate and to solve problems and the greater chance for anxiety disorders to develop. Hildegard Peplau understood that humans existed in interpersonal and physiologic realms; thus, the nurse can better help the client to achieve health by attending to both areas. She identified the four levels of anxiety and developed nursing interventions and interpersonal communication techniques based on Sullivan's interpersonal view of anxiety. Nurses today use Peplau's interpersonal therapeutic communication techniques to develop and to nurture the nurse-client relationship and to apply the nursing process.

Behavioural Theory

Behavioural theorists view anxiety as being learned through experiences. Conversely, people can change or "unlearn" behaviours through new experiences. Behaviourists believe that people can modify maladaptive behaviours without gaining insight into the causes for them. They contend that disturbing behaviours that develop and interfere with a person's life can be extinguished or unlearned by repeated experiences guided by a trained therapist.

DIAGNOSIS

Patients with symptoms of mental sickness should undergo a thorough physical examination and detailed patient history to rule out organic causes (such as brain tumour or head injury). If a neurotic disorder is suspected, a psychologist or psychiatrist will normally conduct an interview with the patient and administer clinical assessments (also called scales, inventories, or tests), to assess mental status. Tests which may be administered for the diagnosis and assessment of neurosis comprise the Neuroticism Extraversion and Openness (NEO-R) scale, the Sixteen Personality Factor Questionnaire (16PF), and the Social Maladjustment Schedule. Neurosis should be treated by a counsellor, therapist, psychologist, psychiatrist, or other mental healthcare professional. Treatment for a neurotic disorder depends on the presenting symptoms and the level of discomfort they are causing the patient. Modes of treatment are similar to that of other mental disorders, and can comprise psychotherapy, cognitive-behavioural therapy, creative therapies (e.g., art or music therapy), psychoactive drugs, and relaxation exercises.

NURSING ASSESSMENT

Nursing assessment of neurotic disorders as the first step of the nursing process is a slightly different than other sickness it involves systematic, thorough consideration of the patient's safety and mental status, together with mood, affect, thought processes, and intellectual processes. It also necessitates careful review of physiologic and psychomotor activities, as well as behavioural and social activities. Suicidality is the priority safety issue and a primary concern for patients suffering from neurotic disorder, but a patient with agitated neurotic disorder may threaten not only to harm self but also others. When evaluating an individual's suicidality, the nurse should remember factors that increase risk for suicide, together with expression of current thoughts or plans about suicide, past history of suicidal attempts or behaviours, formulation of a plan, availability of means for completing suicide, interpersonal conflicts, failure at personal endeavours, and substance abuse.

The assessment of neurotic disorder in elders may call for a slightly different approach because older adults tend to express their symptoms of depression by anxiety and somatic complaints that can mask the depth of ongoing depression. They may be at increased risk for neurotic disorder and suicide because they frequently experience multiple losses (spouse, friends, job), co-morbid medical conditions, cognitive decline, and socioeconomic changes (retirement, limited and fixed income). In older adults, frequently it is difficult to determine whether cognitive symptoms (disorientation, apathy, difficulty concentrating, memory loss) are better accounted for by dementia or by a major depressive episode. A thorough medical evaluation and an evaluation of the onset of the disturbance, temporal sequencing or depressive and cognitive symptoms, course of sickness, and treatment response are helpful in making this determination.

Though the behavioural and cognitive approaches to psychological treatment are theoretically distinct, in practice most interventions involve elements of both. Cognitive-behavioural therapy is of proven effectiveness in the treatment of conditions such as phobias and OCD, in younger adults. Case reports and small series indicate that they are just as effective in the elderly. Anxiety management training, involving instruction, relaxation and other control techniques is a significant approach to anxiety symptoms in the elderly, which can be applied in a wide range of settings to both groups and people. Further research is needed to establish which strategies are most efficient in this age group; while the principles of cognitive-behavioural therapy are the same at all ages, the goals and techniques may need to be modified to make allowance for physical disabilities.

In spite of the effectiveness of behavioural, training and cognitive strategies in the management of neurotic disorders, most elderly patients with these conditions are treated with drugs. Sometimes this is appropriate; for instance, if depression is a prominent feature then a course of antidepressant treatment should always be considered. Nevertheless, the pharmacotherapy of neurotic disorders is frequently merely an easy and convenient means of avoiding a more detailed and painstaking assessment of the patient's symptoms and circumstances.

The greatest problems with inappropriate and excessive drug treatment of neurotic disorders in the elderly have occurred in association with benzodiazepines. Despite the fact that there have been relatively few formal controlled trials of benzodiazepine treatment in elderly patients, old people are the largest consumers of this class of drugs, especially as hypnotics. Due to the altered handling of drugs by the body with increasing age, some benzodiazepines and their metabolites accumulate substantially in some elderly patients, with the result that evidently therapeutic doses can eventually cause pertinacious drowsiness, incontinence, delirium and falls. Other problems in the elderly comprise increased central nervous system sensitivity to the effect of the drug, the presence of physical sickness (especially respiratory disease), interactions with other drugs and alcohol, and non-compliance. At all ages, long-term benzodiazepine use can result in physical dependence, cognitive impairment and paradoxical excitement. In view of all these problems, benzodiazepine prescription in the elderly should be restricted to short courses of short-acting compounds without active metabolites, such as oxazepam. As a rule, long-term benzodiazepine users should be encouraged to withdraw from their medication, especially if they have continuing neurotic symptoms.

There is evidence that some of the new generation of anxiolytics and antidepressants are more effective in providing relief in neurotic disorders without unacceptable side-effects. Buspirone is an azapirone anxiolytic drug whose pharmacokinetics, safety and efficacy in the elderly, are similar to those in younger adults. It is well tolerated by this age group, and it appears that short-term use is not linked with rebound, dependence or misuse. Unlike other anxiolytics it takes two to three weeks to have an effect, so it is not useful in the management of acute anxiety states. Neuroleptic drugs have only a limited role in the management of anxiety due to the danger of disabling extrapyramidal side-effects. Antihistamine drugs such as hydroxyzine have a history of use as anxiolytics in elderly patients, and they may be useful when respiratory depressant drugs are contraindicated.

Neurotic disorders are more common in the elderly than in general realised. Faced with the urgent demands of dementia and depression, it is understandable that some hard-pressed old age psychiatric services might regard the treatment of neurotic disorders as a relatively low priority. While it is true that services should aim to have a limited role in the longterm management of these conditions, they should however be proficient in their assessment and acute treatment, and be able to advise primary care teams, doctors and others responsible for the continuing care of these patients, in appropriate management strategies.

TREATMENT MODALITIES

The diagnosis is always provisional and conditional, because of the time factor involved till the appearance of organic evidence (as in systemic disease). Of importance is the fact that between 25 and 50% of patients diagnosed as conversion, will subsequently be diagnosed with an organic medical condition. This percentage is lower in recent publications, most probably due to increased awareness to the disorder, concurrent with advances in diagnostic techniques.

The possibility that a present symptom is conversion increases, if the patient has a history of un-explained physical complaints (especially conversion) or dissociative symptoms, and if he/she meets the criteria for Somatization Disorder.

The less the patient's medical knowledge, the more he/she appears with inexplicable and irregular symptoms. In contrast, symptoms of educated patients are very similar to genuine ones. In order to reach a right diagnosis a thorough neurological examination is necessary. Prominent suspicious symptoms comprise: jerky sharp movements, unexplained tremor, inconsistency in findings (e.g., muscle strength of quadriceps in standing compared to sitting), bizarre gait pattern, slow motion movements, overflow of emotion during the exam (painful expression, tooth grinding, breath holding, etc).

Other signs comprise normal muscle tone, normal reflexes, flexor plantar reflexes, bizarre movements, and simultaneous contraction of agonist and antagonist muscles (if the patient is asked to flex the elbow, contraction of the triceps, preventing flexion, is noticed. When the examiner attempts to change an abnormal limb position, a resistance in direct relation to the power exerted is felt. If a 'paralyzed' arm is raised above the subject's head and released, it will not fall directly on his head, but to the side.

The sensory examination might reveal changes not related to anatomical dermatomes, inconsistency in repeated examinations, misleading proprioception. Conversion anaesthesia in a hand or foot will have a shape of a glove or sock, affecting all types of sensation, with no determinant level, and with a sharp border, and not as per dermatomal levels.

The autonomic system is normally unaffected with full sphincter control and normal bowel movement. No spinal shock or other typical autonomic signs (e.g., low pulse and blood pressure, dyspnea) are presented in conversion tetraplegia.

GERIATRIC CONSIDERATION

Elderly patients normally have a higher frequency for chronic medical sickness that may coexist with hypochondriasis and which may result in complications in treatment of neurotic disorders.

The nurses should keep in consideration the following points while treating with geriatric patients:

- Talking to the patient may make him or her feel better and then its easy to cope with their emotional reactions and the more effective and healthy relationship with them.
- Clear, frequent communication with other health care providers can help diminish the patient's manipulation.
- Don't take undue flattery or harsh criticism personally, it is a result of the patient's personality disorder.
- Set practical goals and remember that behaviour changes in patients with neurotic disorders take long time progress can be very slow.

FOLLOW-UP AND HOME CARE AND REHABILITATION

In the past, patients were referred to psychiatric departments, but this trend was changed, and because of the functional loss patients are referred to rehabilitation wards. The bulk of papers on the topic are retrospective studies or case reports, authored by psychiatrists or specialists in physical medicine and rehabilitation. There are no long-term follow-up studies. The reference to treatment is minimal, contradicting and vague, offering autosuggestion, placebo, and hypnosis as the main treatments of choice. When the psychological intervention fails, inter-disciplinary rehabilitation treatment becomes even more of an imperative. It is our impression that treatment should be directed towards the symptoms and as such the patients should be hospitalized in the right units as per their physical symptoms, i.e. paraplegic or tetraplegic patients in a rehabilitation spinal unit, hemiplegic patients in a rehabilitation stroke unit etc and not placed in psychiatric units from the offset. Treatment in a rehabilitation system will also address the prevention of secondary disabilities. Those disabled because of conversion have several similarities to those with an organic basis for the disability, with regard to effects on physiology, social and occupational consequences.

Rehabilitation treatment should be introduced as early as possible. There is the need to rule out neurological, orthopedic and other potential medical etiologies. The patients must be screened and diagnosed, and to exclude those with suspected factitious disorder, malingering, or where there is secondary gain. Team members should be educated concerning the unconscious origin of the CS and the type of approach to be used in the treatment. The preferred setting is hospitalization in a rehabilitation ward in order to observe the patients in all activities. When both the medical etiologies and the conscious psychological etiologies are excluded, we are left with those patients disabled because of conversion disorders (impaired vision, balance deficits, difficulty in walking, limb paralysis, etc).

Three main treatment approaches should be considered:

The behaviour modification approach: The objectives underlying this approach are a reduction in the unwanted behaviours and a strengthening of the more desired behaviours. In order to accomplish these objectives it is significant to reward the more desired behaviours. Rather than punishing the unwanted behaviours they should, as much as possible, be ignored or at least not bring the desired focus of attention. A focus on the positive not the negative should be encouraged, and this may be achieved by the use of 'achievement charts' carefully screened obtainable goals, videotape feedback, in order to demonstrate the progress. It is preferable to treat the patient in a quiet place, away from the main treatment area, in order to avoid acquired behaviour.

Treatment utilizing this approach begins even during the initial assessment when a diagnosis of CD is suspected because of the anomalies discovered on physical assessment. The diagnosis given should be vague rather than confrontational, i.e., in the case of hysterical paralysis 'spinal cord concussion', permitting the patient to undergo 'a speedy recovery'.

Communication within the inter disciplinary team is necessary and regular team meetings to document the progress of the patient should be held. Any differences of opinion between team members must be discussed only during these meetings. A case manager, possibly the psychologist, must direct and coordinate all treatments.

The psychotherapeutics approach: The object of this approach is to solve the conflict which has led to the clinical picture of CD. Psychotherapeutic treatment is given on an individual basis and its success will depend, to a large degree, on the cooperation of the patient. Drug therapy in the form of Thiopentone has proven itself to be an effective tool. Others report success with auto-suggestive treatments and hypnosis.

The physical approach: It is useful to combine the above approaches with a physical therapy approach. Exercises according to the 'vague diagnosis' may be prescribed together with functional electrical stimulation (FES), evoked potentials and biofeedback techniques. It is necessary that regular objective measures be taken of the patient's functional abilities and these will have a great impact on the recovery outcome of the patient. Other objective measures in the form of balance testing or gait analysis are also significant, because the results shown by the patient can be compared to the normative data available. As stated earlier the most successful approach to treatment would seem to be a combination of these three approaches.

REFERENCES

Arnold, E., et al. (1999). Interpersonal relationships: Professional communication skills for nurses (3rd ed.). Philadelphia: W. B. Saunders.

Balzer Riley, J. W. (2000). Communications in nursing: Communicating assertively and responsibly in nursing (4th ed.). Philadelphia: Mosby.

Chant, S., Jenkinson, T., Randle, J., & Russell, G. (2002). Communication skills: Some problems in nursing education and practice. Journal of Clinical Nursing, 11(1), 12–21.

Cormier, L. S., Cormier, W. H., & Weisser, R. J. (1997). Interviewing and helping skills for health professionals. Boston: Jones & Bartlett.

deVito, J. A. (2002). Human communication: The basic course (9th ed.). Boston: Allyn and Bacon.

Knapp, M., & Hall, J. (2002). Nonverbal behavior in human interaction (5th ed.). New York: Wadsworth.

Knapp, M. L. (1980). Essentials of nonverbal communication. New York: Holt, Rinehart & Winston.

Kreps, G. L., & Kunimoto, E. N. (1994). Effective communication in multicultural health care settings. Thousand Oaks, CA: Sage Publications.

McGhee P. (1998). Rx: Laughter. RN, 7(3), 50–53.

Morley, W. E., et al. (1967). Crisis: Paradigms of intervention. Journal of Psychiatric Nursing, 5, 537–538.

Peplau, H. (1952). Interpersonal relations in nursing. New York: G. P. Putnam.

Van Servellen, G. (1997). Communication skills for the health care professional: Concepts and techniques. Gaithersburg, MD: Aspen.

Weaver, R. L. (1996). Understanding interpersonal communication (7th ed.). New York: Harper-Collins College Publishers.

9

Management of Patients with Substance Use Disorders

The phrases substance use disorder or disorders because of psychoactive drug use refer to conditions arising from the abuse of alcohol and psychoactive drugs. Alcohol and other substances can have varied physiological and psychological effects. In the short term, the individual may perceive these effects as quite desirable. For instance, the anxiety-relieving properties of alcohol, the alerting effects of caffeine and the sense of well being induced by opioids. Nevertheless, prolonged and heavy usage may result in physical harm, dependency and withdrawal problems and long term psychological damage or social harm.

GENERALLY USED PSYCHOTROPIC SUBSTANCE

ALCOHOL

Forms: Booze, brew, juice, spirits.

Routs: Ingestion.

Action: Depression of major brain functions such as mood, cognition, attention, concentration, insight, judgment, memory, affect and emotional bonding in inter personal relationships. Overdose leads to unconsciousness, coma, depression and death.

Intoxication: signs of intoxication are obvious with blood levels of 150-200 mg%. With blood alcohol levels of 300- 450 mg%, increasing drowsiness followed by coma, and respiratory depression develop. Death occurs with blood alcohol levels between 400-800 mg%.

Withdrawal: Hangover, mild tremors, nausea, vomiting, weakness, irritability, insomnia, and anxiety. The intense forms comprise; delirium tremens, alcoholic seizure, and alcoholic hallucinosis.

BARBITURATES

Forms: Barbs, beans, black beauties, blue angels, candy, downers, goof balls, G.B, nebbies, reds, sleepers, yellow jackets, yellows.

Routs: Ingestion, injection.

Action: Depression of major brain functions such as mood, cognition, attention, concentration, insight, judgment, memory, affect and emotional bonding in inter personal relationships.

Intoxication: confusion, drowsiness, nystagmus, unconsciousness, coma, respiratory depression and death.

Withdrawal: Restlessness, anxiety, insomnia, delirium, convulsions and even death.

AMPHETAMINES

Forms: Benzedrine, Dexedrine, Methedrine

Routs: Ingestion, injection.

Action: It increases release of dopamine from nerve terminals and inhibits the reuptake of dopamine and related transmitters.

Intoxication: Sudden rush of euphoria, abrupt awakening, increased energy, talkativeness, elation, agitation, hyperactivity, irritability, grandiosity, pressured speech.

Withdrawal: Depression with suicidal ideation, apathy, fatigue, hypersomnia alternating with insomnia, agitation and hyperphagia

COCAINE

Forms: Cocaine HCL, free base alkaloid.

Routs: Inhalation, smoking, injection, topical.

Action: CNS stimulant which inhibits the reuptake of dopamine.

Intoxication: Pupillary dilatation, tachycardia, hypertension, sweating, and nausea or vomiting. A hypo manic picture with increased psychomotor activity, grandiosity, elation of mood, hypervigilence and increased speech output may be present. Later, judgment is impaired and there is impairment of social or occupational functioning.

Withdrawal: Depression, anxiety, anhedonia, sleep disturbance, increased appetite, and psychomotor retardation.

OPIATES

Forms: Heroin, morphine, meperidine, codeine, opium, methadone.

Routs: Injection, ingestion, smoking.

Action: Activates receptors called mu and delta opioid receptors

Intoxication: Euphoria, sedation, reduced libido, memory and concentration difficulties, analgesia, constipation, constricted pupils, respiratory depression, stupor, coma.

Withdrawal: Abdominal cramps, rhinorrhea, watery eyes, dilated pupils, yawning, diaphoresis, nausea, diarrhea, anorexia, insomnia, fever.

MARIJUANA

Forms: Smoke.

Routs: Smoking, ingestion.

Action: The main active chemical in marijuana is THC which produces memory and perception problems.

Intoxication: Altered state of awareness, relaxation, mild euphoria, reduced inhibition, red eyes, dry mouth, increased appetite, increased pulse, decreased reflexes, panic reaction.

Withdrawal: Irritability and difficulty in sleeping.

HALLUCINOGENS

Forms: LSD, DMT, MDMA, Mescaline

Routs: ingestion, smoking.

Action: Acts on different brain receptors such as serotonin, glutamate and acetylcholine receptors.

Intoxication: Euphoria or dysphoria, altered body image, distorted visual and auditory perception, depersonalization, bizarre behaviour, confusion, incoordination, impaired judgment and memory, palpitations.

Withdrawal: None

PHENCYCLIDINE (PCP)

Routs: Smoking, ingestion.

Action: NMDA receptor antagonist which blocks the activity of the NMDA receptor.

Intoxication: ataxia, dysarthria, decreased pain perception, hallucinations, paranoia, aggression, adrenergic crisis.

Withdrawal: None.

INHALANTS

Forms: Gasoline, glue, aerosol sprays, paint thinner.

Routs: Inhalation.

Action: Most likely affects inhibitory transmitters.

Intoxication: Euphoria, giddiness, excitation, ataxia, nystagmus, dysarthria, coma and convulsions.

Withdrawal: Anxiety, tremors, hallucinations, and sleep disturbance.

NICOTINE

Routs: Smoking.

Action: Activates nicotinic cholinergic receptors, inhibits dopamine synthesis and release.

Intoxication: Stimulation, alertness, appetite suppression, anxiety.

Withdrawal: Craving, anxiety, poor concentration, sleep disturbances, headaches, gastric distress, and increased appetite.

ETIOLOGY OF DEPENDENCE

Tolerance: It is an adaptive state characterized by a diminished response to the same quantity of a drug or by the fact that a larger dose is required to produce the same degree of pharmacodynamic effect.

Psychological Dependence: It occurs when the drug is central to an individual's thought, emotions and activities. It is difficult for the person to stop thinking of the drug which causes severe craving for it and its effect. It is reduced only on readministration of the drug like in physical dependence.

Physical Dependence: Physical dependence occurs when the drug user's body becomes so accustomed to a specific drug that he can function normally only if the drug is present in his body. Without the drug the user may experience symptoms of mild discomfort to convulsions. These symptoms will only be relieved by readministration of the same drug or of another drug or a similar pharmacological quality. Physical dependence is a powerful factor in reinforcing upon continuing the drug use.

Withdrawal Syndrome: A withdrawal state is characterized by a cluster of symptoms, frequently specific to the drug used, which develop on total or partial withdrawal of a drug, normally after repeated and or high dose use. Basically, the patients reports that the withdrawal symptoms are relieved by further substance use.

DIAGNOSIS

A definite diagnosis of dependence should normally be made only if three or more of the following have been present together at sometime during the previous year.(ICD-10)

- A strong desire or sense of compulsion to take the substance.
- Difficulties in controlling substance-taking behaviour in terms of its onset, termination, or levels of use.
- A physiological withdrawal state when substance use has ceased or been reduced, as evidenced by: the characteristic withdrawal symptom for the substance; or use of the same substance with the intention of relieving or avoiding withdrawal symptoms.
- Evidence of tolerance.
- Progressive neglect of alternative pleasures or interests.
- Persisting with substance use in spite of clear evidence of overtly damaging consequences.

NURSING ASSESSMENT

Nursing assessment of clients with substance abuse disorders focuses on physical status and psychosocial circumstances.

HISTORY

- History of substance use: history of experimentation with any drugs in childhood, age of first use, amount and cost of drug used per day or week, method used to support habit, history of needle sharing.
- Presence of withdrawal symptoms.
- Substances related sickness: hepatitis, pancreatitis, heart complications etc.
- Treatment history: attempts at self detoxification and outcome, names of treatment programs in dates, etc.

- Past medical history.
- Medications: usual dose, amount actually used.
- Family history: history of substance abuse.
- Childhood history: history of physical/sexual/emotional abuse.
- Consequences of substance use: any losses.
- Legal history: arrests, incarcerations, current status.
- Psychiatric history: any known diagnosis, history of suicide, admissions etc.
- Social history: living situation and social support.
- Sexual history.
- Gynecological history.

PHYSICAL AND MENTAL ASSESSMENT

- General observations: blood pressure, pulse, temperature, respiration.
- Appearance: gait, eyes, skin, nose, presence of tremors, grooming.
- Behaviour: speech, attitude, mood and affect, sensorium, perception.
- Height
- Weight
- Skin
- Oral cavity
- Abdomen
- Speech

CAGE SCREENING TEST FOR ALCOHOLISM

- Have you ever felt you ought to cut down on your drinking?
- Have people annoyed you by criticizing your drinking?
- Have you ever felt guilty about your drinking?
- Have you ever had a drink first thing in the morning to steady your nerves or get rid of a hangover (eye-opener)?

DRUG ASSAY

The use of laboratory tests for diagnosing substance abuse continues to become more complex and sophisticated. A large number of variables may affect the results, together with the uniqueness of the drug, the dosage taken, frequency of use, the type of body fluid tested, (urine, blood, stool), differences in drug metabolism, sample collection time and its relationship to time of use, and sensitivity of the test itself.

The most commongenerally used laboratory tests are the blood alcohol level (BAL), the gamma glutamyl transferase (GGT), and the mean corpuscle value (MCV). In most states BAL is used to determine legal intoxication.

TREATMENT

The treatment of substance use disorder patients comprises the following steps:

Detoxification: Detoxification is treatment of alcohol withdrawal symptoms that is symptoms produced by the removal of the toxin (alcohol). The usual duration of uncomplicated withdrawal syndrome is 7-14 days. The aim of detoxification is the symptomatic management of the emergent withdrawal symptoms. The drugs of choice for detoxification are normally benzodiazepines (chlordiazepoxide and diazepam). Vitamins should also be administered.

Antabuse: A long term biological approach to substance abuse is the prescription of disulfiram for alcoholics. When alcohol is ingested by an individual who is on disulfiram, alcohol derived acetaldehyde can't be oxidized to acetate and this leads to an accumulation of acetaldehyde in blood. This causes disulfiram- ethanol reaction, characterized by flushing, tachycardia, hypotension, Tachypnea, palpitations, headache, sweating, nausea, vomiting, giddiness, and a sense of impending doom linked with intense anxiety. The onset of the reaction occurs within 30 minutes, becomes full blown within 1 hour, and subsides normally within 2 hours of ingestion of alcohol.

In sensitive patients or in those who have ingested a large amount of alcohol, the DER can be very intense and life threatening because of one or more of the following: shock, myocardial infarction, convulsions, hypoxia, confusion and coma. Antabuse should never be given without the patients' stated willingness to comply. It is also significant that the patient agree to take antabuse only after careful instruction about the potential consequences of drinking while taking the drug. The instruction should comprise a written list of alcohol containing preparations to be avoided. The usual dose of disulfiram is 250-500 mg per day (before bed time) in the first week and 250 mg per day subsequently for the maintenance treatment. The effect begins within 12 hours of first dose and remains for 7-10 days after the last dose. These patients' should carry a warning card.

Narcotic Antagonist Therapy: An overdose of opioid can be treated with narcotic antagonists (naloxone, naltrexone). Normally an intravenous injection of 2 mg naloxone, followed by a repeat injection in 5-10 minutes, causes reversal of the overdose. But has naloxone has a short half life, repeated dose are needed every 1-2 hours. This should be combined with general care and supportive treatment.

NURSING MANAGEMENT

- Monitor the client's vital signs to establish baseline information about the client's condition.
- Assess the physiological and psychological symptoms of withdrawal and the effects of medications prescribed during the withdrawal process to furnish safe, effective treatment during withdrawal.
- Initiate therapeutic interventions to help the client safely withdraw from the addictive substance.
- Comprise the client in the client's treatment process.
- Furnish a calm, safe, nonthreatening environment for the client.
- Support the client in meeting nutritional needs.
- Initiate the essential vitamin and mineral replacement therapeutic regimen.
- Furnish support to the client in working through denial.
- Intervene with secondary complications exhibited by the client as a result of substance abuse.
- Establish a caring, empathetic relationship through individual and group interactions to help the client improve self esteem and cope with thoughts of guilt.
- Encourage client's efforts to establish family and significant other supports through a variety of measures such as role playing.
- Teach the client, family, and significant others about substance abuse, symptoms, management, and treatment outcomes personally, as a group, or with written material.
- Support the client and family members in maintaining active involvement with patient care.

- Encourage the family to be flexible and patient regarding the client's participation in support groups.
- Teach the client and family about substance abuse and the preventive facets by providing factual informations and suggestions for preventing the use of drugs.
- Support client in establishing a social support system by putting him or her in touch with community organizations.

GERIATRIC CONSIDERATIONS

Substance use disorders in the elderly have been called the "hidden addiction" because one does not normally think of the elderly as having drug problems. Psycho active drug use in the elderly is most likely to involve alcohol or benzodiazepines prescribed for mild worry or sleeplessness. Drugs are metabolized much more slowly than they are at an earlier stage of life. The effect of the drug occur with greater intensity and last longer.

Treatment of the elderly follows therapeutic approaches similar to those used for other chemically dependent populations with regard to detoxification, family interventions, and the need for long term follow up. Additionally, lack of family and occupational supports, lost as the person ages, may call for a greater emphasis on social, financial and medical support services in the community as part of the treatment plan.

FOLLOW-UP AND HOME CARE AND REHABILITATION

The duration of residential treatment should be dictated by the length of time essential for the patient to meet specific criteria that would predict his or her successful transition to a less structured, less restrictive treatment setting (e.g., out-patient care). These criteria may comprise a demonstrated motivation to continue in out-patient treatment, the capability to remain abstinent even in situations where substances are potentially available, the availability of a living situation and linked support system conducive to remaining substance free (e.g., family, substance free peers), sufficient stabilization of any co-occurring general medical or psychiatric disorder so that the patient is regarded as suitable for out-patient aftercare, and the availability of ample follow-up care.

Follow-up visits may also be needed to assess a medication blood level that might increase with cessation. Follow-up visits may also be needed to monitor side effects or plan tapering of antismoking medications. At follow-up, the psychiatrist evaluates whether the patient has smoked and, if so, the number of cigarettes smoked per day; the severity of the patient's withdrawal symptoms; the onset of any psychiatric symptoms; the patient's use of alcohol or other drugs; how the patient dealt with situations in which he or she felt a strong urge to smoke; medication side effects; and other relevant issues and then tailors treatment accordingly. Most but not all studies suggest that brief follow-ups (together with telephone calls) increase quit rates.

REHABILITATION

Planning of leisure time activities is a very significant aspect for patients with substance abuse. It is very significant to counsel the patient to plan their leisure time activities Exercises produce endorphins, which give a pleasant feeling and can help in controlling the withdrawal symptoms. Vocational counselling should be given to the patient regarding what vocation can be taken up by the patient during and after the treatment. These activities also help in increasing the self-esteem of the patients.

MOTIVATIONAL COUNSELLING

Motivation is the key factor in determining the compliance of the patient to treatment and the successful completion of the treatment by the patient. There are different stages of motivation.

- Precontemplation
- Contemplation
- Preparation
- Action
- Maintenance
- During the Precontemplation phase the patient does not consider going for treatment.
- During the contemplation phase patients are ambivalent about going in for treatment.
- During the preparation stage they are prepared for treatment.
- During the action stage patients approach the treatment centre.

The nurse should determine in which phase of the treatment the patient is and should counsel the patient accordingly. A patient seeking treatment is normally in the action stage and should be told about the various options of the treatment and should be reassured that he will be able to complete the treatment and will live a productive life.

FOLLOW UP

'Quality Follow up' is very significant. Every time the patient comes to the out-patient department, the nurse should empathize with the patient and be non judgmental. The nurse should enquire about the progress in his condition and do positive reinforcement for desirable behaviour. The patient should be rewarded for the brave attempt he has taken by continuing the treatment. Ongoing motivational assessment and counselling has to be done from time to time.

The nurse should:

- Educate the patient about various coping strategies
- Teach the patient to drink tea, coffee, or a glass of cold water and get involved in some activities.
- Encourage the patient to go for exercise at the time when he experiences craving.
- Teach the patient to assertively say no when his friend offers him substances/drink.
- Should inform the family members in case there has been a lapse.
- Advise the patient to immediately speak to the relatives if they experience craving.

The nurse should help the patients to identify situations that place them at risk for relapse and to develop alternative reactions other than substance use.

FAMILY COUNSELLING

Substance abuse leads to several problems in the family. Involving the family is very significant as they spend maximum time with the patients. The family should be told to be empathetic and understanding and learn to trust the patient.

REFERENCES

Castledine, G. (2002). Nurses' bedside manner: Is it deteriorating? British Journal of Nursing, 11(10), 723.

Crouch, R. (2002). Communication is the key. Emergency Nurse, 10(3), 3–5.

Kuehn, A. (202). Communication and the nursing shortage. American Nurse, 34(3), 6–7.

Puentas, W. J. (2000). Using social reminiscence to teach therapeutic communication skills. Geriatric Nursing, 21(6), 315–318.

Wallace, L. (2002). More than good manners. Nursing 02, 33(7), 32.

10

Management of Personality, Sexual and Eating Disorders

CLASSIFICATION OF DISORDERS

PERSONALITY

Personality is the total of an individual's internal and external patterns of adjustment to life, determined in part by the individual's genetic make-up and by life experiences. Thus, the dynamics of personality growth become increasingly complex throughout the lifespan as one continually interacts with the environment and experiences various stages of physical and psychological maturation.

Factors influencing psychological maturation comprise genetic endowments such as inherited traits, potentials, and characteristics; environmental stressors together with parental relationships, peer relationships, and cultural and social experiences; individual accomplishments that are the results of learning and adjustment; and one's mental health status at each developmental stage. Thus, a newborn or infant reacts differently to a given environmental stimulus than does an adolescent, a young adult, or an elderly person.

An individualality disorder is described as a non-psychotic sickness characterized by maladaptive behaviour, which the person employs to fulfil his or her needs and bring satisfaction to self. These behaviours begin during childhood or adolescence as a way of coping and remain throughout most of adulthood, becoming less obvious during middle or old age. As a result of his or her inability to relate to the environment, the person acts out his or her conflicts socially. Emotional, economic, social, or occupational problems are frequently seen as a result of such conflicts because of anxiety.

Personality Disorders: Common Descriptive Behaviours

Antisocial personality: Impulsive, aggressive, manipulative

Avoidant personality: Shy, timid "inferiority complex"

Borderline personality: Impulsive, self-destructive, unstable

Dependent personality: Dependent, submissive, clinging

Histrionic personality: Emotional, dramatic, theatrical

Narcissistic personality: Boastful, egotistical, "superiority complex"

Obsessive compulsive personality: Perfectionistic, rigid, controlling

Paranoid personality: Suspicious, distrustful

Schizoid personality: Socially distant, detached

Schizotypal personality: Odd, eccentric

People with personality disorders have several common characteristics. They comprise:

- Inflexible, socially maladaptive behaviours
- Self-centreedness
- Manipulative and exploitative behaviour
- Inability to tolerate minor stress, resulting in increased inability to deal with anxiety or depression
- Lack of individual accountability for behaviour, blaming others for their problems
- Difficulty dealing with reality because of a distorted or superficial understanding of self and the perceptions of others
- Vulnerability to other mental disorders such as obsessive compulsive tendencies and panic attacks

People with personality disorders rarely seek psychiatric help because the person lacks insight regarding his or her behaviours and does not view them to be maladaptive, contributing to a personality disorder.

SEXUAL DISORDERS

Sexual disorders comprise problems of sexual identity, sexual performance, and sexual aim. There are three major categories of sexual disorders: sexual dysfunctions, paraphilia, and gender identity disorders.

Preferences for Nonhuman Objects

There are two types of preferences for nonhuman objects: fetishism and transvestism.

Fetishism: A fetish exists when an individual is sexually aroused by a nonliving object. It can manifest in two ways, one more extreme than the other. One form associates coitus with some object (most often women's panties or other undergarments). It is relatively harmless if the action is taken playfully and is acceptable to the person's partner. Focus on several parts of the body (feet, hair, ears, etc) aside from those part of the pleasurable foreplay, can become fetishistic in its hold on the individual.

The more extreme form of fetishism is when a nonliving object completely substitutes for a human partner, such as underwear, boots, and shoes or such textured objects as velvet or silk. Here, orgasm is achieved when the person is alone, fondling the object.

Transvestism: This paraphilia exists when the person attains sexual excitement by cross-dressing. This is very rarely found in females so the male side of this paraphilia will be used as the example.

Two different purposes seem to be linked with this act in different people. In one aspect the person seeks to intensify sexual excitement in intercourse with a partner by only partially dressing as a woman. In the other form, the male moves about in full female regailia, which suggests some type of gender identity problem but not necessarily homosexuality.

Preferences for Situations Causing Suffering

Sadism and Masochism: The term sadist is derived from the reported violent sexual exploits of the Marquis de Sade. "Sadist" is applied to those who derive sexual excitement from the pain of others. The term masochist was derived from the writing of Leopold von Sacher-Masoch whose characters sought out women who would beat them. "Masochist" is applied to those who derive sexual excitement through their own pain. Hence, sadists and masochists go hand in hand, one depending on the need of the other. The danger of these needs is that each may need succesively more brutal treatment to satisfy their sexual needs.

Preference for Nonconsenting Partners: The three types of this category of paraphilia are exhibitionism, voyeurism, and paedophilia. All three are regarded as crimes in this country and are almost entirely male crimes.

Exhibitionism: Exhibitionism is the exposure of one's genitals in a public place. It is the most prominent sexual offence leading to arrest and makes up one third of all sexual crimes. From the psychological point of view, there are three characteristic features of the exhibition. First, it is always performed for unknown women; second, it always takes place where sexual intercourse is impossible, for instance in a crowded shopping mall; and third, it must be shocking for the unknown woman or it seems to lose its power to produce sexual arousal in the individual. Exhibitionists are not assaultive and are regarded as more of a nuisance than an actual danger.

Voyeurism: Looking at sexually arousing pictures or situations is a relatively common, evidently normal activity. The difference between this and voyeurism is that in normal watching, the viewing is a prelude to normal sexual activity. In the voyeur or "Peeping Tom" the experience replaces normal sexual activity. However, voyeurism may exist in an individual who also engages in normal heterosexual activity.

Paedophilia; Paedophilia is the act of deriving sexual excitement through the physical contact of children. This paraphilia is radically different from exhibitionism and voyeurism in its seriously harmful impact on the nonconsenting partner, a child. Ordinarily, the paedophiliac is someone who has ready access to the child. The child or parent would have no reason to suspect that the individual has a paedophilic orientation.

Gender Identity Disorder

A gender identity disorder exists when an individual, male or female, experiences confusion, vagueness or conflict in their feelings about their own sexual identity. There is a struggle between the individual's anatomical sex gender and subjective feelings about choosing a masculine or feminine style of life.

Children can distinguish the difference between males and females by the age of two and by their fourth birthday can recognize the different roles that each sex plays in society. By the age of fifteen or so an individual can relate to what arouses sexual feelings in themselves. Those with a gender identity disorder may have a problem with one or all of these facets of identity.

EATING DISORDERS

Eating disorders are characterized by intense disturbances in eating behaviour. Three specific diagnoses exist: anorexia nervosa; bulimia nervosa; and eating disorder, not otherwise specified. Obesity is regarded as to be a general medical condition because a consistent association with a psychological or behavioural syndrome has not been established.

When there is evidence that psychological factors are of importance in the etiology or course of a specific case of obesity, the diagnosis is listed under psychological factors affecting medical condition.

Eating disorders are intense disturbances in eating behaviour characterized by preoccupation with weight concerns and unhealthy efforts to control weight. There are two main classes for this disorder; they are anorexia nervosa and bulimia nervosa. Anorexia nervosa is an severe fear of gaining weight, disturbed body image, refusal to maintain normal weight, and dangerous measures to lose weight.

There are two sub classes restricting type anorexia nervosa, where someone drastically reduces their intake of food sometimes almost to the point of starvation. The second sub-class is binge-eating/purging type of anorexia nervosa where someone attempts to lose weight by making their self vomit after eating by laxatives, over exercising, or diuretics. No matter what class someone with this disorder has the main thing is that the person is not happy with the weight they are and always tries to lose more.

This way of weight lose normally leads to other medical health problems such as stomach problems, low blood pressure, lose of bone density, lost of menstrual cycle in females, and others. Bulimia nervosa is out of control over-eating followed by unhealthy compensatory efforts, with the same efforts that anorexics use. The eating binges are normally secret followed by guilt and concern about gaining weight.

Anorexia Nervosa

Anorexia nervosa is deliberate and sustained weight loss driven by a fear of distorted body image. It is not to be confused with anorexia, which is its symptomatic general loss of appetite or disinterest in food. DSM-IV characterizes anorexia nervosa as:

- An abnormally low body weight (the suggested guideline ? 85% of normal for age and height, or BMI ? 17.5).
- For postmenarcheal females, amenorrhea (the absence of three consecutive menstrual cycles).
- An severe fear gaining weight or becoming fat and a preoccupation with body weight and shape.

Most anorexics become so as adolescents, with 76% reporting onset of the disorder between the ages of 11 and 20. The mortality rate for those diagnosed with anorexia nervosa is approximately 6%-the highest of any mental sickness-with roughly half of those because of suicide.

Anorexics are generally perfectionists, driven to succeed; yet they set unattainable standards of performance for themselves. When they fail to meet these standards, they look for a part of their lives they can control; food and weight become that "control" for them. Low self-esteem and constant self-criticism cause anorexics to regularly fear losing control, and even consuming a small amount of food could be regarded as a loss of control.

Bulimia Nervosa

Bulimia nervosa is a cyclical and recurring pattern of binge eating (uncontrolled bursts of overeating) followed by guilt, self-recrimination and overcompensatory behaviour such as crash dieting, overexercising and purging to compensate for the excessive caloric intake.

Bulimics frequently have "binge food," which is the food they basically consume during binges. Some describe their binge episodes as a physical high they feel, numbing out, going into auto-pilot, losing all control, immediate comfort, etc. The reasoning or triggers behind a binge may serve different purposes for different people. This binge episode leads the individual to feel guilt, shame, embarrassment, and complete failure. Bulimics try to regain control of themselves and the situation by purging the food-making up for their mistake. This leads to feeling famished and empty again, and thus, another uncontrollable binge, followed by feeling powerless, and the vicious binge/purge cycle continues. Bulimics have extreme eating and exercising habits, instead of demonstrating moderation. This compulsive behaviour is frequently echoed in similar destructive behaviour such as sexual promiscuity, pathological lying, and shoplifting. Some bulimics not only struggle with the eating disorder, but these other damaging behaviours as well.

Binge Eating

Binge eating is one of the most common eating disorders. It involves the consumption of very large amounts of food in a short period of time. About 3 percent of all adults struggle with binge eating. People at any age can develop this specific order, but it is seen in most adults ranging from age 46 to around age 55. Clinical studies have continued to find that obese binge eaters have much higher levels of depression than other obese people that don't have a binge eating disorder. The individual has feeling of disgust and guilt that leads to depression.

People that struggle with binge eating are likely to have alcohol problems and engage in impulsive behaviour, such as not thinking before acting out. They don't feel that they can control themselves, are basically not close with their community, and have difficulty discussing their problems and feelings. They also have more health problems, a hard time sleeping at night, joint pain, muscle pains, menstrual problems, and headaches. These people frequently have suicidal thoughts, struggle digesting their food, and are stressed. People that have a binge eating disorder are normally very ashamed and become very good at hiding the fact that they have it. They become so good at hiding their disorder that most people around them, together with close friends and family members, don't even know about their struggle.

Orthorexia Nervosa

Orthorexia Nervosa is a recently discovered disease because it was thought to be Anorexia earlier on. This type of disorder is an obsession with eating only healthy types of foods. This disease normally occurs when people are so driven to become thin that they start to become obsessed with everything that they are consuming. Someone who struggles with Orthorexia Nervosa will do things like planning out their meals for the next day. This means that they will have a strict planned schedule of breakfast, lunch and dinner. This person will try to be regularly limiting the amount of food that he/she is eating in order to maintain a several weight. People who have Orthorexia Nervosa are frequently critical of what others eat, and normally isolate themselves from environment.

Compulsive Exercising

Compulsive exercising is another type of eating disorder. One that struggles with this disorder takes part of vigorous physical activity to the point that it is not healthy and unsafe. It is frequently referred to as obligatory exercise or anorexia athletic. The individual normally starts to feel compelled to exercise and has problems with anxiety and guilt if he/she does not get their exercises in. Someone that has compulsive exercising disorder will still force themselves to work out even if he/she is sick or injured.

They frequently calculate how much they have eaten and exercise on the amount of calories they have eaten and normally have low energy due to all the calories they have burned. People who struggle with this disorder normally do it to have more control in their life. Praise is frequently given to the individual about how in shape he/she may look which gives that person more of a drive to continue to work out. Females most commongenerally have compulsive exercising disorder and measure their self worth through their performance. They frequently take out their emotions like anger, depression, or frustration when exercising by pushing their bodies to the limit.

ETIOLOGY, PSYCHOPATHOLOGY, CHARACTERISTICS, DIAGNOSIS

ETIOLOGY OF PERSONALITY DISORDER

During the process of personality growth, the person establishes several traits that enable him or her to observe, interact with, and think about the environment and one's self. If the person develops a positive self-concept, body image, and sense of self-worth, and is able to relate to others openly and honestly, she or he is said to have characteristics of a healthy personality. Should the person develop inflexible, maladaptive behaviours (e.g., manipulation, hostility, lying, poor judgment, and alienation) that interfere with social or occupational functioning, the person exhibits signs and symptoms of a personality disorder.

Personality disorders exist on a continuum. They can range from mild to more intense based on how pervasive the symptoms of a specific personality disorder are, and to what degree an individual exhibits these symptoms. Though most people can live fairly normal lives with mild symptoms of personality disorders, during times of increased stress or external pressures (e.g., because of work, family, or a new relationship), the symptoms will be exacerbated and begin to seriously interfere with the individual's emotional and psychological functioning.

The potential causes of personality disorders are as numerous as the people who suffer from them. Genetic and biologic factors, as well as a combination of one's personality, social growth, and parental upbringing, are linked with these disorders. Quite a few factors, classified as genetic, biologic, or psychoanalytic, may contribute to the growth of a personality disorder.

PSYCHOPATHOLOGY OF PERSONALITY DISORDER

In practice, mental health professionals rarely treat psychopathic personality disorders as they are regarded as untreatable and no interventions have proved to be effective. In England and Wales the diagnosis of dissocial personality disorder is grounds for detention in secure psychiatric hospitals under the Mental Health Act if they have committed serious crimes, but since such people are disruptive for other patients and not responsive to treatment this alternative to prison is not frequently used.

Because an individual's scores may have significant consequences for his or her future, the potential for harm if the test is used or administered incorrectly is considerable. The test should only be regarded as valid if administered by a suitably qualified and experienced clinician under controlled conditions.

Hare wants the Diagnostic and Statistical Manual of Mental Disorders to list psychopathy as a distinctive disorder, saying that psychopathy has no precise equivalent in either the DSM-IV-TR, where it is most strongly correlated with the diagnosis of antisocial personality disorder, or the ICD-10, which has a partly similar condition called dissocial personality disorder. Both organisations view the terms as synonymous. But only a minority of what Hare and his followers would diagnose as psychopaths who are in institutions are violent offenders. The manipulative skills of some of the others are valued for providing audacious leadership. It is argued that psychopathy is adaptive in a highly competitive environment, because it gets results for both the individual and the corporations or, frequently small political sects that they represent. Nevertheless, these people will frequently cause long-term harm, both to their co-workers and the organization as a whole, because of their manipulative, deceitful, abusive, and frequently fraudulent behaviour.

Hare describes people he calls psychopaths as "intraspecies predators who use charm, manipulation, intimidation, sex and violence to control others and to satisfy their own selfish needs. Lacking in conscience and empathy, they take what they want and do as they please, violating social norms and expectations without guilt or remorse". "What is missing, putting differently, are the very qualities that allow a human being to live in social harmony."

CHARACTERISTICS OF PERSONALITY DISORDER

Patients with personality disorders share several characteristics:

- Except those suffering from the Schizoid or the Avoidant Personality Disorders, they are insistent and demand preferential and privileged treatment. They complain about numerous symptoms, although they often second guess the diagnosis and disobey the doctor, his treatment recommendations and instructions.
- They feel unique, are affected with grandiosity and a diminished capacity for empathy. Consequently, they regard the doctor as inferior to them, alienate him and bore him with their self-preoccupation.

- They are manipulative and exploitative, trust no one and find it difficult to love or share. They are socially maladaptive and emotionally labile.
- Disturbed cognitive and, mainly, emotional growth peaks in adolescence.
- Personality disorders are stable and all-pervasive - not episodic or transient. They affect all the dimensions of the patient's life: his career, his interpersonal relationships, his social functioning.
- Although the patient is sometimes depressed and suffers from mood and anxiety disorders - defences - splitting, projection, projective identification, denial, intellectualization - are so strong, that the patient is unaware of the reasons for his distress. The character problems, behavioural deficits and emotional deficiencies and instability encountered by the patient with personality disorder are, mostly, ego-syntonic. This means that the patient does not, on the whole, find his personality traits or behaviour objectionable, unacceptable, disagreeable, or alien to his self.
- The patient is prone to suffer from other psychiatric disturbances, both personality disorders and Axis I disorders ("co-morbidity"). Substance abuse and reckless behaviours are also common ("dual diagnosis").
- Defences are alloplastic: patients tend to blame the external world for their misfortune and failures. In stressful situations, they try to preempt a (real or imaginary) menace, change the rules of the game, introduce new variables, or otherwise influence the external world to conform to their needs.
- The personality-disordered are not psychotic. They have no hallucinations, delusions or thought disorders (except those who suffer from a Borderline Personality Disorder and who experience brief psychotic "microepisodes", mostly during treatment). They are also fully oriented, with clear senses (sensorium), good memory and general fund of knowledge.

DIAGNOSIS

Diagnosis of personality disorders is complicated by the fact that affected individuals rarely seek help till they are in serious trouble or till their families (or the law) pressure them to get treatment. The reason for this slowness is that the problematic traits are so deeply entrenched that they seem normal (ego-syntonic) to the patient. Diagnosis of a personality disorder depends in part on the patient's age. Though personality disorders originate during the childhood years, they are regarded as adult disorders. Some patients, in fact, are not diagnosed till late in life because their symptoms had been modified by the demands of their job or by marriage. After retirement or the spouse's death, nevertheless, these patients' personality disorders become fully evident. Generally, nevertheless, if the onset of the patient's problem is in mid- or late-life, the physician will rule out substance abuse or personality change caused by medical or neurological problems before considering the diagnosis of a personality disorder. It is unusual for people to develop personality disorders "out of the blue" in mid-life.

There are no tests that can furnish a definitive diagnosis of personality disorder. Most physicians will assess a patient on the basis of quite a few sources of information collected over a period of time in order to determine how long the patient has been having difficulties, how several areas of life are affected, and how intense the dysfunction is. These sources of information may comprise:

Interviews

The physician may schedule two or three interviews with the patient, spaced over many weeks or months, in order to rule out an adjustment disorder caused by job loss, bereavement, or a similar problem. An office interview allows the physician to form an impression of the patient's overall personality as well as obtain information about his or her occupation and family.

During the interview, the physician will note the patient's appearance, tone of voice, body language, eye contact, and other significant non-verbal signals, as well as the content of the conversation. In some cases, the physician may contact other people (family members, employers, close friends) who know the patient well in order to assess the accuracy of the patient's perception of his or her difficulties. It is quite common for people with personality disorders to have distorted views of their situations or to be unaware of the impact of their behaviour on others.

Psychologic Testing

Physicians use psychologic testing to help in the diagnosis of a personality disorder. Most of these tests call for interpretation by a professional with specialized training. Physicians normally refer patients to a clinical psychologist for this type of test.

Personality Inventories

Personality inventories are tests with true/false or yes/no answers that can be used to compare the patient's scores with those of people with known personality distortions. The single most commongenerally used test of this type is the Minnesota Multiphasic Personality Inventory, or MMPI. Another test that is frequently used is the Millon Clinical Multiaxial Inventory, or MCMI.

Projective Tests

Projective tests are unstructured. Unstructured means that instead of giving one-word answers to questions, the patient is asked to talk at some length about a picture that the psychologist has shown him or her, or to supply an ending for the beginning of a story. Projective tests allow the clinician to assess the patient's patterns of thinking, fantasies, worries or anxieties, moral concerns, values, and habits. Common projective tests comprise the Rorschach, in which the patient responds to a set of ten inkblots; and the Thematic Apperception Test (TAT), in which the patient is shown drawings of people in different situations and then tells a story about the picture.

TREATMENT

At one time psychiatrists thought that personality disorders didn't react very well to treatment. This opinion was derived from the notion that human personality is fixed for life once it has been molded in childhood, and from the belief among people with personality disorders that their own views and behaviours are right, and that others are the ones at fault.

More recently, nevertheless, physicians have recognized that human beings can continue to grow and change throughout life. Most patients with personality disorders are now regarded as to be treatable, though the degree of improvement may vary. The type of treatment recommended depends on the personality characteristics linked with the specific disorder.

Hospitalization

In-patient treatment is rarely required for patients with personality disorders, with two major exceptions: borderline patients who are threatening suicide or suffering from drug or alcohol withdrawal; and patients with paranoid personality disorder who are having psychotic symptoms.

Psychotherapy

Psychoanalytic psychotherapy is suggested for patients who can benefit from insight-oriented treatment. These patients basically comprise those with dependent, obsessive-compulsive, and avoidant personality disorders. Physicians normally recommend individual psychotherapy for narcissistic and borderline patients, but frequently refer these patients to therapists with specialized training in these disorders. Psychotherapeutic treatment for personality disorders may take as long as three to five years.

Insight-oriented approaches are not recommended for patients with paranoid or antisocial personality disorders. These patients are likely to resent the therapist and see him or her as trying to control or dominate them.

Supportive therapy is regarded as the most helpful form of psychotherapy for patients with schizoid personality disorder.

Cognitive-behavioural Therapy

Cognitive-behavioural approaches are frequently recommended for patients with avoidant or dependent personality disorders. Patients in these groups basically have mistaken beliefs about their competence or likableness. These assumptions can be successfully challenged by cognitive-behavioural methods. More recently, Aaron Beck and his coworkers have successfully extended their approach to cognitive therapy to all ten personality disorders as defined by DSM-IV.

Group Therapy

Group therapy is often useful for patients with schizoid or avoidant personality disorders because it helps them to break out of their social isolation. It has also been recommended for patients with histrionic and antisocial personality disorders. These patients tend to act out, and pressure from peers in group treatment can motivate them to change. Because patients with antisocial personality disorder can destabilize groups that comprise people with other disorders, it is normally best if these people meet exclusively with others who have APD (in homogeneous groups).

Family Therapy

Family therapy may be suggested for patients whose personality disorders cause serious problems for members of their families. It is also sometimes recommended for borderline patients from overinvolved or possessive families.

Medications

Medications may be prescribed for patients with specific personality disorders. The type of medication depends on the disorder. Generally, nevertheless, patients with personality disorders are helped only moderately by medications.

Antipsychotic Drugs

Antipsychotic drugs, such as haloperidol (Haldol), may be given to patients with paranoid personality disorder if they are having brief psychotic episodes. Patients with borderline or schizotypal personality disorder are sometimes given antipsychotic drugs in low doses; nevertheless, the efficacy of these drugs in treating personality disorder is less clear than in schizophrenia.

Mood Stabilizers

Carbamazepine (Tegretol) is a drug that is generally used to treat seizures, but is also helpful for borderline patients with rage outbursts and similar behavioural problems. Lithium and valproate may also be used as mood stabilizers, especially among people with borderline personality disorder.

Antidepressants and Anti-anxiety Medications

Medications in these classes are sometimes prescribed for patients with schizoid personality disorder to help them manage anxiety symptoms while they are in psychotherapy. Antidepressants are also generally used to treat people with borderline personality disorder.

Treatment with medications is not recommended for patients with avoidant, histrionic, dependent, or narcissistic personality disorders. The use of potentially addictive medications should be avoided in people with borderline or antisocial personality disorders. Nevertheless, some avoidant patients who also have social phobia may benefit from monoamine oxidase inhibitors (MAO inhibitors), a specific class of antidepressant.

ETIOLOGY OF SEXUAL DISORDERS

Sexual disorders are in general classified as sexual dysfunctions, paraphilias, and sexual addiction. Few systematic epidemiologic data are available regarding the prevalence of various sexual disorders. Two major factors that impact sexual performance are the presence or absence of normal sexuality (i.e., feelings of desire and pleasure to engage in the sexual act) and the presence or absence of an adequate sexual response cycle.

PSYCHOPATHOLOGY OF SEXUAL DISORDERS

Sexual Dysfunction or Sexual difficulties can begin early in a person's sex life or they may develop after an individual has formerly experienced enjoyable and satisfying sex. A problem may develop gradually over time, or may occur abruptly as a total or partial inability to partake in one or more stages of the sexual act. The causes of sexual difficulties can be physical, psychological, or both.

Emotional factors affecting sex comprise both interpersonal problems such as marital/relationship problems, or lack of trust and open communication between partners and psychological problems within the individual (depression, sexual fears or guilt, past sexual trauma, sexual disorders, and so on).

Physical factors comprise drugs (alcohol, nicotine, narcotics, stimulants, antihypertensives, antihistamines, and some psychotherapeutic drugs); injuries to the back, problems with an enlarged prostate gland, problems with blood supply, nerve damage (as in spinal cord injuries); or disease (diabetic neuropathy, multiple sclerosis, tumours, and, rarely, tertiary syphilis); failure of various organ systems (such as the heart and lungs); endocrine disorders (thyroid, pituitary, or adrenal gland problems); hormonal deficiencies (low testosterone, estrogen, or androgens); and some birth defects. Sexual dysfunction disorders are in general classified into four classes: sexual desire disorders, sexual arousal disorders, orgasm disorders, and sexual pain disorders.

CHARACTERISTICS

The characteristics of sexual disorders comprise:

- Low sexual desire disorders. Patients may have an extremely low desire for sex. Low sexual desire disorder occurs when patients are not in general interested in sex, but may perform adequately after sexual activity has begun. Sexual aversion disorder is marked by a feeling of disgust toward the notion of sexual activity.
- Sexual arousal disorders. Patients are interested in sex, but not enough to complete a sex act. In female sexual arousal disorder, a woman may not attain adequate levels of lubrication to permit vaginal sex. In male erectile disorder, the penis may not attain an erection sufficient to begin or complete sex.
- Orgasmic disorders. Patients are partially or completely unable to experience sexual climax. This may occur in spite of adequate

sexual interest and arousal. Female orgasmic disorder occurs when a woman experiences either a delayed or nonexistent climax, whereas male orgasmic disorder involves the same criteria for males. In addition, males may experience premature ejaculation, which involves repeated climaxes before, during or shortly after penetration.

- Sexual pain disorders. These disorders involve pain during the sex act. In dyspareunia, either a woman or man feels genital pain at some point during intercourse, especially during insertion. Vaginismus is a intense spasm of the vagina that prevents penetration.
- Secondary and other sexual dysfunctions. Sexual dysfunction because of a general medical condition (involving anatomical or other physical problems) and substance-induced sexual dysfunction (caused by intoxication or withdrawal from alcohol or drugs) may feature symptoms listed in the disorders above. Sexual dysfunction not otherwise specified is used when the sexual disturbances don't meet criteria for any specific sexual dysfunction. A lack of sexual interest may be caused by another mental disorder, such as somatotization disorder, depression or schizophrenia.

DIAGNOSIS

The diagnostic criteria for sexual addiction are derived from the behaviourally nonspecific criteria for addictive disorder, by replacing "behaviour" with "sexual behaviour." A definition of sexual addiction, which facilitates preliminary diagnosis of the disorder, can likewise be derived from the simple definition of addiction. Accordingly, sexual addiction is defined as a condition in which some form of sexual behaviour is employed in a pattern that is characterized by two key features: (1) recurrent failure to control the sexual behaviour, and (2) continuation of the sexual behaviour in spite of significant damaging consequences. Consequently, sexual addiction is a syndrome in which some form of sexual behaviour relates to and affects an individual's life in such a manner as to accord with the simple definition of addiction or to meet the diagnostic criteria for addictive disorder.

Significantly, no form of sexual behaviour in itself constitutes sexual addiction. Whether a pattern of sexual behaviour qualifies as sexual addiction is determined not by the type of behaviour, its object, its frequency or its social acceptability, but by the relationship between this behaviour pattern and an individual's life, as indicated in the definition and specified in the diagnostic criteria. The key features that distinguish sexual addiction from other patterns of sexual behaviour are: (1) the individual is not reliably able to control the sexual behaviour, and (2) the sexual behaviour has significant damaging consequences and continues in spite of these consequences.

Differential Diagnosis

The paraphilic and hypersexual behaviours that characterize sexual addiction also can occur as manifestations of underlying organic pathology. Paraphilic or hypersexual behaviour can be a symptom of a brain lesion, a side effect of medication or a symptom of endocrine abnormality.

The differential diagnosis is normally facilitated by the presence of additional symptoms or circumstances that suggest the underlying etiology. Clues that invite an organic evaluation comprise: onset in middle age or later, regression from formerly normal sexuality, excessive aggression, report of auras or seizure-like symptoms prior to or during the sexual behaviour, abnormal body habitus and presence of soft neurological signs.

Also of value in determining whether a case of paraphilia or hypersexuality represents sexual addiction are the diagnostic criteria for sexual addiction. Tolerance, psychophysiological withdrawal symptoms on discontinuation of the sexual behaviour (normally affective discomfort, irritability or restlessness), and a pertinacious desire to cut down or control the behaviour are in general not observed in patterns of paraphilic or hypersexual behaviour that are not part of the sexual addiction syndrome.

ETIOLOGY OF EATING DISORDERS

The prevalence of eating disorders is at an all-time high. A wide range of psychological influences contributing to the growth of an eating disorder have been suggested. One theory addresses the theme of starvation as a form of self-punishment, with the unacknowledged purpose of pleasing an introjected or internalized parent. This parent is seen as imposing harsh restrictions on the otherwise well-behaved, orderly, perfectionistic, hypersensitive individual.

A second theory suggests that fasting restores a sense of order to a female who fears the independence of adult femininity (e.g., social and sexual functioning) and fears becoming like her mother. Fasting allows the client to exert control over herself and others. The capability to lose weight is a substitute for independence as well as an avoidance of acknowledging one's sexual desires. A third theory notes that people starve themselves to suppress or control feelings of emotional emptiness. They struggle for perfection to prove that they don't depend on others to validate their self-concept or self-esteem.

A final theory postulates that females develop an eating disorder because they believe their parents have never responded adequately to their initiatives or recognized individualities. Anorectic females have difficulty distinguishing personal wants from those of others and fear abandonment if they take independent action. Rather than permitting outside influences, together with food, to invade them, anorectics deny their needs and will not permit anyone else to control them.

PSYCHOPATHOLOGY OF EATING DISORDERS

With more an more people turning to healthy eating there is always going to be those that go to extremes. Women desperately trying to look good by losing weight are always at danger of developing Anorexia Nervosa through excessive dieting. Women aren't the only sex at risk as more and more men are developing Anorexia Nervosa too.

Anorexics see themselves as obese no matter how much they weigh or how thin they look in the mirror. Sadly, they can not see themselves as anything other and refuse to seek help or accept it when offered, and simply diet till, for 10 to 20 percent of Anorexia Nervosa suffers they eventually die from related complications.

Most sufferers are frequently perfectionists that can be very strict with themselves and set high and unrealistic goals that will not lead to anything other than failure. Frequently what leads to this behaviour is a lack of control in some other part of their life.

They realize that they can gain some control back or the power they feel from being in control of at least one part of their life, by dieting. This slowly turns into an obsession as they self monitor their food intake and their weight, as they gain satisfaction from finally being in control of something.

This obsession or focus on constant monitoring of calories and weighing themselves helps them block out unwanted feelings and emotions. So it can be seen as a symptom of possible mental health problems, especially around self-esteem or what I prefer to refer to as self-acceptance. This need for control doesn't help them as they live in denial and refuse to seek help basically because they do not feel they deserve the attention and most feel they do not deserve to eat this tying into problems with self-acceptance.

Nevertheless bleak the picture painted in this article so far, remember that the bulk of Anorexia Nervosa suffers don't succumb to the sickness and help is at hand for all. There are a number of treatments available to sufferers. Medical care especially for those with intense anorexia is available along with psychotherapy. Cognitive Behaviour Therapy (CBT) is proving very affective in tackling helpful thoughts and behaviour that are at the core of the eating disorder. Recognizing triggers and developing coping strategies that patients can use to help take control of their anorexia can be very effective.

CHARACTERISTICS OF EATING DISORDERS

Anorexia nervosa is characterized by emaciation, a relentless pursuit of thinness and unwillingness to maintain a normal or healthy weight, a distortion of body image and severe fear of gaining weight, a lack of menstruation among girls and women, and extremely disturbed eating behaviour. Some people with anorexia lose weight by dieting and exercising excessively; others lose weight by self-induced vomiting, or misusing laxatives, diuretics or enemas. More characteristics of anorexia nervosa comprise:

- Significant weight loss
- Continual dieting
- Severe fear of gaining weight or becoming fat, even if underweight
- Undue influence of body weight or shape on self-evaluation
- Preoccupation with food calories or nutrition
- Preference to eat alone
- Compulsive exercise
- Bingeing and purging
- Brittle hair or nails
- Depression
- Infrequent or absent menstrual periods (in females who have reached puberty)
- Growth of fine hair over body
- Mild anemia, and muscle weakness and loss
- Intense constipation
- Low blood pressure, slowed breathing and pulse

- Drop in internal body temperature, causing an individual to feel cold all the time
- Lethargy

Several people with anorexia also have coexisting psychiatric and physical illnesses, together with depression, anxiety, obsessive behaviour, substance abuse, cardiovascular and neurological complications, and impaired physical growth.

Bulimia Nervosa

Bulimia nervosa is characterized by recurrent and frequent episodes of eating unusually large amounts of food (binge-eating), and feeling a lack of control over the eating. This is followed by some type of behaviour that compensates for the binge, such as purging (vomiting, excessive use of laxatives or diuretics), fasting and/or excessive exercise. Normally, bulimic behaviour is done secretly. Additional symptoms comprise:

- Recurrent episodes of binge eating
- Purging by strict dieting, fasting, vigorous exercise or vomiting
- Abuse of laxatives or diuretics to lose weight
- Frequent use of bathroom after meals
- Reddened fingers
- Swollen cheeks
- Self-evaluation is unduly influenced by body shape and weight
- Depression or mood swings
- Irregular menstrual periods
- Dental problems, like tooth decay
- Heartburn or bloating
- Intestinal distress and irritation from laxative abuse
- Kidney problems from diuretic abuse
- Intense dehydration from purging of fluids

Binge-Eating Disorder

Binge-eating disorder is characterized by recurrent binge-eating episodes during which an individual feels a loss of control over her eating. Unlike bulimia, binge-eating episodes are not followed by purging, excessive exercise or fasting. As a result, people with binge-eating disorder frequently are overweight or obese. Characteristics comprise:

- Eating much more rapidly than normal
- Eating till feeling uncomfortably full
- Eating large amounts of food when not hungry
- Eating alone due to embarrassment caused by how much is eaten
- Marked distress about the binge-eating behaviour
- Binge-eating occurs, on average, at least 2 days a week for 6 months
- Binge-eating not linked with regular use of compensatory behaviours (purging, fasting, excessive exercise)

DIAGNOSIS

Eating disorders can be treated and a healthy weight can be restored. The sooner these disorders are diagnosed and treated, the better the outcomes are likely to be. Due to their complexity, eating disorders call for a complete treatment plan involving medical care and monitoring, professional interventions, nutritional counselling and, when appropriate, medication management.

Treatment of anorexia calls for a specific program that involves three main phases: restoring the person to a healthy weight lost to intense dieting and purging; treating psychological disturbances such as distortion of body image, low self-esteem, and interpersonal conflicts; and reducing or eliminating behaviours or thoughts that lead to disordered eating, and preventing relapse.

Some research suggests that the use of medications, such as antidepressants, antipsychotics or mood stabilizers, may be modestly effective in treating patients with anorexia by helping to solve mood and anxiety symptoms that frequently co-exist with anorexia. Recent studies, nevertheless, have suggested that antidepressants may not be effective in preventing some patients with anorexia from relapsing. In addition, no medication has shown to be effective during the critical first phase of restoring a patient to healthy weight. Overall, it is unclear if and how medications can help patients conquer anorexia, but research is ongoing.

Different forms of psychotherapy, together with individual, group and family-based, can help address the psychological reasons for anorexia nervosa. Some studies suggest that family-based therapies in which parents assume responsibility for feeding their afflicted adolescent are the most efficient in helping an individual with anorexia gain weight and improve eating habits and moods. Others have noted that a combined approach of medical attention and supportive psychotherapy designed especially for anorexia patients is more effective than just psychotherapy. But the effectiveness of a treatment depends on the person involved and her situation.

Hospital based care (together with in-patient, partial hospitalization, intensive out-patient and/or residential care in an eating disorders specialty unit or facility) is essential when an eating disorder has led to physical problems that may be life-threatening, or when it is linked with intense psychological or behavioural problems.

The course and outcome of anorexia nervosa differ across people: some fully recover after a single episode; some fluctuate between weight gain and relapse; and others chronically deteriorate over several years. The mortality rate among people with anorexia has been estimated at56 percent per year which is about 12 times higher than the annual death rate because of all causes of death among females ages 15-24 in the general population. The most common causes of death are complications of the disorder, such as cardiac arrest or electrolyte imbalance, and suicide.

The primary goal of treatment for bulimia is to reduce or eliminate binge-eating and purging behaviour. Nutritional rehabilitation, professional intervention and medication management are frequently employed. As with anorexia, treatment for bulimia frequently involves a combination of options and depends on the needs of the individual.

To reduce or eliminate binge and purge behaviour, a patient may undergo nutritional counselling and psychotherapy, especially cognitive behavioural therapy (CBT), or be prescribed medication. Some antidepressants, such as fluoxetine (Prozac), which is the only medication sanctioned by the FDA for treating bulimia, may help patients who also have depression and/or anxiety.

It also appears to help reduce binge-eating and purging behaviour, reduces the chance of relapse, and improves eating attitudes. CBT that has been tailored to treat bulimia also has shown to be effective in changing binging and purging behaviour, and eating attitudes. Therapy may be personally oriented or group-based.

The treatment goals and strategies for binge-eating disorder are similar to those for bulimia. Fluoxetine and other antidepressants may reduce binge-eating episodes and help alleviate depression in some patients. Patients with binge-eating disorder also may be prescribed appetite suppressants. Psychotherapy, especially CBT, is also used to treat the underlying psychological issues linked with binge-eating, in a person or group environment.

People with eating disorders frequently don't recognize or admit that they are sick. As a result, they may strongly resist getting and staying in treatment. Family members or other trusted persons can be helpful in ensuring that the person with an eating disorder receives needed care and rehabilitation.

NURSING ASSESSMENT

PERSONALITY DISORDER

A thorough assessment, together with a nursing history and physical examination, is especially significant for clients with personality disorders, to determine the severity of the disorder and ascertain the presence of comorbid, potentially treatable syndromes. Because the disorder frequently manifests in adolescence, a detailed history of the client's childhood and adolescent behavioural patterns is necessary.

As per the diagnostic criteria for a personality disorder, disturbances of cognition, affect, interpersonal functioning, and impulse control are present and deviate markedly from the expectations of the individual's culture. These criteria furnish the guidelines for a systematic assessment.

Disturbance of Cognition: Patients with personality disorders are in contact with reality, but may have difficulty coping with stress. Cognitive capability may be difficult to assess if the client is suspicious or distrustful; exhibits distorted perceptions of self, other people, or events; or exhibits impoverished thoughts. Illusions or feelings of depersonalization (complaint of feeling strange or unreal) may be exhibited by clients with schizotypal personality disorder. Insight and judgment may be impaired because maladaptive coping behaviours have become a way of life. Anticipate the need to obtain additional data from family or friends, because clients may exhibit denial and minimize clinical symptoms.

Disturbance of Affect: Pay specific attention to the intensity, degree of lability, and appropriateness of the client's affect. He or she may be irritable; indifferent; exhibit emotional coldness such as flat affect or detachment; exhibit anger; or exhibit dysphoria. Clinical symptoms of anxiety or depression may be present. Obtaining information about the onset of symptoms and history of any previous treatment is significant. Also inquire whether the client has ever attempted suicide or exhibited self-mutilation and whether the client relies on alcohol or drugs to "feel good."

Disturbance of Interpersonal Functioning: Collect data regarding the client's interpersonal functioning. He or she may be reserved, introverted, socially withdrawn, lonely, lack close friends or confidants, or exhibit indifference toward others. Pose questions to family members and friends such as "Has the patient ever been able to maintain a satisfactory interpersonal relationship?" to help furnish insight into the client's interpersonal skills.

Dysfunctional Behaviour: Exhibits of unpredictable behaviour by the client with a personality disorder are possible. Thus, perform the assessment in a structured environment. Focus the assessment on the client's behaviour, such as:

- Which maladaptive behaviours does the client exhibit that lead to lack of impulse control?
- Does the client have a history of being aggressive, disrespectful, reckless, or destructive?
- Are any legal charges pending because of illegal activities such as gambling, shoplifting, or dealing in drugs?
- Has the client been arrested in the past?

Persons with histrionic behaviour are prone to conflict with the law, given their inappropriate sexually seductive or provocative behaviour. Clients with antisocial behaviour are often treated in forensic settings because they fail to comply with social norms when meeting their needs for immediate gratification.

Transcultural Considerations: Culture is a significant variable in the growth of personality. To understand an ethnic group and work effectively with clients or family members, be aware of a culture's unique qualities and the lifestyles, values, and structures within it that influence the growth of personality. Poor communication, interpersonal worry, the inability to work effectively, and a poor assessment of health problems can result if cultural differences are ignored. Thus, pay attention to the client's racial identity, religious preferences, and distinctive cultural experiences.

As stated in the DSM-IV-TR, judgments about personality functioning must take into account the individual's ethnic, cultural, and social background. Don't confuse personality disorders with problems linked with acculturation following immigration, or with the expression of habits, customs, or religious and political values professed by the individual's culture of origin. For instance, members of ethnic minority groups, immigrants, or political and economic refugees who exhibit guarded or defensive behaviours because of unfamiliarity with, or in response to the perceived neglect or indifference of, the bulk of society may be labeled as having paranoid personality disorder. Others may exhibit defensive behaviour and interpersonal styles similar to that of schizoid personality disorder. Always obtain additional information from informants who are knowledgable about the client's cultural background and determine whether behaviours are culturally approved.

NURSING DIAGNOSES

Nursing diagnoses also focus on disturbances of cognition, affect, interpersonal functioning, and impulse control.

SEXUAL DISORDERS

"In a perfect world, health care providers would be both trained and proficient in all areas of care. In reality, sexual health is frequently the exception. This statement was made regarding the lack of emphasis placed on together with a sexual history as part of the assessment phase of the nursing process.

Sexual History: Obtaining a sexual history in a nonthreatening, quiet, and private environment is necessary. Too frequently, the discomfort of both the nurse and the client interferes with communication during this time. By focusing on the universal facets of human sexuality, together with the need for acceptance, personal bias can be overcome and compassionate interaction with clients can occur.

During the assessment, ask the client's permission to discuss his or her "sex life," emphasizing that all client information provided is confidential. Be professional when approaching the subject about sexuality and furnish support without appearing judgmental. Keep in mind the client's educational level and familiarity with terminology. Use easy words and phrases when asking questions to avoid any misunderstanding or confusion.

Gather data regarding the client's earliest sexual behaviour and experiences, attitude about sex, and gender identity. Pres questions in order of least sensitive to most sensitive material. Be sure to word the questions in a closed-ended style to elicit a specific response. Examples of questions may comprise "Are you married?" or "Are you living with a partner?" Allow the information revealed to guide the discussion.

Explore the client's role in sexual relationships, both past and present. Also obtain information about the client's perception of any sexual issues in the relationships. Be especially sensitive with questions regarding the history of any sexual trauma. Also explore any history of substance abuse and legal problems and pay specific attention to any cultural and religious influences affecting the client's sexuality.

As the assessment progresses, determine whether additional data, together with a history and physical, genital or pelvic examination, and laboratory tests, are indicated; whether the client is willing to involve a family member or significant other in the collection of data; whether the client would benefit from a referral to a support group; or whether the client and spouse or significant other would benefit from a referral to a knowledgeable family or sex therapist who understands the dynamics of sexual problems.

Transcultural Considerations: A client's ethnic, cultural, religious, and social back ground influences sexual attitude, desire, and expectations. Andrews and Boyle (2003) comment about cultural norms related to appropriate male-female and same-sex relationships. Failure to adhere to cultural codes is regarded as to be a serious transgression. For instance, in some cultures, the sexual desires of the woman are not regarded as relevant; fertility is the primary function of the woman. Also, what is regarded as deviant sexual behaviour in one cultural setting may be an acceptable practice in another culture. Thus, be as familiar as possible with the customs of each client's culture.

EATING DISORDER

It is not uncommon for a client with clinical symptoms of a psychiatric disorder (e.g., depression, delusions, delirium, or eating disorder) to refuse to eat, be uninterested in eating, or be unaware of the need or desire to eat. A client may be experiencing physical or psychological problems that interfere with appetite or that make it difficult for the client to eat.

The assessment of clients with clinical symptoms of an eating disorder is a complex process focusing on the client's medical status, physical appearance, capability to meet basic needs, mood and affect, cognitive abilities, interpersonal skills, and behavioural manifestations. Skill is needed in eliciting feelings and thoughts from clients who are in general secretive about their sickness and who frequently use intellectualization to defend their behaviours. A firm but caring approach is used. Utilizing an assessment tool is helpful in determining whether a psychiatric problem underlies the individual's abnormal eating habits, inability to eat, or refusal to eat.

Assessment Tools: Many assessment guides can be used to collect data about the client with an eating disorder. Conant (1996) and Muscari (1998) have developed assessment guides to use when collecting biopsychosocial data about clients with anorexia nervosa, bulimia nervosa, or obesity. Regardless of the specific tool used, the focus is on the following:

- Weight history and what the client thinks an ideal weight would be
- Perception of body appearance, together with self-concept and sexuality
- Lifestyle, together with living arrangements, meal preparation, financial resources, neighborhood resources, occupation, and available support
- Eating habits or pattern, together with kinds, amounts, and frequency of food used or avoided
- Dieting history, together with date of onset and what prompted dieting
- Bingeing and purging rituals surrounding food consumption such as the use of diet pills, diuretics, laxatives, or herbal remedies
- Physical activities or exercise used to attain ideal weight
- Sleep-rest pattern, together with the use of sleep remedies
- Interpersonal relationships with family, peers, or authority figures, together with history of physical or sexual abuse
- Spiritual difficulties because of excessive preoccupation with food or body
- Behavioural changes such as the presence of mood swings or withdrawal from others to eat or starve
- Psychiatric history regarding any prior treatment for an eating disorder as well as the absence or presence of a comorbid psychiatric disorder (e.g., depression, anxiety, obsessive-compulsive behaviour, substance abuse, or suicide attempts)

A new tool, the SCOFF questionnaire (acronym for Sick, Control, One, Fat, and Food), can be used to assess a client for an eating disorder. The client is asked five questions:

- Do you make yourself sick because you feel uncomfortably full?
- Do you worry that you have lost control over how much you eat?
- Have you recently lost more than 14 pounds in a 3-month period?
- Do you believe yourself to be fat when others say you are too thin?
- Would you say that food dominates your life?

If the client answers yes to two or more questions, a referral is essential for further evaluation to determine the presence of an eating disorder.

Physical Examination: A physical examination is conducted to rule out any serious or potentially life-threatening medical complications. Record data about the client's height and weight and assess the client's BMI. Clients with a history of anorexia nervosa may wear layered clothing to conceal weight loss. The physical examination may reveal clinical symptoms of cachexia (e.g., malnourishment and emaciation) because of extreme weight loss. Conversely, clients with a history of bulimia nervosa in general appear to be within their ideal body weight range or even slightly above ideal body weight.

Muscari (1998) suggests that a systems review address symptoms specific to eating disorders such as cold intolerance, fatigue, irregular menses, constipation, lethargy, dental problems (e.g., discolouration, dental caries), and a history of electrolyte or fluid imbalances. Be alert for possible medical complications of anorexia nervosa, bulimia nervosa, and obesity.

Laboratory Tests: Additional tests may be essential depending on the client's medical status. They comprise:

- Electrocardiogram (ECG)
- Comprehensive metabolic panel (together with serum sodium, potassium, amylase, blood urea nitrogen [BUN], magnesium and phosphate levels)
- Haemogram
- Endocrine studies such as growth hormone level, cortisol level, and thyroid profile
- Ultrasonography to rule out gallstones

- Electroencephalogram (EEG)
- Drug screen such as for benzodiazepine or psychostimulant use

In the assessment of obesity, if Cushing's syndrome is suspected, a 24-hour urine cortisol level assessment followed by a low-dose dexamethasone suppression test may be beneficial. Clients with signs, symptoms, or laboratory studies consistent with a secondary cause for obesity may be referred to a specialist such as an endocrinologist or specialist in internal medicine for a more complete evaluation to rule out a comorbid medical condition.

Transcultural Considerations: As with any assessment, be sure to address the client's cultural and ethnic background. Keep in mind that anorexia nervosa is prevalent in industrialized societies with an abundance of food and where physical attractiveness is linked to being thin.

Bulimia nervosa occurs with roughly similar frequencies as anorexia nervosa in the industrialized societies listed above. This disorder affects mainly white persons but has been reported among other ethnic groups.

TREATMENT MODALITIES

There are several treatment options for eating disorders. The correct approach for each individual depends on his or her specific symptoms, issues, and strengths, as well as the severity of the disorder. To be most efficient, treatment for an eating disorder must address both the physical and psychological facets of the problem. The goal is to treat any medical or nutritional needs, promote a healthy relationship with food, and teach constructive ways to deal with life and its challenges.

Frequently, a combination of therapy, nutritional counselling, and group support works best. In some cases, residential treatment or hospitalization may be essential.

- Psychotherapy - Individual and group therapy can help your loved one explore the issues underlying the eating disorder, improve self-esteem, and learn healthy ways of responding to stress and emotional pain. Family therapy is also effective for dealing with the impact the eating disorder has on the entire family unit.
- Nutritional counselling - Dieticians or nutritionists are frequently involved in the treatment of eating disorders. They can help your loved one design meal plans, set dietary goals, and attain

a healthy weight. Nutritional counselling may also involve education about basic nutrition and the health consequences of eating disorders.

- Support groups - Attending an eating disorder support group can help your loved one feel less alone and ashamed. Run by peers rather than professionals, support groups furnish a safe environment to share experiences, advice, encouragement, and coping strategies.
- Residential treatment - Residential or hospital-based care may be required when there are intense physical or behavioural problems, such as a resistance to treatment, medical issues that call for a physician's supervision, or continuing weight loss.

GERIATRIC CONSIDERATIONS

PERSONALITY DISORDER

Following are the considerations which the nurse should keep in mind while treating or taking care of a geriatric patient:

Little experience being interviewed

Less open then today's younger generation

Need to understand why information is needed and that it will be kept in confidence

Chief complaint may seem trivial or vague

- May fail to report significant symptoms
- Need to distinguish patient's chief complaint from their primary problem
- Suffer from more than one disease at a time
- Chronic problems make it difficult to assess acute problems
- Multiple medications can interact and cause side effects
- Age changes reactions to sickness or injury
- Pain may be diminished or absent leading to underestimating the severity of the sickness
- Temperature regulation altered or depressed
- May have absence of fever or a minimal fever even with a intense infection

- Depression
- Inhibits cooperation
- May mimic dementia
- May be mistaken for other diseases

Assessment Tips

- Allow more time
- Allow for slower reflexes
- Allow for review of longer history they possess
- May need hints (memories can be poor)
- Ask if ever got sick or a rash from food or medications rather than asking if they have any allergies
- Make eye contact
- Determine if hard of hearing-several are not
- If they are speak directly at them, they may need to read your lips
- Speak distinctly and slowly
- Do not dwell on unanswered questions
- Return to question later

SEXUAL DISORDERS

During the aging process, the brain decreases in weight and volume; nevertheless, there is no significant loss of higher cortical functioning. Elderly patients may have a slower response time to questions, and new learning is slower. Recent memory may be decreased, but long term memory is not affected. Age-related changes in sensory perception (e.g., hearing loss) can affect the results of the mental status examination, and the elderly person may appear to be confused. The elderly person has more potential for loss of loved ones, job status, prestige, income, and physical health. Coping with both current and potential losses puts added stress on the elderly person.

Older patients who have functioned well in the past but are having difficulty adjusting to age-related physical changes frequently react well to educationally oriented counselling with their health care provider. If counselling is not effective, they may react to brief psychosexual therapy with a specialist in this discipline. A sex therapist will normally meet with a couple together, though individual sessions may also be scheduled. Sex therapists may come from a variety of fields, together with psychiatry, psychology, social work, nursing, or the clergy. They have received additional training in sex therapy and are normally certified in that discipline.

After obtaining a detailed sexual history, the therapist prescribes behavioural homework assignments that especially address the couple's sexual problems. The couple then carries out the assignments at home and reports back on the next visit.

In interviewing patients who are past midlife, it helps to keep a nonjudgmental attitude and to convey that it is normal and desirable to have sex in the later years. At the same time, it is significant not to give the impression that remaining sexually active is necessary to maintaining quality of life, because several older persons prefer to be celibate. It also helps when the clinician is comfortable with discussing sexual functioning in some detail.

The guide for sexual history taking described in the companion piece to this column can be adapted for men. It frequently helps for the clinician to echo the patient's own language in describing sexual activity rather than to use clinical terms with which the patient may not be comfortable. When discussing sexuality with patients, it is significant not to assume anything, especially about sexual orientation or preferred activities.

EATING DISORDERS

The most common eating disorder in the elderly in both community and hospital settings is food refusal. This may lead to weight loss and malnutrition with all the adverse consequences on independence and function. The management of disorders of eating in the elderly is a diagnostic and therapeutic challenge, requiring the combined skills of the medical and nursing staff. The causes are frequently multifactorial and call for careful and repeated assessment of the patient's social, psychological, and medical history. Approach to treatment involves these factors, as well as ethical and cultural considerations. Eating is the most basic biological drive for survival in nature. In human societies there are additional cultural and social facets that may override this instinct, as in the case of hunger strikes for political motives. In the elderly, food is one of the major sources of possible pleasure and it is the challenge for health patients.

When formulating nursing diagnoses, consider quite a few factors such as the client's physical health, nutritional status, developmental level, coping skills, emotional status, behavioural reactions, and family dynamics.

A coexisting psychiatric disorder such as substance abuse or alcoholism may be present.

FOLLOW UP AND HOME CARE AND REHABILITATION

Nursing staff and allied health professionals can assist in the treatment of any kind of patient having disorders by being aware of the symptoms of each cluster. Since the sickness related to any type of disorders frequently present as relationship difficulties, nursing staff and allied health professionals may recognize personality disorders in especially problematic patients. During the treatment phase, nursing staff and allied health professionals can help patients by providing them with appropriate educational materials and referrals for ongoing psychotherapy or group therapy, if applicable.

REFERENCES

Andrews, M. M., & Boyle, J. S. (2003). Transcultural concepts in nursing care (4th ed.). Philadelphia: Lippincott Williams & Wilkins.

Bandura, A. (1997). Insights: Self-efficacy. Harvard Mental Health Letter, 13(9), 4–6.

Bechtel, G., Giger, J. N., & Davidhizar, R. (1998). Case managing patients from other cultures. Journal of Care Management, 4(5), 87–91.

Benishek, L. A., & Lopez, F. G. (1997). Critical evaluation of hardiness theory: Gender differences, perception of life events, and neuroticism. Work & Stress, 11(3), 33–45.

Buchanan, J. (1995). Social support and schizophrenia: A review of the literature. Archives of Psychiatric Nursing, 9(2), 68–76.

Calvert, W. J. (1997). Protective factors within the family, and their role in fostering resiliency in African American adolescents. Journal of Cultural Diversity, 4(4), 110–117.

Campinha-Bacote, J. (2002). The process of cultural competence in the delivery of health care services: A model of care. Journal of Transcultural Nursing, 13(3), 181–184.

Chin, P. (1996). Chinese Americans. In J. G. Lipson, S. L. Dibble, & P. A. Minarik (Eds.), Culture & nursing care: A pocket guide (pp. 74–81). San Francisco: UCSF Nursing Press.

11

Management of Childhood and Adolescent Disorders

Psychiatric disorders are not diagnosed as easily in children as they are in adults. Children normally lack the abstract cognitive abilities and verbal skills to describe what is happening. Because they regularly are changing and developing, children have no sense of a stable, normal self to allow them to discriminate unusual or unwanted symptoms from normal feelings and sensations.

Additionally, behaviours that are normal in a child of one age may indicate problems in a child of another age. For instance, an infant who cries and wails when separated from her mother is normal. If the same child at 5 years of age cries and shows extreme anxiety when separated from her or his mother, nevertheless, this behaviour would warrant investigation.

Children and adolescents experience some of the same mental health problems as adults, such as mood and anxiety disorders, and are diagnosed with these disorders utilizing the same criteria as for adults. Eating disorders, especially anorexia, normally begin in adolescence and continue into adulthood. Discussions of mood, anxiety, and eating disorders are presented in separate chapters of this text.

CLASSIFICATION OF DISORDERS

MENTAL RETARDATION

The necessary feature of mental retardation is below average intellectual functioning (IQ less than 70) accompanied by significant restrictions in areas of adaptive functioning such as communication skills, selfcare, home living, social or interpersonal skills, use of community resources, self-direction, academic skills, work, leisure, and health and safety. The degree of retardation is based on IQ and greatly affects the person's capability to function:

- Mild retardation: IQ 50 to 70
- Moderate retardation: IQ 35 to 50
- Intense retardation: IQ 20 to 35
- Profound retardation: IQ less than 20

LEARNING DISORDER

A learning disorder is diagnosed when a child's achievement in reading, mathematics, or written expression is below that expected for age, formal education, and intelligence. Learning problems interfere with academic achievement and life activities requiring reading, math, or writing. Reading and written expression disorders normally are identified in the first grade; math disorder may go undetected till the child reaches fifth grade.

MOTOR SKILLS DISORDER

The necessary feature of developmental coordination disorder is impaired coordination intense enough to interfere with academic achievement or activities of daily living. This diagnosis is not made if the problem with motor coordination is part of a general medical condition such as cerebral palsy or muscular dystrophy. This disorder becomes apparent as a child attempts to crawl or walk or as an older child tries to dress independently or manipulate toys such as building blocks. Developmental coordination disorder frequently coexists with a communication disorder.

Its course is variable; sometimes lack of coordination persists into adulthood. Schools furnish adaptive physical education and sensory integration programs to treat motor skills disorder. Adaptive physical education programs emphasize inclusion of movement games such as kicking a football or soccer ball. Sensory integration programs are specific physical therapies prescribed to target improvement in areas where the child has difficulties. For instance, a child with tactile defensiveness (discomfort at being touched by another person) might be involved in touching and rubbing skin surfaces.

COMMUNICATION DISORDERS

A communication disorder is diagnosed when a communication deficit is intense enough to hinder growth, academic achievement, or

ADLs together with socialization. Expressive language disorder involves an impaired capability to communicate through verbal and sign language.

The child has difficulty learning new words and speaking in complete and right sentences; his or her speech is limited. Mixed receptive-expressive language disorder comprises the problems of expressive language disorder along with difficulty understanding (receiving) and determining the meaning of words and sentences.

Both disorders can be present at birth (developmental) or they may be acquired as a result of neurologic injury or insult to the brain. Phonologic disorder involves problems with articulation (forming sounds that are part of speech). Stuttering is a disturbance of the normal fluency and time patterning of speech. Phonologic disorder and stuttering run in families and occur more often in boys than in girls.

Communication disorders may be mild to intense. Difficulties that prevail into adulthood are related most closely to the severity of the disorder. Speech and language therapists work with children who have communication disorders to improve their communication skills and to teach parents to continue speech therapy activities at home.

PERVASIVE DEVELOPMENTAL DISORDERS

Pervasive developmental disorders are characterized by pervasive and normally intense impairment of reciprocal social interaction skills, communication deviance, and restricted stereotypical behavioural patterns. This class of disorders also is called autism spectrum disorders and comprises autistic disorder (classic autism), Rett's disorder, childhood disintegrative disorder, and Asperger's disorder. Approximately 75% of children with pervasive developmental disorders have mental retardation.

AUTISTIC DISORDER

Autistic disorder, the best known of the pervasive developmental disorders, is more prevalent in boys than in girls and is identified no later than 3 years of age. Children with autism exhibit little eye contact with and make few facial expressions toward others; they don't use gestures to communicate. They don't relate to peers or parents. They lack spontaneous enjoyment, have evidently no moods or emotional affect, and can't engage in play or make-believe with toys. There is little intelligible speech. These children engage in stereotyped motor behaviours such as handflapping, body-twisting, or head-banging.

RETT'S DISORDER

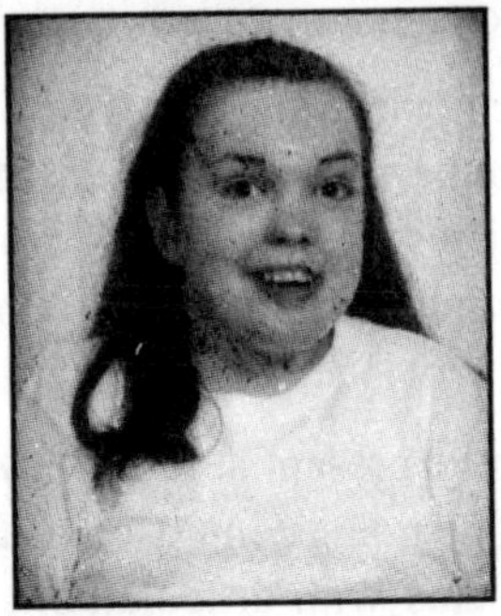

Fig. Rett's Disorder

Rett's disorder is a pervasive developmental disorder characterized by the growth of multiple deficits after a period of normal functioning. It occurs exclusively in girls, is rare, and persists throughout life. Rett's disorder develops between birth to 5 months of age. The child loses motor skills and begins showing stereotyped movements instead. She loses interest in the social environment, and intense impairment of expressive and receptive language becomes apparent as she grows older. Treatment is similar to those for autism.

CHILDHOOD DISINTEGRATIVE DISORDER

Childhood disintegrative disorder is characterized by marked regression in multiple areas of functioning after at least 2 years of evidently normal development and growth. Typical age of onset is 3 to 4 years. Children with childhood disintegrative disorder have the same social and communication deficits and behavioural patterns seen with autistic disorder. This rare disorder occurs slightly more frequently in boys than in girls.

ASPERGER'S DISORDER

Asperger's disorder is a pervasive developmental disorder characterized by the same impairments of social interaction and restricted, stereotyped behaviours seen in autistic disorder but there are no language or cognitive delays. This rare disorder occurs more frequently in boys than in girls; the effects are in general life-long.

ATTENTION DEFICIT HYPERACTIVITY DISORDER

Attention deficit hyperactivity disorder (ADHD) is characterized by inattentiveness, overactivity, and impulsiveness. ADHD is a common disorder, especially in boys, and probably accounts for more child mental health referrals than any other single disorder. The necessary feature of ADHD is a persistent pattern of inattention and/or hyperactivity and impulsivity more common than in general observed in children of the same age.

FEEDING AND EATING DISORDERS OF INFANCY AND EARLY CHILDHOOD

The disorders of feeding and eating included in this class are persistent in nature and are not explained by underlying medical conditions. They comprise pica, rumination disorder, and feeding disorder.

TIC DISORDERS

A tic is a sudden, rapid, recurrent, nonrhythmic, stereotyped motor movement or vocalization. Tics can be suppressed but not indefinitely. Stress exacerbates tics, which diminish during sleep and when the person is engaged in an absorbing activity. Common simple motor tics comprise blinking, jerking the neck, shrugging the shoulders, grimacing, and coughing. Common simple vocal tics comprise clearing the throat, grunting, sniffing, snorting, and barking. Complex vocal tics comprise repeating words or phrases out of context, coprolalia (use of socially unacceptable words, often obscene), palilalia (repeating one's own sounds or words), and echolalia (repeating the last-heard sound word or phrase). Complex motor tics comprise facial gestures, jumping, or touching or smelling an object. Tic disorders tend to run in families. Abnormal transmission of the neurotransmitter dopamine is thought to play a part in tic disorders.

SEPARATION ANXIETY DISORDER

Separation anxiety disorder is characterized by anxiety exceeding that expected for developmental level related to separation from the home or those to whom the child is attached. When apart from attachment figures, the child insists on knowing their whereabouts and may need frequent contact with them such as phone calls. These children are miserable away from home and may fear never seeing their homes or loved ones again.

They frequently follow parents like a shadow, will not be in a room alone, and have trouble going to bed at night unless someone stays with them. Fear of separation may lead to avoidance behaviours such as refusal to attend school or go on errands. Separation anxiety disorder frequently is accompanied by nightmares and multiple physical complaints such as headaches, nausea, vomiting, and dizziness.

Separation anxiety disorders are thought to result from an interaction between temperament and parenting behaviours. Inherited temperament traits, such as passivity, avoidance, fearfulness, or shyness in novel situations, coupled with parenting behaviours that encourage avoidance as a way to cope with unfamiliar or unknown situations are thought to cause anxiety in the child. Depending on the severity of the disorder, children may have academic difficulties and social withdrawal if their avoidance behaviour keeps them from school or relationships with others. Children may be described as demanding, intrusive, and in need of constant attention, or they may be compliant and eager to please. As adults, they may be slow to leave the family home or overly worried about and protective of their own spouses and children. They may continue to have marked discomfort when separated from home or family. Parent education and family therapy are necessary components of treatment; 80% of children experience remission at 4-year follow-up.

SELECTIVE MUTISM

Selective mutism is characterized by pertinacious failure to speak in social situations where speaking is expected, such as school. Children may communicate by gestures, nodding or shaking the head, or some times one-syllable vocalizations in a voice different from their natural voice. These children are frequently excessively shy, socially withdrawn or isolated, and clinging; they may have temper tantrums. Selective mutism is rare and slightly more common in girls than in boys. It normally lasts only a few months but may prevail for years.

REACTIVE ATTACHMENT DISORDER

Reactive attachment disorder involves a markedly disturbed and developmentally inappropriate social relatedness in most situations. This disorder normally begins before 5 years of age and is linked with grossly pathogenic care such as parental neglect, abuse, or failure to meet the child's basic physical or emotional needs. Repeated changes in primary caregivers, such as multiple foster care placements, also can prevent the formation of stable attachments. The disturbed social relatedness may be evidenced by the child's failure to initiate or react to social interaction (inhibited type) or indiscriminate sociability or lack of selectivity in choice of attachment figures (disinhibited type). In the first type, the child will not cuddle or desire to be close to anyone. In the second type, the child's response is the same to a stranger or to a parent.

Initially, treatment focuses on the child's safety, together with removal of the child from the home if neglect or abuse is found. Individual and family therapy (either with parents or foster caregivers) is most efficient. With early identification and effective intervention, remission or considerable improvements can be attained. Otherwise the disorder follows a continuous course with relationship problems persisting into adulthood.

STEREOTYPIC MOVEMENT DISORDER

Stereotypic movement disorder is linked with several genetic, metabolic, and neurologic disorders and frequently accompanies mental retardation. The precise cause is unknown. It involves repetitive motor behaviour that is nonfunctional and either interferes with normal activities or results in self-injury requiring medical treatment. Stereotypic movements may comprise waving, rocking, twirling objects, biting fingernails, banging the head, biting or hitting oneself, or picking at the skin or body orifices. In general speaking, the more intense the retardation, the higher the risk for self-injury behaviours. Stereotypic movement behaviours are relatively stable over time but may diminish with age.

ETIOLOGY

Though much research is taking place, the definitive causes of ADHD remain unknown. A combination of factors, such as environmental toxins, prenatal influences, heredity, and damage to brain structure and functions, is likely responsible. Prenatal exposure to alcohol, tobacco, and lead and intense malnutrition in early childhood increase the likelihood of ADHD. Though the relation between ADHD and dietary sugar and vitamins has been studied, results have been inconclusive. Brain images of people with ADHD have suggested decreased metabolism in the frontal lobes, which are necessary for attention, impulse control, organization, and sustained goal-directed activity. Studies also have shown decreased blood perfusion of the frontal cortex in children with ADHD and frontal cortical atrophy in young adults with a history of childhood ADHD.

Another study showed decreased glucose use in the frontal lobes of parents of children with ADHD who had ADHD themselves. Evidence is not conclusive, but research in these areas seems promising. There seems to be a genetic link for ADHD that is most likely linked with abnormalities in catecholamine and possibly serotonin metabolism. Having a first-degree relative with ADHD increases the danger of the disorder by four to five times that of the general population. In spite of the strong evidence supporting a genetic contribution, there are also sporadic cases of ADHD with no family history of ADHD; this furthers the theory of multiple contributing factors.

Risk factors for ADHD comprise family history of ADHD; male relatives with antisocial personality disorder or alcoholism; female relatives with somatization disorder; lower socioeconomic status; male gender; marital or family discord, together with divorce, neglect, abuse, or parental deprivation; low birth weight; and various kinds of brain insult.

PSYCHOPATHOLOGY

Medications frequently are effective in decreasing hyperactivity and impulsiveness and improving attention; this enables the child to partake in school and family life. The most common medications are methylphenidate (Ritalin) and an amphetamine compound

(Adderall). Methylphenidate is effective in 70% to 80% of children with ADHD; it reduces hyperactivity, impulsivity, and mood lability and helps the child to pay attention more appropriately. Dextroamphetamine (Dexedrine) and pemoline (Cylert) are other stimulants used to treat ADHD. The most common side effects of these drugs are insomnia, loss of appetite, and weight loss or failure to gain weight. Methylphenidate, dextroamphetamine, and amphetamine compound are also available in sustained-release form taken once daily; this eliminates the need for additional doses when the child is at school. Because pemoline can cause liver damage, it is the last of these drugs to be prescribed.

Giving stimulants during daytime hours normally effectively combats insomnia. Eating a good breakfast with the morning dose and substantial, nutritious snacks late in the day and at bedtime will help the child to maintain an adequate dietary intake. When stimulant medications are not effective or their side effects are intolerable, antidepressants are the second choice for treatment. Atomoxetine (Strattera) is a nonstimulant drug sanctioned in 2002 by the Food and Drug Administration for treatment of ADHD. It is an antidepressant, especially a selective norepinephrine reuptake inhibitor. The most common side effects in children during clinical trials were decreased appetite, nausea, vomiting, tiredness, and upset stomach. In adults, side effects were similar to other antidepressants together with insomnia, dry mouth, urinary retention, decreased appetite, nausea, vomiting, dizziness, and sexual side effects.

CHARACTERISTICS

- Psychiatric disorders are more difficult to diagnose in children than in adults because their basic growth is incomplete and children may lack the capability to recognize or to describe what they are experiencing.

- Children and adolescents can experience some of the same mental health problems seen in adults such as depression, bipolar disorder, and anxiety.
- The disorders of childhood and adolescence most frequently encountered in mental health settings comprise pervasive developmental disorders, attention deficit hyperactivity disorder, and disruptive behaviour disorders.
- Mental retardation involves below-average intellectual functioning (IQ below 70) and is accompanied by significant restrictions in adaptive functioning such as communication, selfcare, self-direction, academic achievement, work, and health and safety. The degree of impairment is directly related to the IQ.
- Learning disorders comprise classes for substandard achievement in reading, mathematics, and written expression. They are treated through special education in schools.
- Communication disorders may be expressive or receptive and expressive. They mainly involve articulation or stuttering and are treated by speech and language therapists.
- Pervasive developmental disorders are characterized by intense impairment of reciprocal social interaction skills, communication deviance, and restricted stereotyped behavioural patterns.
- Children with autism, the best known of the pervasive developmental disorders, seem detached with little eye contact and few facial expressions toward others. They don't relate to peers or parents, lack spontaneous enjoyment, and can't engage in play or make-believe with toys. Autism frequently is treated with behavioural approaches. Months or years of treatment may be needed before positive outcomes appear.
- The necessary feature of ADHD is a pertinacious pattern of inattention and/or hyperactivity and impulsivity. ADHD, the most common disorder of childhood, results in poor academic performance, strained family relations, and rejection by peers.
- Interventions for ADHD comprise a combination of medication, behavioural interventions, and parental education. Frequently special educational aid is needed to help with academic achievement. Conduct disorder, the most common disruptive behaviour disorder, is characterized by aggression to people

and animals, destruction of property, deceitfulness and theft, and serious violation of rules.

- Interventions for conduct disorder comprise decreasing violent behaviour, increasing compliance, improving coping skills and self-esteem, promoting social interaction, and training and supporting parents.
- Feeding and eating disorders of infancy and childhood comprise pica, rumination, and feeding disorders of infancy or early childhood. Pica and rumination frequently improve with time, and most cases of feeding disorders can be successfully treated.
- Tic disorders involve various combinations of involuntary vocal and/or motor tics. Tourette's disorder is most common. Tic disorders are normally treated successfully with atypical antipsychotic medications.
- Elimination disorders cause impairment for the child based on the response of parents, the level of self-esteem, and the degree of ostracism by peers.

DIAGNOSIS

Asperger's Syndrome: Asperger's Disorder is a separate Autistic Spectrum disorder which does not meet criteria for other Pervasive Developmental Disorders or Schizophrenia. Features of Asperger's Disorder are intense and sustained impairment in social interaction and the growth of repetitive patterns of behaviour, interests and activities, and significant impairment in social, occupational and other significant areas of functioning. Because there are no significant language delays or cognitive deficits, Asperger's is regarded as a form of high functioning autism.

Attention Deficit Hyperactivity Disorder: Attention Deficit Hyperactivity Disorder (ADHD), sometimes inaccurately referred to as ADD (There is no clinical term by this name) is a disorder normally first diagnosed in infancy, childhood or adolescence. There are 4 recognized types of ADHD. They are: Predominantly Inattentive type; Predominantly Hyperactive-Impulsive type; Combined type (inattention and hyperactivity-impulsivity); and ADHD - Not Otherwise Specified. There is a high level of correlation between children with ADHD and other psychiatric illnesses. This included illnesses ranging from behavioural, mood, family, anxiety, cognitive, social to school functioning, with the greatest increase in those with the ADHD - combined subtype.

Autism: Autism may manifest in early infancy, with the infant shying away from the parent's touch, not responding to a parent who returns after an absence, and inappropriate gaze behaviour. The Autistic child may fail to meet early language and other developmental milestones. And there can be as much as a 3-year delay between the report of symptoms and the diagnosis, which is normally made at around age five.

Childhood Disintegrative Disorder: Childhood Disintegrative Disorder strikes children who have developed normally through at least their first two years of life. They then become impaired in at least two of the following major functional areas: social, communication, restricted receptive language, or stereotyped movements. Although the age of onset is later, in the most intense cases, these children can resemble autistic children, though the severity is in general less.

Childhood Disorder NOS: This diagnosis is used for disorders with onset in infancy, childhood, or adolescence that don't meet the criteria for any specific disorder. As per the ICD-10, there are two sub-classes: (1) Other specified behavioural and emotional disorders normally taking place during in childhood and adolescence and (2) Unspecified behavioural and emotional disorders with onset normally taking place in childhood and adolescence.

Childhood Eating Disorders: There are 3 feeding and eating disorders of infancy or early childhood. The first is Pica, in which the child pertinaciously eats non-nutritive substances for at least one month. The behaviour must be developmentally inappropriate, and not culturally approved. It appears more often in young children than adults.

The second disorder is rumination disorder, in which the infant or child repeatedly regurgitates and rechews food, after a period of normal functioning. The symptoms must last for at least one month. The last disorder is feeding disorder of infancy or early childhood, in which there is a feeding disturbance evidenced by pertinacious failure to eat enough food and a significant failure to gain weight or weight loss.

Conduct Disorder: Conduct Disorder is essentially a disorder where the person violates the social norms and rights of others. Those with this disorder are habitually in trouble, either with parents, teachers or peers. In spite of presenting a tough image to those around them, they have a low self-esteem. Their frustration tolerance, irritability, temper outbursts and recklessness are hallmarks. Conduct Disorder may lead to adult antisocial personality disorder.

Disruptive Behaviour Disorder NOS: Disruptive Behaviour Disorder NOS (not otherwise specified) is utilized when there are conduct or oppositional-defiant behaviours that don't meet the diagnostic criteria for either conduct disorder or oppositional defiant disorder, but in which there is notable impairment.

Dyslexia: Dyslexia is a specific learning disability that is neurological in origin. It is characterized by difficulties with accurate and/or fluent word recognition and by poor spelling and decoding abilities. These difficulties basically result from a deficit in the phonological component of language that is frequently unexpected in relation to other cognitive abilities and the provision of effective classroom instruction.

Learning Disorders: Learning Disorders occur in three major classes: reading, mathematics, and written expression. Reading problems in general occur before the age of 7. This is followed normally by problems with spelling and written language expression by the age of 8. Mathematical learning disorders frequently are not detected till after rote memorization mathematics work has ended, and application of more abstract skills is essential. These diagnoses are given only after standardized testing in the specific area is significantly below that expected by the child's chronological age, IQ, and educational level.

Mental Retardation: Mental Retardation is based on both IQ and deficits in functioning. It is not a single, simple syndrome, but rather a state of impairment. By definition, to have the label Mental Retardation, the person must have an IQ below 70, and impairments in adaptive functioning in at least two of the following areas: communication, selfcare, home living, social/interpersonal skills, use of community resources, self-direction, functional academic skills, work, leisure, health, and safety. Finally, the onset must be before age 18. There are 4 levels of Mental Retardation, based on IQ: Mild, with a mental age of 8.5 to 11.0 years; Moderate, with a mental age of 6.0 to 8.5 years; Intense, with a mental age of 3.75 to 6.0 years, and Profound, with a mental age of 0 to 3.75 years.

Mixed-Receptive-Expressive Language Disorder: In this disorder, children are impaired in both the understanding and expressing of language. The receptive and expressive disorders may be either acquired, congenital or developmental.

Oppositional Defiant Disorder: Oppositional Defiant Disorder (ODD) is a disorder in which children ignore or defy adults' requests and rules. They may be passive, finding ways to annoy others, or active, verbally saying "No". They tend to blame others for their mistakes and difficulties. When asked why they are so defiant, they may say that they are only acting against unreasonable rules. They are different from children with conduct disorders in that they don't violate the rights of others. These behaviours are present at home, but not necessarily in other situations, such as school, or with other adults.

Pervasive Developmental Disorder NOS: This indicates a intense, pervasive impairment in social interaction or communication skills, or the presence of stereotyped behaviour, interests and activities. The criteria for a specific PDD, schizophrenia and schizotypal and avoidant personality disorders are not med. This diagnosis in general has a better outcome than does autistic disorder.

Reactive Attachment Disorder: Reactive Attachment Disorder is characterized by the breakdown of social capability of a child. It is linked with the failure of the child to bond with a caretaker in infancy or early childhood. This can be caused by several factors, ranging from child neglect to the child being hospitalized for intense medical problems. The children may exhibit either indiscriminate social extroversion as they grow older (treating all people as though they were their best friend) or showing mistrust of nearly everyone.

Rett's Disorder: Rett's Disorder is a disorder that is exclusive to females. For the first 6 months of life, growth is normal. At that point, they begin to exhibit several of the symptoms of autism, such as stereotyped movements, poor social interaction, and impaired communication. In addition, they also have problems with both expressive and receptive language, psychomotor retardation, and poorly coordinated gait and/or trunk movements, along with decreased head growth. They will, as they mature, nevertheless, gain back a degree of positive social interaction.

Selective Mutism: Selective Mutism is a disorder in which children may talk at home but because of intense anxiety, are unable to speak in several social situations. Their anxiety may affect their capability to communicate in other ways as well. For a diagnosis of Selective Mutism to be made the communication problem must last at least one month, without treatment SM can prevail for years. Onset is normally quite slow, with children showing inhibited temperaments as infants, frequently displaying Separation Anxiety through their toddler years. SM is frequently not diagnosed till the child begins school, and sometimes even later because of a lack of awareness in Pediatricians and other Healthcare workers.

Separation Anxiety Disorder: Separation Anxiety Disorder is a disorder that affects children who are afraid to be separated from the main caretakers in their lives, even to go to a friend's house or school. When separated, they are regularly afraid that something horrible will happen to either themselves or to their primary caretaker (they or the caretaker will die, for example). When the subject of separating is brought up, the child begins to present with somatic symptoms ranging from headaches to nausea and vomiting, with anxiety.

Stuttering: Stuttering is a disturbance in the fluency and time patterning of speech that is inappropriate for the patient's age. It may contain sound repetitions, prolongations, interjections, pauses in words, word substitutions to avoid blocking, and audible or silent blocking.

NURSING ASSESSMENT

During assessment, the nurse gathers information from the child's parents, day care providers (if any), and teachers as well as through direct observation. Evaluating the child in a group of peers is likely to yield useful information because the child's behaviour may be subdued or different in a centred one-to-one interaction with the nurse. It is frequently helpful to use a checklist when talking with parents to help focus their input on the target symptoms or behaviours their child exhibits.

TREATMENT MODALITIES

Treatment is based on a combination of psychotherapy, medication, and nutritional counselling. Goals comprise restoration of healthy body weight, correction of medical complications, adoption of healthful eating habits and treatment of maladaptive food-related thought processes, treatment of coexisting psychiatric conditions, and prevention of relapse. Depending on the severity of the sickness, therapy may be conducted on an out-patient, day treatment, or in-patient basis.

Out-patient therapy: Out-patient therapy provided by practitioners specializing in eating disorders is appropriate for highly motivated patients within 20 percent of their normal body weight and whose sickness is mild or just developing. Treatment consists of cognitive-behavioural therapy, intensive nutritional counselling, support-group referrals, and medical monitoring. At the outset of treatment, a contract is established, outlining an anticipated rate of weight gain (normally between 0.5 and 2 pounds per week), target goal weight, and consequences if weight gain is not achieved. Vitamin and mineral supplementation and the use of liquid supplements to facilitate weight gain may also be indicated.

Day treatment programs: Day treatment programs are being used with increasing frequency in place of in-patient hospitalization. This form of therapy provides an intermediate level of care for patients who call for frequent monitoring but don't call for treatment twenty-four hours a day. It may be used for patients who are not responding to out-patient therapy or who are stepping down from in-patient hospitalization. Treatment, which may take place four or five days per week from morning till evening, is similar in structure to out-patient therapy, but is provided on a more intensive level.

In-patient hospitalization: In-patient hospitalization is indicated for patients whose eating disorder has reached life-threatening status. Criteria for admission to such programs are weight loss of 25 percent or more of ideal body weight or the presence of an eating disorder in a child or adolescent. It may also be essential for persons who are medically unstable. Normally, participants in in-patient programs are anorexic, though hospitalization for bulimia may be essential if there is serious deterioration of vital signs, uncontrollable vomiting, or concurrent psychiatric sickness. The immediate goals of in-patient treatment are weight gain and stabilization of vital signs. In several cases, the patient is so fragile that complete bed rest is required. Eating is gently encouraged. In extreme medical situations refusal may be met with tube feeding or, in rare instances, intravenously.

Medication: Medication is increasingly becoming a routine part of treatment for eating disorders. Antidepressants, especially the selective serotonin reuptake inhibitors (SSRIs), are the most efficient and most commongenerally used medication in treating this spectrum of illnesses. They are found to be of greatest benefit when used in combination with therapy, and are of little value if offered on their own. In the case of anorexia, these medications are most efficient if employed after successful weight restoration is achieved, at which time they can be useful for relapse prevention and the treatment of coexisting psychiatric conditions. SSRIs are also used in preventing binge relapses among bulimics, though their effectiveness ceases once the medication is discontinued. Though antidepressants have also been employed in the treatment of binge eating disorder, outcomes have not been sufficiently positive to warrant recommendations for their use.

Outcomes: Persons are normally regarded as to be ready to terminate therapy once they have achieved a healthy body weight and can eat all foods free of guilt or anxiety. For a complete recovery, extensive treatment may be required from six months to two years, and for as long as three to five years in cases where other psychiatric conditions are present. For some, eating disorders will be a lifelong struggle, with stressful or traumatic events triggering relapses that may call for occasional check-in therapy to restore healthful eating patterns.

FOLLOW-UP AND HOME CARE AND REHABILITATION

The function of the nurse in the provision of home care has been categorized into three activities: making home visits, making referrals of patients to home care agencies, and participation in the multidisciplinary team providing care to adults and MFTD children at home. Doctors also serve as medical directors of home health and hospice agencies. Primary care and internal medicine physicians make regular but infrequent home visits, especially in rural areas, but specialists such as chest physicians and pulmonologists may also make home visits to supervise home management of mechanical ventilation or other care.

Medicare and other payers call for that the doctor direct the provision of home health care by the interdisciplinary care team through on-going oversight of the treatment plan. The doctor determines the patient's medical needs, approves a treatment plan and orders that meet those needs, and monitors implementation of the plan. The doctor may assume the function of case coordinator, but is more likely to delegate this role to the home health nurse or other home care agency personnel. Most doctors, together with specialists, report that they work with home health agency or hospital staff to determine home health services needed by patients.

Regular communication between the doctor, the case coordinator, and other home care agency personnel is critical to assure that patients receive appropriate clinical care, and that treatment plans are updated and sanctioned when the patient's condition changes. Home care agencies are increasing their use of technology and telemedicine programs to send reports and treatment plan changes to doctors. Effective electronic modes of communication, telemedicine, and other home care technologies exist but are beyond the scope of this statement.

REFERENCES

Dirksen, S. R. (2000). Predicting well-being among breast cancer survivors. Journal of Advanced Nursing, 32(4), 937–943.

Evanikoff, L. J. (1996). Russians. In J. G. Lipson, S. L. Dibble, & P. A. Minarik (Eds.), Culture & nursing care: A pocket guide (pp. 239–249). San Francisco: UCSF Nursing Press.

Fallot, R. D. (2001). Spirituality and religion in psychiatric rehabilitation and recovery from mental illness. International Review of Psychiatry, 13(2), 110–116.

Juarbe, T. (1996). Puerto Ricans. In J. G. Lipson, S. L. Dibble, & P. A. Minarik (Eds.), Culture and nursing care: A pocket guide (pp. 222–238). San Francisco: USCF Nursing Press.

Kobasa, S. C. (1979). Stressful life events, personality, and health: An inquiry into hardiness. Journal of Personality & Social Psychology, 37(1), 1–11.

Kennedy, M. G. (1999). Cultural competence and psychiatric-mental health nursing. Journal of Transcultural Nursing, 10(1), 11.

Krafcik, K. A. (2002). Predictors of resourcefulness in school aged children. Issues in Mental Health Nursing, 23(4), 385–407.

Lease, S. H. (1999). Occupational role stressors, coping, support, and hardiness as predictors of strain. Research in Higher Education, 40(3), 285–307.

12

Management of Organic Brain Disorders

Agitated patients with organic brain disorders represent relatively common diagnostic and management problems. Therapeutic failures normally result from a failure to understand the patient's disturbed behaviour, the staff's emotional response to the patient's behaviour, or neglect of the biological cause and ineffective use of medication. Effective management depends on continued monitoring of the patient's mental status and physical condition.

The central clinical feature of most organic psychiatric disorders is impaired cognitive functioning. Cerebral dysfunction can nevertheless also cause organic mood states, personality change as well as organic psychotic and even neurotic states. The cerebral dysfunction may be caused by a disruption of brain structures or by alterations in neurophysiology. A vast array of medical and surgical conditions are capable of producing this disruption, they may be systemic or originate within the brain.

CLASSIFICATION: ICD

Disorders linked with organic brain disorder comprise:

- Brain injury caused by trauma
  - Bleeding into the brain (intracerebral haemorrhage)
  - Bleeding into the space around the brain (subarachnoid haemorrhage)
  - Blood clot causing pressure on brain (chronic subdural hematoma)
  - Concussion

- Breathing conditions
  - Low oxygen in the body (hypoxia)
  - High carbon dioxide levels in the body (hypercapnia)
- Cardiovascular disorders
  - Abnormal heart rhythm (arrhythmias)
  - Brain injury because of high blood pressure (hypertensive brain injury)
  - Dementia because of several strokes (multi-infarct dementia)
  - Heart infections (endocarditis, myocarditis)
  - Stroke
  - Transient ischemic attack (TIA)
- Degenerative disorders
  - Creutzfeldt-Jacob disease
  - Diffuse Lewy Body disease
  - Huntington's disease
  - Multiple sclerosis
  - Normal pressure hydrocephalus
  - Parkinson's disease
  - Pick's disease
  - Senile dementia, Alzheimer's type
- Dementia because of metabolic causes
- Drug and alcohol-related conditions
  - Alcohol withdrawal state
  - Intoxication, drug abuse, or alcohol use
  - Long-term effects of alcohol, Wernicke-Korsakoff syndrome
  - Withdrawal from drugs (especially sedative-hypnotics and corticosteroids)
- Infections
  - Any sudden onset (acute) or long-term (chronic) infection
  - Blood poisoning (septicemia)
  - Swelling of the brain (encephalitis)
  - Swelling of the lining of the brain and spinal cord (meningitis)

- Other medical disorders
  - Cancer
  - Kidney disease
  - Liver disease
  - Thyroid disease (high or low)
  - Vitamin deficiency (B12 and others)

Other conditions that may be related to organic brain disorder comprise:

- Depression
- Neurosis
- Psychosis

ETIOLOGY

Very frequently the etiology, or cause, of a specific type of mental disorder is unknown or is understood only to a very limited degree. The situation is complicated by the fact that a mental disorder such as schizophrenia may be caused by a combination and interaction of quite a few factors, together with a probable genetic predisposition to develop the disease, a postulated biochemical imbalance in the brain, and a cluster of stressful life events that help to precipitate the actual onset of the sickness. The predominance of these and other factors probably varies from person to person in schizophrenia. A likewise complex interaction of constitutional, developmental, and social factors can influence the formation of mood and anxiety disorders.

No single theory of causation can explain all mental disorders or even all those of a specific type. Moreover, the same type of disorder may have different causes in different individuals: e.g., an obsessive-compulsive disorder may have its origins in a biochemical imbalance, in an unconscious emotional conflict, in faulty learning processes, or in a combination of these. The fact that quite different therapeutic approaches can produce equal improvements in different patients with the same type of disorder underscores the complex and ambiguous nature of the causes of mental sickness.

PSYCHOPATHOLOGY

Organic explanations of mental sickness have normally been genetic, biochemical, neuropathological, or a combination of these.

The study of the genetic causes of mental disorders involves both the laboratory analysis of the human genome and the statistical analysis of the frequency of a specific disorder's occurrence among persons who share related genes-i.e., family members and especially twins. Family risk studies compare the observed frequency of occurrence of a mental sickness in close relatives of the patient with its frequency in the general population. First-degree relatives (parents, siblings, and children) share 50 percent of their genetic material with the patient, and higher rates of the sickness in these relatives than expected indicate a possible genetic factor. In twin studies the frequency of occurrence of the sickness in both members of pairs of identical (monozygous) twins is compared with its frequency in both members of a pair of fraternal (dizygous) twins.

A higher concordance for disease among the identical than the fraternal twins suggests a genetic component. Further information on the relative importance of genetic and environmental factors accrues from comparing identical twins reared together with those reared apart. Adoption studies comparing adopted children whose biological parents had the sickness with those whose parents didn't can also be useful in separating biological from environmental influences.

If a mental disease is caused by a biochemical abnormality, investigation of the brain at the site where the biochemical imbalance occurs should show neurochemical differences from normal.

In practice such a simplistic approach is fraught with practical, methodological, and ethical difficulties. The living human brain is not readily accessible to direct investigation, and the dead brain undergoes chemical change; moreover, findings of abnormalities in cerebrospinal fluid, blood, or urine may have no relevance to the question of a presumed biochemical imbalance in the brain. It is difficult to study human mental illnesses using animals as analogs, because most mental disorders either don't occur or are not recognizable in animals. Even when biochemical abnormalities have been found in individuals with mental disorders, it is difficult to know whether they are the cause or the result of the sickness, or of its treatment, or of other consequences. In spite of these problems, progress has been made in unravelling the biochemistry of mood disorders, schizophrenia, and some of the dementias.

CLINICAL FEATURES

The clinical features of organic brain disorders is reduced level of consciousness, though mild degrees of this can be easy to in clinical practice. The patient is confused and disoriented, frequently restless, overactive, and fearful, but sometimes underactive and withdrawn. Inattention, together with reduced capability to focus, sustain, or shift attention, is common. Illusions; hallucinations of visual, auditory, or tactile type; and changeable paranoid delusions may be present. Severity fluctuates, normally being worse at night, because when there is less light, the environment is more likely to be misinterpreted, curtains appearing as threatening monsters.

DIAGNOSIS AND DIFFERENTIAL DIAGNOSIS

Diagnosis is made on clinical grounds from the history and mental state examination together with simple cognitive testing. In taking the history if there is a suspicion of dementia, it will be appropriate to do cognitive testing early in the interview. This will give guidance as to whether the patient can give a proper history or not (so as not to spend too much time, and annoy the patient, by inappropriately persisting in trying to take a history that must ultimately be coherent).

Disorientation may be unsuspected by examiner unless tested; short-term memory will normally be abnormal. Formal psychometric tests can be used to confirm the diagnosis and specify the type of defects present, and repeated at intervals to monitor progress.

NURSING ASSESSMENT

An organic brain disorder patient's history can be obtained if the patient is alert enough and oriented to person, place, and time. If the person appears to be disoriented or confused upon questioning, ask family members and friends to confirm the information. The person should be questioned as to previous history of seizures, loss of consciousness, anaesthesia (an absence of normal sensation - especially to pain), paresthesia (numbness and tingling; a "pins and needles" feeling), neuralgia, twitches, tremors, personality changes, memory deficits, mental deterioration, nervousness, anxiety, history of psychiatric problems, vertigo, sensory disturbance, phobias, hallucinations, delusions, illusions, nightmares, insomnia, and/or grandiose ideas.

DIFFERENCES AMONG HALLUCINATIONS, DELUSIONS, AND ILLUSIONS

Hallucinations: A sensory perception not resulting from external stimuli. An example would be someone who is hearing voices.

Delusions: A pertinacious belief although illogical. An example would be someone who is feeling controlled by external sources.

Illusions: A false interpretation of external stimuli. Examples of illusions comprise seeing mirages or hearing the ocean in a sea shell.

PHYSICAL ASSESSMENT

A complete organic brain disorder assessment consists of five steps:

- Mental status exam
- Cranial nerve assessment
- Reflex testing
- Motor system assessment
- Sensory system assessment

Mental Status Exam

The mental status exam really evaluates the patient's cerebral function. Remember that the cerebrum controls sophisticated mental functions such as speech, problem solving, and memory. As you perform this portion of the neurological assessment, pay special attention to the patient's speech and language abilities. His speech should be clear, coherent, and spoken at an appropriate rate. The language used should be appropriate for the education and socioeconomic levels of the person. Altered speech patterns can alert you to the possibility of organic brain disorder problems.

Intellect: (Memory, Orientation, Recognition, Calculations)

Orientation: Assess time, place, person. Organic brain disorders lose time first, then place, rarely person.

Attention span: Should be able to focus on examiner's questions and respond. Impaired in anxiety, fatigue, intoxication.

Recent memory: Ask for 24 hour diet recall and other easily verifiable information. Impaired in organic brain syndromes and Alzheimer's.

Remote memory: Ask for past health, birthdays, anniversary, relevant history. Lost in Alzheimer's, cortical injury, but not in normal aging or most organic brain syndromes.

New learning: Assess 4-word recall (should be able to recall all four at 10 minutes and three words at 30 minutes). Use the word groups "brown, honesty, tulip, eyedropper" or "fun, carrot, ankle, loyalty". Four-word recall is impaired in Alzheimer's, anxiety, and depression.

Judgement: Ask questions such as "What would you do if your house caught fire?" or "What are your plans for the future?". Judgement is impaired in mental retardation, emotional dysfunction, schizophrenia, and organic brain disease.

Perception: Visual hallucinations are frequently linked with medications and organic syndromes. Auditory hallucinations are linked more with psychiatric disorders.

Neurological Assessment

The following guide will furnish a quick overview of each cranial nerve's function.

Cranial Nerve I (Olfactory): After evaluating patency of both nares, have client close eyes, obstruct one nare, and sniff. Use common, easily identifiable substances such as coffee, toothpaste, orange, vanilla, soap, or peppermint. Use different substances for each side. Bilateral decreased sense of smell occurs with age, tobacco smoking, allergic rhinitis, cocaine use. Unilateral loss of sense of smell (neurologic anosmia) can indicate a frontal lobe lesion.

Cranial Nerve II (Optic): Check visual acuity (have the patient read newspaper print) and visual fields for each eye. Unilateral blindness can indicate a lesion or pressure in the globe or optic nerve. Loss of the same half of the visual field in both eyes (homonymous hemianopsia) can indicate a lesion of the opposite side optic tract as in a CVA.

Cranial Nerve III (Oculomotor): Assess pupil size and light reflex. A unilaterally dilated pupil with unilateral absent light reflex and/or if the eye will not turn upwards could indicate an internal carotid aneurysm or uncal herniation with increased intracranial pressure.

Cranial Nerve IV (Trochlear) and Cranial Nerve VI (Abducens): Have patient turn eyes downward, temporally, and nasally. If the eyes will not do this the patient may have a fracture of the eye orbit or a brain stem tumour. (Note: Cranial Nerves III, IV, and VI are examined together because they control eyelid elevation, eye movement, and pupillary constriction.)

Cranial Nerve V (Trigeminal)

Motor - Palpate jaws and temples while patient clenches teeth.

Sensory - Have patient close eyes, touch cotton ball to all areas of face.

Unilateral deficit seen with trauma and tumours.

Cranial Nerve VII (Facial)

- Motor
- Check symmetry and mobility of face by having patient frown, close eyes, lift eyebrows, and puff cheeks.
- Sensory Asses the patient's capability to identify taste (sugar, salt, lemon juice)
- An asymmetrical deficit can be found in trauma, Bell's palsy, CVA, tumour, and inflammation.

Cranial Nerve VIII (Acoustic or Vestibulocochlear)

- This tests hearing acuity. Impairment indicates inflammation or occlusion of the ear canal, drug toxicity, or a possible tumour.
- Cranial Nerve IX (Glossopharyngeal) and X (Vagus)
- Motor
- Depress the tongue with a tongue blade and have the patient say "ahh" or yawn. Uvula and soft palate should rise. Gag reflex should be present and the voice should sound smooth.
- Deficits can indicate a brain stem tumour or neck injury.

Cranial Nerve XI (Spinal Accessory): Have the patient rotate the head and shrug shoulders against resistance. If the patient is unable to do this it may indicate a neck injury.

Cranial Nerve XII (Hypoglossal)

- Motor
- Assess tongue control.
- Wasting of the tongue, deviation to one side, tremors, and an inability to distinctly say l,t,d,n sounds can indicate a lower or upper motor neuron lesion.

Reflex Testing

When you strike a slightly stretched tendon with a reflex hammer, a simple muscle contraction occurs. DTRs assist with evaluation of !ower motor neurons and fibers. For instance, if the patient's biceps reflex is normal, you know that the lower motor neurons and fibers at levels C5 and C6 are intact.

There are five reflexes to check which comprise:

Biceps: With the patient sitting, flex his arm at the elbow and rest his forearm on his thigh with the palm up. Place your thumb firmly on the biceps tendon in the antecubital fossa. Strike your thumb with the hammer. The elbow and forearm should flex, and the biceps muscle should contract.

Triceps: The triceps tendon is tested with the patient's arm flexed at a 90° angle. Supporting the arm with your hand, strike the triceps tendon on the posterior arm just above the elbow. The tendon should contract and the elbow extend.

Brachioradialis: Have the patient rest his slightly flexed arm on his lap with the palm facing downward. Strike the posterior arm about two inches above the wrist on the thumb side. The forearm should rotate laterally and the palm turn upward.

Patellar: Dangle the patient's legs over the side of the bed. Place your hand on the patient's thigh and strike the distal patellar tendon just below the kneecap. (If the patient must remain supine, flex each leg to a 45° angle and place your dominant hand behind his knee to support it.) The normal response is contraction of the quadriceps muscle with extension of the knee.

Achilles: Have the patient dorsiflex (point downward) his foot slightly and lightly tap the Achilles's tendon on the posterior ankle area. A slight jerking of the foot should be seen.

TREATMENT MODALITIES

In distinguishing PTSD from organic brain dysfunction, the neuropsychological assessment becomes key. Through neuropsychological assessment cognitive abilities are basically evaluated through a variety of testing. Because the criteria for diagnosis of dementia calls for impairment in "occupational" or "social functioning", and because there must be a "decline from a formerly higher level of functioning", neuropsychological assessment greatly aids in the diagnostic process.

In general, the cause of PTSD is thought to be functional or psychologically based. In contrast, the cause for organic brain injury involves an actual change in the brain tissue itself.

Treatment modalities differ markedly between the two. PTSD is generally treated through psychotherapy or through the use of medications to control anxiety and stress. Depending upon the pre-existing characteristics of the individual, treatment for PTSD can be prolonged and the progression gradual.

In contrast, maximum recovery from organically based brain injury, at least in terms of thinking skills, basically occurs soon after the event in question, with gradual recovery continuing throughout the first year to two years post-injury. Though technology changes with each day, treating cognitive problems because of brain tissue changes with medications has not proved highly fruitful thus far.

Perhaps the easiest manner of determining whether a specific victim is suffering from PTSD - related symptoms only, versus organically based brain impairments involves analyzing the overall pattern of neuropsychological assessment results. For instance, if the victim demonstrates problems with motor or sensory abilities isolated on one side of the body (or other abilities governed by one hemisphere of the brain), such injuries are more likely to be the result of actual organic brain damage than because of interference in efficiency of thinking because of PTSD or other emotional distress.

The problem is frequently times not nearly so clear. Making matters worse, a victim may be experiencing both PTSD and organic brain injury. In these cases, a synergistic result can occur heightening dysfunction both in everyday life and on formal testing.

What must be recognized is that deficits can result from either organic brain injury or post-traumatic stress syndrome. Neuropsychological assessment can do much to identify the etiology of the deficits thereby permitting prompt treatment to ensue.

It should also be recognized that several mild TBI patients experience emotional distress, fatigue, depression and anxiety. After all, as the individual sustaining the traumatic brain injury becomes a more self-aware of the restrictions imposed by the injury, why would the individual not become depressed or experience emotional depress and anxiety? Fatigue in and of itself can cause of emotional alterations. Add processing speed slowness together with fatigue and a recipe for a emotional distress exists. Processing speed difficulties required deliberate effort of the victim to accomplish what was premorbidly accomplished automatically. The additional concentration required to accomplish even the simplest of tasks overwhelms and compounds to cause fatigue in the individual sustaining mild TBI. Irritability sets in.

It should also be recognized that the plethora of symptomology experienced by individual's sustaining mild TBI can similarly cause the onset of depression and anxiety. Awareness of changes in cognitive efficiency distinctly result in anxiety to the patient. Depression in virtually all minor TBI cases occurs within six months of the trauma, but may be delayed as self recognition of the injury develops. Depression severity results in a functional disability and can contribute to cognitive impairments. The simple fact that one has sustained and organic brain injury does not preclude the growth of emotional disorders. It is not one or the other. In virtually all cases, it is both. Unfortunately, a synergy of response to the awareness of organic brain injury can heighten anxiety, depression, a emotional distress and fatigue. Similarly, the symptoms of depression, anxiety, and emotional distress can exacerbate the cognitive deficits resulting from the organic brain injury. This circle of incapacitation renders the victim helpless.

In the litigation arena, it is similarly frequently forgotten that we injure the brains we already have. Any and all "personality flaws" pre-existing the trauma will likely be amplified following the traumatic brain injury. These "flaws" certainly will not improve with the traumatic brain injury. It has unfortunately become the defence of choice for the defence bar to argue that the cognitive deficits displayed by the plaintiff resulted not from the trauma but from pre-existing emotional disorders. It is thus absolutely essential that premorbid levels of function be determined and verified with all corroboration possible.

GERIATRIC CONSIDERATIONS

Organic Brain disorder may be because of a long-standing psychotic sickness that has persisted into older age or may present for the first time in later life in association with underlying medical conditions, especially dementia. Estimates of schizophrenia in the elderly population range from 0.1-0.5%. The prevalence of other psychotic syndromes such as paranoid ideation is higher, estimated at 4-6% in the elderly population, and is often linked with dementia. Patients with Alzheimer's disease have a especially high incidence of psychosis; 50% manifest psychotic symptoms within three years of diagnosis.

FOLLOW-UP AND HOME CARE AND REHABILITATION

When patients are discharged from a psychiatric hospital nurses furnish support and rehabilitation for the patient. Several of these patients call for only minimal support, with weekly or biweekly individual or family therapy and medication evaluation. Most of these clients, nevertheless, represent the chronically mentally sick population. They experience repeat hospitalizations and call for various support functions from the treatment team at the nurses. One of the most efficient and novel approaches community mental health care providers use is the programme for assertive community treatment. The key (e.g., psychopharmacology; individual supportive therapy; mobile crisis intervention), rehabilitation (e.g., behaviourally oriented skill teaching, support services for resuming education), and support services (e.g., legal and advocacy services, financial support, transportation). This approach has been described as a hospital without walls. The goal of this integrated program is to help patients with schizophrenia and related disorders, such as depression or substance abuse, stay out of psychiatric hospitals and live independently.

REFERENCES

Borge, L., Martinsen, E. W., Ruud, T., Watne, O., & Friis, S. (1999). Quality of life, loneliness, and social contact among long-term psychiatric patients. Psychiatric Services, 50(1), 81–84.

Finley, L. Y. (1998). The cultural context: Families coping with severe mental illness. Psychiatric Rehabilitation Journal, 21(3), 230–40.

Jordan, J. B. (1997). Mental health considerations with the Yupik Eskimo. Alaska Medicine, 39(3), 67–70.

Low, J. (1996). The concept of hardiness: A brief but critical commentary. Journal of Advanced Nursing, 24, 588–590.

Meadows, M. (1997). Mental health and medicine: Cultural considerations in treating Asians. Minority Nurse Newsletter, 4(4), 1–2.

Sims, E. M., Pernell-Arnold, A., Graham, R., et al. (1998). Principles of multicultural psychiatric rehabilitation services. Psychiatric Rehabilitation Journal, 21(3), 219–223.

Solomon, P., & Draine, J. (1995). Adaptive coping among family members of persons with serious mental illness. Psychiatric Services, 46(11), 1156–1160.

Tuck, I. (1997). The cultural context of mental health nursing. Issues in Mental Health Nursing, 18(3), 269–281.

13

Psychiatric Emergencies

A psychiatric emergency is an acute disturbance of behaviour, thought or mood of a patient which if untreated may lead to harm, either to the individual or to others in the environment. Thus the definition of a psychiatric emergency differs from other medical emergencies in that the danger of harm to the society is also taken into account. Emergencies may be classified as major, where there is a danger to life either of the patient or to others in his environment or minor where there is no menace to life but causes intense incapacitation.

TYPES OF PSYCHIATRIC EMERGENCIES AND THEIR MANAGEMENT

SUICIDE

The suicide risk is highest for primary psychiatric disorder and least for organic disorders with substance use disorders falling in between. Indian studies show that most people attempting suicide are in the age group of 15-30 years and are predicted to increase further in the coming years. Suicide is common in the unmarried (in the married the loss of spouse increases the risk during the first year of the loss). Rates are also high in the unemployed and in those suffering from a concurrent medical sickness. More men than women commit suicide although more women attempt it. Psychosocial factors that predispose to suicide, comprise, chaotic home environment, sudden loss (death, divorce, job, finances), recent humiliating life event, unfaithful partner, HIV and legal problems. In the young, suicides are common after declaration of the results of the board exams. The most common symptom in patients is hopelessness i.e. the belief that no action can save the patient from the trauma that he or she may be undergoing. A majority (56%) attempt suicide as an escape from an unbearable situation, 13% do so to produce a change in others or the environment and the rest have a combination of escape and manipulative motives. 50 to 80% of suicide attempters have communicated their intent to the family or to their treating psychiatrist.

All psychiatric patients need to be asked about suicidal ideation as a part of routine assessment. Self destructive behaviours and previous attempts are the most powerful predictors of a future suicidal attempt. It needs to be distinctly understood that asking about suicidal attempt does not provoke the patient to commit suicide or instil the idea of committing suicide. Several patients feel relieved on being asked about suicidal ideation and being explained that their ideas are part of a sickness. In case the patient has arrived in the emergency department with history of an attempt, then, first the medical condition of the patient needs to be assessed for risk to life and admitted to the ICU under escort till the medical condition stabilizes. At the earliest opportunity he is referred for assessment by a psychiatrist.

Seriously suicidal patients who are depressed need to be treated with electro-convulsive therapy (ECT). In Schizophrenia, apart from ECT, atypical antipsychotics such as clozapine are reported to be having a specific antidepressant and anti-suicidal effect. Crisis intervention centres and helplines are available in most cities all over the world. They furnish an avenue for the person contemplating suicide to ventilate his problems and enable the counsellor to persuade the patient to seek professional help. Nevertheless, a scientific validity of their usefulness is still lacking.

AGITATED AND VIOLENT PATIENTS

Violence is a danger frequently faced in the emergency room setting. The danger of violence is especially high in those societies where there is easier access to firearms and alcohol/drug abuse. The use of alcohol also predisposes to violence. Specific psychiatric and medical disorders have also been linked with violent behaviour. Several characteristics predict an assault in the emergency setting. Signs predicting an impending assault are anger, demanding immediate attention, loud voice, excitement, staring eyes, flared nostrils, flushed face, hands clenched or gripping, pacing about in the room, possessing weapons, pushing furniture, uncooperativeness and suspiciousness, slamming objects and sudden movements.

Drugs used for controlling aggression Nonspecific sedation may be required to first bring the patient under control before an assessment can be made. Emergency staff should be knowledgably about the administration of these drugs which should readily be available. If the patient is willing, drugs may be given orally, nevertheless, normally the parenteral route is essential. The most commongenerally used drug is haloperidol 10 mg given as a single intramuscular dose and can be safely repeated at intervals of every half hour to a maximum of 60 mg. Once the patient is under control, it is mandatory to carry out a careful physical examination and laboratory studies to exclude the common causes of violent behaviour enumerated earlier. Frequently, if the patient is accompanied by relatives or friends, the diagnosis may be revealed by history.

DELIRIUM

Delirium is managed with environmental manipulation to help orient the patient (e.g. leaving a light on at night, frequent orientation to time, place, and person) and with drugs. Drugs should be prescribed only after the underlying disorder has been diagnosed or the process of determining the diagnosis has been initiated. Haloperidol in low doses (0.5 to 2 mg) is often the drug of choice. Lorazepam 0.5 to 2 mg can reduce agitation and is preferable when substance withdrawal is the cause. Anticholinergic drugs (e.g., benztropine) should be used with caution in delirious patients, especially the elderly, because anticholinergic toxicity (atropine psychosis) can occur.

SUBSTANCE INTOXICATION AND WITHDRAWAL

It may occur with a psychiatric disorder or as a primary presenting complaint. Alcohol, cocaine and phencyclidine are the substances that most commongenerally lead to violent behaviour. Patients should be placed under observation in a secure room away from stimulation; attempting to talk the patient down is not recommended. Physical restraints or sedation may be essential for violent patients. Lorazepam 2 to 4 mg stat or diazepam 10 to 20 mg stat is recommended to treat agitation. Withdrawal from barbiturates, other sedatives and hypnotics (together with benzodiazepines) and alcohol are similar clinically.

When symptoms are intense, treatment in a hospital is safest and is mandatory if the patient is febrile (>38.3°C or 101°F), can't hold down fluids to prevent dehydration, or has a intense underlying physical disorder. Alcohol withdrawal can be life threatening. Seizures can occur. Delirium tremens, a withdrawal syndrome that starts within 7 days of withdrawal (normally within 24 to 72 h), is a medical emergency and should be treated in an ICU. Management is normally with high doses of benzodiazepines, parenteral thiamine and maintenance of fluid and electrolyte balance.

OVERDOSE OF PRESCRIBED PSYCHOACTIVE DRUGS

It can also pose a menace to life apart from causing intoxication. Hence, the patient should be jointly managed by a doctor and a psychiatrist. If the patient has taken a toxic dose and is awake, treatment consists of inducing emesis followed by administering activated charcoal. Overdose with tricyclic antidepressants or carbamazepine calls for cardiac monitoring. Overdose with barbiturates or benzodiazepines and alcohol may cause respiratory arrest. Antipsychotic drugs, at therapeutic as well as toxic doses, can cause acute extrapyramidal adverse effects together with dystonia, oculogyric crisis, torticollis, and akinesia. Akathisia is a common adverse effect of high-potency antipsychotics, when intense, it is accompanied by extreme anxiety or terror. Acute onset of oculogyric or orofacial dystonia in an otherwise healthy person may suggest meaningful or inadvertent ingestion of an antipsychotic. Immediate relief may be provided with a parenteral antihistaminic such as promethazine 25 mg IM.

NEUROLEPTIC MALIGNANT SYNDROME

It is a hypermetabolic reaction to dopamine antagonists, mainly antipsychotic drugs, such as phenothiazines and butyrophenones. It normally occurs early in treatment and rarely during maintenance treatment. It develops in up to 3% of patients began on antipsychotics. Risk is increased in agitated male patients who have received large and rapidly increased doses. No genetic component is evident. Its pathophysiologic basis is believed to be blockade of central dopamine receptors. Characteristic signs are muscle rigidity, hyperpyrexia, tachycardia, hypertension, tachypnea, change in mental status and autonomic dysfunction. Laboratory abnormalities comprise respiratory and metabolic acidosis, myoglobinuria, elevated CK and leucocytosis. Mortality rates are between 10 to 20%. Treatment comprises cessation of antipsychotic drugs, supportive care, and aggressive treatment of myoglobinuria, fever, and acidosis. The dopamine agonist bromocriptine 2.5 to 20 mg tid or dantrolene up to 10 mg/kg IV q 4 h may be used as a muscle relaxant. Treatment is normally in an ICU. After recovery, reintroduction of the antipsychotic drug retriggers the syndrome in up to 1/3 of patients.

SEROTONIN SYNDROME

It occurs when serotonergic agents are used in combination with MAOI inhibitors. A sudden build up of serotonin systemically may lead to a life threatening condition manifesting in hyperthermia, diaphoresis, excitement or confusion, hyperreflexia, hypotension, tremor. The condition may progress to DIC, rhabdomyolysis and cardiovascular collapse. Urgent medical management is essential. Drugs like dantrolene, a potent muscle relaxant and periactin, which is also a serotonin antagonist are useful.

The increasing incidence of alcohol and substance abuse in our country as well as the rise in levels of unipolar depression, have led to an increased number of patients reporting to the emergency care unit. It is essential for all clinicians to be knowledgable about common psychiatric emergencies especially suicide attempts and violent behaviour and other psychiatric emergencies so as to improve the level of care offered to the patients.

STRESS ADAPTATION MODEL

In psychiatry the stress adaptation model is a significant model of treating psychotic patients. Stuart has developed a model of stress adaptation that incorporates several of the ideas presented in stress theories and applies these ideas to nursing care.

This model comprises five components: predisposing factors, precipitating stressors, appraisal of stressor, coping resources or strategies, and coping mechanisms. Each factor plays a significant role in the continuum of coping reactions - some adaptive and others maladaptive- that the patient experiences. The goal is to assist the patient toward development and goal achievements by strengthening these five components:

1. Predisposing factors: Predisposing factors are biological, psychological, and sociocultural. They are "conditioning factors that influence both the type and amount of resources the person is able to use to handle stress."
2. Precipitating stressors: Precipitating stressors are "stimuli that the individual perceives as challenging, threatening, or demanding. They call for energy and produce a state of worry and stress with the individual. Stressors may be biological, psychological, or sociocultural, and for each patient they are internal and external.
   - For each patient, the timing of the experience is a critical factor- especially when the stressor occurs, its duration, and its frequency.
   - The number of stressors is also a critical factor. Some patients can tolerate several stressors at one time or over

a period of time; nevertheless, if the patient is in pain or confused, the patient may have less capability to deal with stress.

3. Appraisal of stressor: The appraisal of the stressor is the assessment of the stress experience. How the patient appraises the event is the key to understanding the patient's coping and the nature and intensity of the stress response. There is a danger in presuming to know how the patient is appraising a stressful event. This may lead to mistakes in the selection of interventions, and the patient may feel that the home care nurse is not really listening to the patient and together with the patient in the treatment process. Basically, reactions fall into the following classes:
   - Cognitive reactions: The patient's decision making is influencing by several factors such as emotions, physiological status, and beliefs and values. In general, the patient views a stressful event as a loss, a menace, or a challenge.
   - Affective reactions: The most frequent affective response to stress is anxiety. Depression and anger may also be experienced.
   - Physiological reactions: The fight-or-fight physiological response stimulates the sympathetic division of the autonomic nervous system and increases activity of the pituitary-adrenal axis. For patients with some medical problems (e.g., cardiac or respiratory), these reactions may have a direct effect on their physical status.
   - Behavioural reactions: The patient looks for the meaning of stressful event, and search for cause. These reactions are significant as the patient assesses his or her need for support.
4. Coping resources of strategies: There are quite a few critical questions related to coping resources: What options are available? What they accomplish? Can the patient use resources or strategies successfully? These coping resources comprise personal abilities, social support, material assets, positive beliefs, social skills, problem solving, health, and energy.
5. Coping mechanisms: Coping mechanisms can be constructive or destructive. The home care nurse should help the patient use constructive coping mechanisms. It is significant to

remember that different patients react to different interventions. Examples of simple interventions that might be used to increase constructive coping comprise the following:

- Assertiveness training
- Time management
- Anger management
- Conflict management
- Social problem solving
- Relaxation training

Another intervention approach is to use many types of interventions that combine behavioural, cognitive, and relaxation techniques. Diversion and relaxation might be used to deal with chaemotherapy, cancer, pain management, preparation for surgery or with a stressful medical procedure. Other techniques that might be used are teaching healthy eating and exercise, enhancing health-related treatment adherence, and controlling smoking and substance abuse.

GRIEF

Grief refers to the subjective emotions and affect that are a normal response to the experience of loss. Grieving, also known as bereavement, refers to the process by which an individual experiences the grief. It involves not only the content (what an individual thinks, says, and feels) but also the process (how an individual thinks, says, and feels). All people grieve when they experience life's changes and losses. Frequently, grieving is one of the most difficult and challenging processes of human existence; rarely is it comfortable or pleasant. Anticipatory grieving is when people facing an imminent loss begin to grapple with the very real possibility of the loss or death in the near future. Mourning is the outward expression of grief. Rituals of mourning-comprise having a wake, sitting shivah, holding religious ceremonies, and arranging funerals.

THEORIES OF GRIEVING

Kubler-Ross's Stages of Grieving

Elisabeth Kubler-Ross (1969) established a basis for understanding how loss affects human life. As she attended to clients with terminal illnesses, a process of dying became evident to her. Through observations of and work with dying clients and their families, Kubler-Ross developed a model of five stages to explain what people experience as they grieve and mourn:

- Denial is shock and disbelief regarding the loss.
- Anger may be expressed toward God, relatives, friends, or health care providers.
- Bargaining occurs when the person asks God or fate for more time to delay the inevitable loss.
- Depression results when awareness of the loss becomes acute.
- Acceptance occurs when the person shows evidence of coming to terms with death.

This model became a prototype for care providers as they looked for ways to understand and assist their clients in the grieving process.

Bowlby's Theory of Attachment Behaviours

John Bowlby, a British psychoanalyst, proposed a theory that human beings instinctively attain and retain affectional bonds with significant others through attachment behaviours, which are crucial to the growth of a sense of security and survival. Examples of attachment behaviours comprise following, clinging, calling out, and crying. Bowlby saw that human beings modified these attachment behaviours as they matured from childhood into adulthood, but that patterns of attachment behaviour formed early endure throughout the life cycle.

People experience the most severe emotions when forming a bond such as falling in love; maintaining a bond such as loving someone; disrupting a bond such as in a divorce; and renewing an attachment such as resolving a conflict or renewing a relationship. An attachment that is maintained is a source of security; an attachment that is renewed is a source of joy. When a bond is threatened or broken, nevertheless, the person responds with anxiety, protest, and anger. Actual loss leads to sorrow. As per Bowlby, these emotions reflect affectional bonds. Loss strongly activates or arouses attachment behaviours. Thus the clinical picture of increased anxiety, sorrow, anger, looking for the lost person or object, calling out, crying, and protesting is an attempt to restore the lost affectional bond through attachment behaviours.

PRINCIPLES

Nurses interact with clients responding to a myriad of losses along the continuum of health and sickness. Regardless of the type of loss, nurses must have a basic understanding of what is involved to meet the challenge that grief brings to clients. By understanding the phenomena that clients experience as they cope with the discomfort of loss, nurses may promote the expression and release of emotional as well as physical pain, thus supporting the grieving process. Supporting this process means ministering to psychological as well as physical needs.

The therapeutic relationship and therapeutic communication skills such as active listening are paramount when assisting grieving clients. Recognizing the verbal and nonverbal communication content of the various stages of grieving can help nurses to select interventions that will meet the client's psychological and physical needs.

TECHNIQUES OF COUNSELLING

Because the strong emotional attachment created in a significant relationship is not released easily, the loss of that relationship is a major crisis with momentous consequences. Aquilera and Messick (1982) developed a broad approach to assessment and intervention in their work on crisis intervention. The state of disequilibrium that a crisis produces causes great consternation, compelling the person to return to homeostasis, a state of equilibrium or balance. Factors that influence the grieving person's return to homeostasis are adequate perception of the situation, adequate situational support, and adequate coping. These factors help the person to regain balance and return to previous functioning or even to use the crisis as an opportunity to grow. Because any loss may be perceived as a personal crisis, it seems appropriate for the nurse to link understanding of crisis theory with the nursing process.

For the nurse to support and facilitate the grief process for clients, he or she must observe and listen for cognitive, emotional, spiritual, behavioural, and physiologic cues. Though the nurse must be knowledgable about the phases, tasks, and dimensions of human response to loss, he or she must realize that each client's experience is distinctive. Skilled communication is key to performing assessment and providing interventions. To meet clients' needs effectively, the nurse must examine his or her own personal attitudes, maintain an attentive presence, and furnish a psychologically safe environment for deeply intimate sharing. Awareness of one's own beliefs and attitudes is necessary so that the nurse can avoid imposing them on the client. Attentive presence is being with the client and focusing intently on communicating with and understanding him or her. The nurse can maintain attentive presence by utilizing open body language such as standing or sitting with arms down, facing the client, and maintaining moderate eye contact especially as the client speaks. Creating a psychologically safe environment comprises assuring the client of confidentiality, refraining from judging or giving specific advice, and permitting the client to share thoughts and feelings freely.

TYPES OF CRISIS

A crisis in life frequently appears like a bolt out of the blue. The sudden onset of sickness, the loss of a job or a death in the family can visit a man any time. These can throw a man's stable life into a chaotic state with no evident positive solution.

A crisis can be distinguished from a stressful event that may pass swiftly, such as exam. The most common defining features of a crisis are as follows:

- There is a triggering stress event or long-term stress.
- The individual experiences distress.
- There is a loss, danger or humiliation.
- There is a sense of uncontrollability.
- The events feel unexpected.
- There is a disruption of routine.
- There is uncertainty about the future.
- The distress continues over time (from about two to six weeks).

CRISIS INTERVENTION

Crisis intervention refers to the methods used to offer immediate, short-term help to persons who experience an event that produces emotional, mental, physical, and behavioural distress or problems. A crisis can refer to any situation in which the individual perceives a sudden loss of his or her capability to use effective problem-solving and coping skills. A number of events or circumstances can be regarded as a crisis: life-threatening situations, such as natural disasters (such as an earthquake or tornado), sexual assault or other criminal victimization; medical sickness; mental sickness; thoughts of suicide or homicide; and loss or drastic changes in relationships (death of a loved one or divorce, for instance).

- Mobilize a crisis intervention team in response to a significant critical incident, then actively implement the most appropriate crisis intervention tactics in response to observable signs or reported symptoms (evidence of need) of distress and/or dysfunction. It will be recalled that a crisis is a response, not an event. This phenomenological differentiation has direct tactical ramifications. Especially, the direct implementation of crisis intervention tactics is predicated upon evidence of human distress and/or dysfunction, not merely the occurrence of an event (critical incident). Distinctly some persons possess a natural resistance to extreme stress. Furthermore, several persons who are traumatized possess natural recovery mechanisms sufficient enough to preclude external psychological support.

- Not all signs and symptoms of acute distress are pathognomonic! It is significant that those implementing the crisis intervention be cognizant of putative criteria for psychological triage. More especially, it is significant to differentiate the signs and symptoms of acute stress which predict PTSD and those which don't.
- Tailor the crisis intervention to the needs of the individual(s). The great Johns Hopkins' doctor Sir William Osler once said "Where malignant disease is concerned, it may be more significant to understand what kind of person has the disease, rather than what kind of disease the person has." Once again it is argued that the most significant element of the critical incident - crisis response complex is the person and that person's idiosyncratic reaction to the critical incident. Cognitively oriented persons tend to call for emotional distance, information, and aid in problem-solving and re-establishing control as they recover from a crisis. Conversely, affectively oriented persons tend to prosper from cathartic ventilation and empathetically based interventions.
- Timing for crisis intervention is based upon psychological readiness, rather than the actual passage of time. A useful model for understanding the "timing" of crisis intervention is the model developed by Faberow and Gordon (1981). These authors describe four phases of a disaster:
  - Heroic Phase: This phase begins immediately upon the onset of the disaster and may even begin in anticipation of the impact of the event itself. It consists of efforts to protect lives and property.
  - Honeymoon Phase: This phase is characterized by optimism and thanksgiving. There is a sigh of relief as the realization of survival is appreciated. Congratulatory behaviour is common.

— Disillusionment Phase: This phase, which may begin as early as 3 - 4 weeks post disaster, is replete with the realization that something "disastrous" has really taken place. There is a great deal of "second-guessing" wherein anger, frustration, and even efforts to place blame are revealed. The question, "Why did this have to happen?" is frequently posed. Religious beliefs may be challenged. Here the mourning process actually begins. The development and growth of persons and communities is arrested. Stagnation is apparent. This phase may last weeks, months, or even years. For some, the phase never ends. It is the goal of crisis intervention to facilitate the transition from this disillusionment phase to the final phase.

— Reconstruction Phase: In this final phase, restoration of "normal" routine functioning is achieved. Memories of the disaster are not erased, but life does continue on. The development of persons and communities is continued. While the model described above was developed for understanding the human response to disasters, it will prove useful in understanding how persons psychologically progress through any crisis reaction. Obviously, the duration of each of these phases may be drastically constricted. However, the goal of crisis intervention remains the same whether in response to a mass disaster or an acute, isolated event.

— The final principle of crisis intervention is to select the best crisis intervention strategies and tactics:

- For the specific event,
- For the specific population affected, and
- Applied at the best respective times.

The Critical Incident Stress Management (CISM) approach to crisis intervention represents a complete, integrated, multicomponent crisis intervention system ideally suited to meet the demands of numerous and various critical incidents, experienced by numerous and various populations, anytime a crisis is in evidence.

The need for crisis intervention services is clear. Yet the efforts to furnish those services must well-timed and well measured. Crisis intervention services must complement and augment natural recovery and restorative mechanisms. They must not interfere with said mechanisms. This is true for wherever the crisis response is in evidence, whether for persons, organizations, or entire communities. Consideration of the aforementioned principles may assist the crisis worker in the most efficient application of crisis intervention strategies and tactics.

GERIATRIC CONSIDERATIONS

Among patients who are seen in the psychiatric emergency department, geriatric patients-defined as patients aged 65 years and older-are statistically underrepresented. Geriatric individuals account for only 5 to 6 percent of all psychiatric emergency service visitors-although they account for about 12 percent of the population at large and represent the fastest growing segment of the population.

In addition to differences in demographic characteristics-such as the gender imbalance (more females than males) or the preponderance of patients with a fixed income-other special considerations exist for geriatric patients in the psychiatric emergency service. First is the high rate of comorbid medical and neurological problems, which can be chronic or acute. Behavioural disturbances can result from major medical problems, such as stroke, and from relatively minor problems, such as urinary tract infection. The increased danger of medical problems carries with it a danger of adverse drug reactions from the simultaneous use of multiple medications. The psychiatric consultant must be vigilant in screening for medical and neurological problems or be confident that the other doctors in the emergency department have already addressed them.

Geriatric patients are also at danger of pharmacological emergencies-medical emergencies that are related to psychiatric medications. Possible problems comprise agranulocytosis secondary to antipsychotics, hypotension or cardiac conduction disturbances that are caused by the use of antipsychotics or antidepressants, neuroleptic malignant syndrome, lithium toxicity, anticholinergic delirium, and acute dystonia.

Another critical factor in evaluating geriatric patients in the psychiatric emergency service is the danger of suicide, which is much higher among geriatric patients than younger patients. The suicide rate for white men aged 80 to 84 years is six times that of the general adult population. Clinicians in the psychiatric emergency service need to calibrate their index of concern about the danger of completed suicide for elderly psychiatric emergency service patients who present with depression, alcohol abuse, or other risk factors for suicide.

ROLE AND RESPONSIBILITIES OF NURSE

- Establishing the situational context: It is no accident that more patients from nursing homes are referred to the emergency psychiatric service on Friday nights than on any other night of the week. Normally, Friday evening is when staffing levels and programming decline for the weekend, which leads to an increased likelihood that nursing home residents will become symptomatic and that staff members will worry about their capacity to handle residents' problem behaviours. Only 5 percent of individuals who are aged 65 years and older live in nursing homes; nevertheless, the prevalence of psychiatric disorders in these settings is at least 80 percent. Resources to take care of patients with psychiatric sickness-together with training and supervising caregivers as well as having access to psychiatric consultation-may be lacking. The same resource shortages could be true for caregivers in the home.
- Communicating with third parties: Taking the presenting complaint of the referral source seriously. In the evaluation of children, the involvement of parents, teachers, and other persons is taken for granted-if only for legal reasons. Nevertheless, in the evaluation of an older person, family members' or caregivers' input is frequently invaluable in determining a pattern of behavioural change-such as threatening or assaultive behaviours toward caregivers or roommates-that easily escapes a one-point observation. Obtaining consent and calling family members, primary care physicians, visiting nurses, adult protective workers, and other parties should be part of the protocol for evaluating geriatric patients. Most elderly patients don't come to the psychiatric emergency service on their own but are brought in by family members or others. Elderly patients may minimize or outright deny significant issues, such as environmental problems-together with changes in the home environment-and psychiatric symptoms.
- Determining the accompanying psychopathology: Rarely will an older person develop new psychiatric symptoms without precipitants. For example, a new onset of psychotic symptoms demands an evaluation of cognitive functions to determine whether underlying dementia or delirium exists. Attention to the milieu interne and milieu externe is critical. An infectious disease, a transient ischemic episode, a change of cardiovascular

medication, the loss of a pet, or the death of a roommate in the nursing home can trigger a psychiatric crisis. As with younger patients, it is appropriate to screen for affective and anxiety symptoms-such as changes in sleep, appetite, energy, and mood-as well as psychotic symptoms-such as auditory hallucinations and paranoid ideation.

- Assessing cognitive functioning: The Folstein Mini-Mental State Examination is a brief objective screen for cognitive impairment. Although behavioural problems, not memory problems, lead to admission to the psychiatric emergency service, a cognitive evaluation is mandatory for each geriatric patient. The presenting complaint of the referral source should be taken seriously. Nursing home staff members are all too swiftly accused of "dumping" patients. Nevertheless, nursing home staff members can't rationally be expected to manage an agitated patient with dementia who threatens to assault staff or his roommate. Combativeness among elderly people with dementia is dangerous and calls for a high level of staff monitoring as well as access to psychopharmacological medication, seclusion rooms, and restraints, which are available only in a hospital setting.
- Suspecting extrinsic substances: Elderly patients receive a disproportionate number of prescribed medications. Polypharmacy is probably the most common reason for delirium in the elderly patient, and a review of all medications in the patient's nursing home chart or in the home medicine cabinet is essential. Older individuals have a reduced tolerance for the central nervous system effects of prescribed medications and of alcohol and street drugs. Although substance abuse seems to be less common among elderly individuals, intoxication and withdrawal should be regarded as in the differential diagnosis for patients who present in a psychiatric emergency service, irrespective of their age. Also, a breath analysis and urine drug screens should be obtained if substance abuse is suspected.
- Screening carefully for suicidal ideation and behaviour: Among geriatric patients, compared with other age groups, suicidal action is highly correlated with lethal outcomes. Mood disorders are common among older psychiatric patients, and the presenting affect, even in a manic state, is more frequently dysphoric compared with that of younger patients. Other risk

factors for suicide, such as being unmarried and having a chronic medical sickness, are also common in this population.

- Considering the situation that awaits the patient after discharge from the psychiatric emergency service; Questions to be considered comprise: Did this patient's home situation contribute to admission to the psychiatric emergency service? If so, has the home situation changed? Evaluators should try to put themselves in the patient's and caregiver's shoes. For example, the case should be handled as it would if it involved a family member. The presence of an outreach team can dramatically alter the disposition options.
- Considering the possibility of elder abuse: The patient may be the carrier of symptoms for a dysfunctional social unit. The elderly person with "failure to thrive" or with multiple falls shouldn't be too swiftly seen as depressed. Memory impairment or intimidation can disguise recent abuse by the spouse, adult children or grandchildren, and others. The patient should be interviewed separately from the caregivers after the initial part of the interview and screened for abuse.
- Getting a second opinion when in doubt: Older patients may not be routinely seen in the psychiatric emergency service. So that a significant aspect of a geropsychiatric assessment will not be missed, a consultation with a colleague may be helpful. An internist or family practitioner with experience in geriatrics may be especially helpful in dealing with medical and psychosocial problems.
- Documenting the dispositional decision and its rationale, and communicate it to the referral source: An attempt should be made to give the patient's caregivers and primary care doctor a copy of any notes relating to the dispositional decision and its rationale. The failure to communicate across institutional or disciplinary boundaries creates specific problems for older individuals who are served by a variety of systems or agencies.

REFERENCES

Chow, T. W., & Cummings, J. L. (2000). Neuropsychiatry: Clinical assessment and approach to diagnosis. In B. J. Sadock & V. A. Sadock (Eds.), Comprehensive textbook of psychiatry, Vol. 1 (7th ed., pp. 221–253). Philadelphia: Lippincott Williams & Wilkins.

Hanna, D. R. & Roy, Sr. C. (2001). Roy adaptation model and perspectives on family. Nursing Science Quarterly, 14(1), 9–13.

McBride, L. & Walden-McBride, D. (1995). Balancing the heart of patient care. Home Healthcare Nurse, 13(4), 46–49.

Schultz, J. M., & Videbeck, S. (2002). Lippincott's manual of psychiatric nursing care plans (6th ed.). Philadelphia: Lippincott Williams, & Wilkins.

Schutle, N. S. & Malouff, J. M. (1995). Sourcebook of adult assessment strategies. New York: Plenum Press.

14

Legal Issues in Mental Health Nursing

Nurses, therapists, and other health care workers are expected to make informed and effective patient care decisions swiftly by using rational problem solving skills. Historically, the care of those deemed mentally sick included questionable practices and involved the loss of individual rights. Ethical and legal issues concerning nurse-client relationships were identified and subsequently addressed by the nursing profession. For instance, nursing as a profession is influenced in each state by legislative acts referred to as Nurse Practice Acts.

The everyday practice of psychiatric mental health nursing is full of value-laden decisions requiring the use of critical thinking skills. Such decisions demand knowledge of the law, especially the rights of clients, their legal status, and the prescribed quality of their care.

THE MENTAL HEALTH ACT, 1987

Aim: To consolidate and amend the law relating to the treatment and care of mentally ill person, to make better provisions with respect to their property and affairs and for matters connected therewith or incidental thereto.

It has 10 Chapters

Chapter I: Preliminary

Chapter II: Mental Health Authorities

Chapter III: Psychiatric Hospitals and Psychiatric Nursing Homes

Chapter IV: Admission and Detention in Psychiatric Hospital or Psychiatric Nursing Home

Chapter V: Inspection, Discharge, Leave of Absence and Removal of Mentally Ill Persons.

Chapter VI: Judicial Inquisition Regarding Alleged Mentally Ill person Possessing Property, custody of his Person & Management of his Property.

Chapter VII: Liability to meet cost of maintenance of Mentally Ill persons detained Psychiatric Hospital or Psychiatric Nursing Home.

Chapter VIII: Protection of Human Rights of Mentally Ill Persons.

Chapter IX: Penalties and Procedure.

Chapter X: Miscellaneous.

V. It is called the Mental Health Act 1987 & came into force with effect from 1.4.93 in all the States and Union Territories.

VI. Mental Health Authorities:

i. Central Authority for Mental Health Services: - established by the Central Government.

ii. State Authority for Mental Health Services - established by the State Government.

Authority shall-

5. Be in charge of regulation development, direction and Coordination with respect to Mental Health Services under the Central Government and all other matters Concerning Central Government/authority/sub. ordinate to Central Government.
6. Supervise Psychiatric Hospital/Psychiatric Nursing Homes/other Mental Health Service agencies under the Control of Central Government/State Government respectively.
7. Advice the Central Government/State Government in all matters relating to Mental Health.
8. Discharge such other functions with respect to matters relating to mental health as the Central Government/State Government may require.

VII. Psychiatric Hospitals and Psychiatric Nursing Homes:

i. Establishment or maintenance of psychiatric hospital/ nursing home by the Central Government/State Government. Within the limits of its jurisdiction for the admission, treatment and care of mentally ill persons at such places as it may think fit.

ii. Establishment or maintenance of psychiatric hospital/ nursing home only with license under this Act.

iii. Application for license:

4. Every person holding a license under this act; if wishes to continue after the expiry of person the nursing home/hospital should apply at least one month before the date of expiry to issue a fresh license.
5. A person who intends to establish or maintain such nursing home/hospital shall apply to the licensing authority for the grant of license.
6. Every application should be of the prescribed format with the prescribed fee.

iv. Grant or refusal of license:

The licensing authority should be satisfied in matters relating to

4. Establishment/maintenance
5. Minimum facilities provided which are proscribed for the admission, treatment and care for mentally ill persons &
6. The hospital/nursing home should be under the control of medical officers.

If not satisfied on the above aspects the licensing authority can cancel the orders after giving a reasonable chance for hearing.

Duration of renewal of license:

The psychiatric hospital/nursing home shall be maintained in accordance with conditions laid down in the Act.

The licensing authority can revoke the license by an order in writing if it is satisfied that the hospital/nursing home is not maintained in accordance with the Act. If it is against the moral, mental or physical well being of the inpatients thereof after giving a reasonable opportunity of being heard.

An appeal can be made on such revocation with such period of time.

The appeal can be made in a prescribed format with a prescribed fee.

VIII. It has got 3 parts. The first part being admission

c. On voluntary basis - Requisition by major for admission as voluntary patient. So any person who considers himself as mentally ill can apply to a medical officer-in-charge for being admitted as voluntary patient in the hospital/ nursing home.

d. Requisition made by the Guardian for admission of a ward whom he considers as mentally ill to be admitted in a hospital or nursing home. In both the cases the medical officer on receipt of such application conduct an enquiry within a period of 24 hrs may admit such an applicant. The patient should abide by the regulations made by the medical officer.

I. Admission under special circumstance: So if a mentally ill person is unable to express his willingness for admission, he may be admitted on an application made by a relative of such a person in a prescribed format accompanied by two medical certificates by two medical practitioners.

II. Reception orders on application - A medical officer in charge of a hospital/nursing home, husband, wife or any relative of such person shall apply to the magistrate for the detention of such a person and a reception order.

Chapter V deals with inspection, discharge, leave of absence and removal of mentally ill person.

The State government/Central Government shall appoint not less than five visitors for the inspection of hospital/nursing home. Not less than 3 visitors shall make a joint inspection of every part of the hospital/ nursing home at least once in every month. If such a visitor does not participate in such an inspection for 3 consecutive months, he shall cease to hold the office.

In case of inspection of mentally ill prisoners all the 3 visitors should visit at least once in three months in the place where he is detained.

Part II deals with discharge of mentally ill person.

The medical officer in charge may direct the discharge of any person other than a voluntary patient by an order in writing based on the recommendations made by two medical practitioners. In case if a person is admitted by the application made under this Act, shall be discharged only if an application is made to the medical officer by the concerned person.

Any person not being ill prisoner who feels that he has recovered from his mental illness may make an application for his discharge.

Part III deals with leave of absence of medically ill person from a psychiatrist hospital may be made by an application by the husband or wife or relatives or any other person related to the medical officer. If the medical officer refuses to grant leave of absence, the applicant may apply to the magistrate within the local limit.

The application should be of the prescribed format.

Chapter VI deals with the property of the mentally ill person.

If a mentally ill person possess a property, it can be taken care of by any of his relatives or by public curator or by the advocate general of the state concerned or by the collector of the district in case the property is a land, by means of an application to the district court which shall pass order after examining the concerned mentally ill person personally. If the district court finds the mentally ill person incapable of maintaining his property may appoint a guardian to take care of the person and a manager for his property who shall within a period of six months from the date of appointment gives a statement of all claims due and all debts and liabilities due by such mentally ill person. He should also within a period of three months from the close of the financial year an account of property, sums received and disbursed.

Chapter VII deals with the cost of maintenance of a mentally ill person.

The cost of maintenance unless otherwise provided by the law should be borne by the state. In case of a mentally il person having an estate or the person bound to maintain a mentally ill person has a means to maintain shall apply to the concerned government or to the district court for a direction to tear the cost of maintenance of such mentally ill person.

Chapter VIII deals with the protection of human rights of mentally ill person.

No mentally ill person should be treated with indignity or cruelty during the treatment. No mentally ill person shall be used for research unless otherwise for the benefit of such person or with the acceptance of such person in writing. In case of the person is incompetent because of minority or otherwise, with the consent of the guardian.

Chapter IX deals with penalties and procedures:

Any person establishes or maintains such nursing home or hospital in contravention of the Act, shall be punishable with an imprisonment of 3 months or with fine or with both.

Any person who detains mentally ill person otherwise than in accordance with the Act, shall be punishable with imprisonment for two years or with a fine of Rs. 1000/- or with both.

Any other person who contravenes any of the provision of the Act for which no penalty is expressly provided shall be punishable with an imprisonment for a period of 6 months or with a fine of Rs. 500/- or with both.

AIM

The main object of the Mental Health Act 1987 is to implement and regulate:

i. Admission to psychiatric hospitals or psychiatric nursing homes of mentally ill-persons who do not have sufficient understanding to seek treatment on a voluntary basis, and to protect the rights of such persons while being detained;

ii. To protect society from the presence of mentally ill persons who have become or might become a danger or nuisance to others;

iii. To protect citizens from being detained in psychiatric hospitals or psychiatric nursing homes without sufficient cause;

iv. To regulate responsibility for maintenance charges of mentally ill persons who are admitted to psychiatric hospitals or psychiatric nursing homes;

iv. To provide facilities for establishing guardianship or custody of mentally ill persons who are incapable of managing their own affairs;

vi. To provide for the establishment of Central Authority and State Authorities for Mental Health Services;

vii. To regulate the powers of the Government for establishing, licensing and controlling psychiatric hospitals and psychiatric nursing homes for mentally ill persons;

viii. To provide for legal aid to mentally ill persons at State expense in certain cases.

As per section 5 of the Act the Central Government may, in any part of India, or the State Government may, within the limits of its jurisdiction, establish or maintain psychiatric hospitals or psychiatric nursing homes for the admission, treatment and care of mentally ill persons at such places as it thinks fit and separate psychiatric hospitals and psychiatric nursing homes may be established or maintained for: (a) those who are under the age of sixteen years; (b) those who are addicted to alcohol or other drugs which lead to behavioural changes in a person; (c) those who have been convicted of any offence and (d) those belonging to such other class or category of persons as may be prescribed.

Section 6 of the Act stipulates that no person shall establish or maintain a psychiatric hospital or psychiatric nursing home unless he holds a valid license granted to him under this Act but this clause is not applicable to a psychiatric hospital or psychiatric nursing home established or maintained by the Central Government or a State Government.

Does this mean that all general hospitals and general nursing homes that also treat psychiatric patients have to be registered under the Mental Health Act? The answer to this question lies in section 2(q) of the Act which defines the words 'psychiatric hospital' and 'psychiatric nursing home'. A 'psychiatric hospital' or 'psychiatric nursing home' means a hospital or as the case may be, a nursing home established or maintained by the Government or any other person for the treatment and care of mentally ill persons and includes a convalescent home established or maintained by the Government or any other person for such mentally ill reasons; but does not include any general hospital or general nursing home established or maintained by the Government and which provides also for psychiatric services.

If this definition is analysed it is very clear that any general hospital or general nursing home established or maintained ONLY by the Government which provides also for psychiatric services is considered not to be a 'psychiatric hospital' or 'psychiatric nursing home'. Here the words 'or any other person' has been expressly omitted by the statute. Therefore all non-government general hospital or general nursing homes which also cater to psychiatric patients do not fall within the ambit of the exclusion clause. Hence they have to be registered under the Act as they are deemed to be 'psychiatric hospitals' or 'psychiatric nursing homes'.

The next question that automatically comes up is whether the hospitals created and maintained by the municipal corporations need to be registered under the Act?

If the Act is minutely read the word 'Government' refers to the Central or the State Government and does not refer to the municipal corporation. In statues, municipal corporations are expressly referred to 'Local Self-Governing Bodies'. There is no such reference any where in the Act. Therefore hospitals and nursing homes run by such local self-governing bodies or Municipal Corporations also need to be registered under the Act. What happens when the Hospitals and Nursing Homes have only OPDs catering to psychiatric patients and do not have any psychiatric wards? Do they need to be registered under the Act?

Section 2(q) clearly states that hospitals and/or nursing homes where mentally ill patients are treated or cared for, in the eyes of law, are 'psychiatric hospitals/nursing homes'. In OPDs mentally ill patients are not only examined and diagnosed but are also treated inasmuch as electro-convulsive therapy is also given on OPD basis. Therefore such hospitals and nursing homes also need to be registered.

Any person who establishes or maintains a psychiatric hospital or psychiatric nursing home in contravention of the provisions of the Act shall, on conviction, be punishable with imprisonment for a term which may extend to three months, or with fine which may extend to two hundred rupees, or with both, and in the case of a second or subsequent offence, with imprisonment for a term which may extend to six months, or with fine which may extend to one thousand rupees, or with both.

Whoever, after conviction continues to maintain a psychiatric hospital or psychiatric nursing home in contravention of the provisions of the Act shall, on conviction, be punishable with fine which may extend to one hundred rupees, for every day after the first day during which the contravention is continued.

INDIAN LUNACY ACT. 1912

Lunatic Asylum act, Act 36 of 1856 was modified to form Indian Lunacy Act, Act 4 of 1912. The enactment of act resulted in opening of new asylums and improvement in the condition of asylums. The name lunatic asylum was changed to mental hospital in 1920. In 1946, the Bhore committee recommended changes in Indian Lunacy Act 1912, as it had become outdated. Indian Psychiatric Society formed in January 1947 quickly acted on the recommendation and a committee consisted of Dr. J. Roy, major R. B Davis, Dr. Hasib was formed. It was finally enacted on 22nd May 1987.

RIGHTS OF MENTALLY ILL CLIENTS

Since the dawn of human civilization, mentally sick patients have received the scant care and concern of the community due to their unproductive value in the socio-economic value system. They have not only been neglected but received step motherly treatment from the health planners especially in the developing countries. It was only after the plea of progressive incorporation of the norms of human rights and liberal jurisprudence in the respective legal system of nation states that has created the urgency and necessity of initiating appropriate steps for the care and treatment of mentally sick individuals. Thus as a result of the development of humanistic values it is now admitted on all hands that a mentally sick person needs more care and concern for his treatment and well being. Due to the social interests involved in ameliorating their conditions, the founding fathers of the Constitution directed the future government to continuously work for improving public health.

The provisions relating to the human rights of mentally sick patients have hitherto been neither especially documented in any code nor been prescribed or elaborated by Judiciary in India. But it is admitted on all hands that barring few exceptions, the mentally sick person deserves the same privileges as enjoyed by any other human being. They comprise a right to better and more accessible care, to good recovery and increased hopes of reintegration into society. Nevertheless, the Stigma, residual disability and its intolerance, and more importantly the inability of the mentally sick to protest against exploitation, have all made basic human rights of the mentally sick a major cause of growing concern. The term human rights in a broad sense mean "those claims which every individual has or should have upon the society in which he/she lives.

As per Richard Wasserstorm it means, one ought to be able to claims as entitlements (i.e. human rights) those minimal things without which it is impossible to develop ones capabilities and to live life as human beings. Thus Human Rights is about balancing the rights of all of us as individual within the community. In the context of mentally sick individuals, it not only refers to their privileges but remedial right of protection against infringement of their human and other statutory rights. Nevertheless, the Human Rights of mentally sick individuals can be discussed under the following heads:

1. Right to Health and the Constitution of India

As Citizens of India, they are entitled to all those human and fundamental rights which are guaranteed to each and every citizen by the Constitution of India, to the degree their disability don't prevent them from enjoying those rights or their enjoyment is expressly or impliedly barred by the Constitution or by any other statutory law. The fundamental right to life and liberty as interpreted by the Supreme Court of India in number of landmark cases comprises the right to live with human dignity and the right to health. The Supreme Court has also laid down the maintenance and improvement of public health is one of the obligations that flow from Article 21 of the Constitution. This means that mentally sick have the fundamental/human right to receive equality mental health care and to humane living conditions in the mental hospitals. The right to life in Article 21 of the Constitution means something more than survival of animal existence. It would comprise within its ambit the right to live with human dignity, right to health, right to potable water, right to pollution free environment and right to education etc., which have been held to be part of right to life. In the context of mentally sick person, apart from above narrated rights, it also comprises right to live, work as far as possible in the community, to privacy and to lead a normal family life. The seriously mentally sick are a very special group with disabilities. The concern with this group are two folds not only providing the privileges to live in society along with other citizens but also ensuring their right to protection from exploitation.

2. i. Right to Health as a Basic Human Right and International Covenant:

The United Nations has defined human rights to mean in general as "those rights, which are inherent in our nature and without which we can't live as human beings. Section 2(d) of the protection of Human Rights Act, 1993 has defined the human rights to mean the rights relating to life, liberty, equality and dignity of the individual guaranteed under the Constitution or embodied in the international covenants and enforceable by the courts in India. In 1948, the United Nations through its Declaration of Human Rights affirmed the basic principle that a mentally sick person should at all times be treated with humanity and respect for the inherent dignity of the person. Every person with a mental sickness should have the right to exercise all civil, political, social and cultural rights. The Declaration of the Rights of the disable, which comprises person with mental sickness was adopted by the United Nations in 1975.

Article 12 of the International Covenant on Economic, Social and Cultural Rights, 1966 also provides "that the state parties to the present Covenant recognize the rights of everyone to the enjoyment of highest attainable standards of physical and mental health. As far as women mentally sick patients are concerned, Article 12 of the Convention on the Elimination of all forms of discrimination against women provides that state parties shall take all appropriate measures to eliminate discrimination against women in the discipline of health. In the area of providing access to free medical services to mentally sick patients Article 19 of 969 Declaration on Social progress and Growth could be relied upon, which calls for the provision of free health services of the whole population and of adequate preventive and curative facilities and welfare medical services accessible to all.

ii. The 1971 Declaration on the Rights of Mentally Retarded Persons:

This Declaration was adopted by the General Assembly on 20th December 1971, keeping in view the necessity of providing help to mentally retarded persons in order to enable them to develop their abilities and promoting their integration in the normal life. The Declaration provides a model within which national and international actions should be initiated for the advancement of rights set forth in the Declaration

The Declaration lays down following principles:

1. The mentally retarded persons has to the maximum degrees of feasibility the same rights as other human beings.
2. The mentally retarded person has a right to proper medical care and physical therapy and to such education, training, rehabilitation and guidance as will enable him to develop his ability and maximum potential.
3. The mentally retarded person has a right to economic security and to a decent standard of living. He has a right to perform productive work or to engage in any other meaningful occupation to the fullest possible degree of his capabilities.
4. The mentally retarded person, whenever possible should live with his own family, or with foster parents and partake in different forms of community life. The family with which he lives should be provided with aid.
5. The mentally retarded person has a right to qualified guardian when this is required to protect his personal well being and interests.
6. Disabled persons are entitled to have their special need taken into consideration at all stage of economic and social planning.
7. Disabled persons have the right to live with their families or with foster parents an to partake in all social, creative or recreational activities.
8. Disabled persons shall be protected against all exploitation, and treatment of a discriminatory, abusive or degrading nature.
9. Disabled persons shall be able to avail themselves of qualified legal aid when such aid proves indispensable for the protection

of their person and property. If judicial proceeding are instituted against them, the legal procedure applied shall take their physical and mental condition fully into account.

iii. International Year of Disabled Persons(1981)

The General Assembly on 16th December 1978, decided to observe the Year 1981 as International Year for Disabled persons with the following objective:

1. Helping disabled persons in their physical and psychological adjustment to society.
2. Promoting all national and international efforts to furnish disabled persons with proper assistance, training, care and guidance, to make available to them opportunities for suitable work and to ensure their full integration in society.
3. Encouraging study and research projects designed to facilitate the practical participation of disabled persons in daily life, for instance, for improving their access to public buildings and transportation systems.
4. Training and informing the public of the rights of disabled persons to partake in and contribute to various aspect of economic, social and political life.
5. Promoting effective measures for the prevention of disability for the rehabilitation of disabled persons.

3. Human Rights and Mental Health Act, 1987

Chapter VIII of this Act contains a very novel and explicit provision of protection of human rights of mentally sick persons. Section 81 provides that-

1. No mentally sick persons shall be subjected during treatment to any indignity whether physical or mental or cruelty.
2. No mentally sick person under treatment hall be used for the purpose or research unless (i) such research is of direct benefit to him for the purpose of diagnosis or treatment, or (ii) such person being a voluntary patient has given his consent in writing or where such person is incompetent by reason of minority or otherwise to give valid consent, on his behalf, has given his consent in writing, for such research.
3. Subject to any rules made in this behalf under Section 94 for the purpose of preventing vexatious or defamatory.

Communication or Communications pre-judicial to the treatment of mentally sick persons, no letter or other communications sent by or to a mentally sick persons under treatment shall be intercepted, detained or destroyed. The doctrine of informed consent is partially recognized under the Mental Health Act 1987, when a patient voluntarily admits himself in the hospital or accepts treatment without any admission.

When a mentally sick patient detained as an in-patient and does not have property to bear the cost of treatment, in such cases his expenses shall be borne by the Government of the State. (Sec. 78) If a mentally sick patient owns a property and he is not in a position to manage his property, the Court may entrust the management of such property to the Court of wards, Section 54(1). Under Section 97 of the Act when a mentally sick person is not represented by a legal practitioner in any proceedings under Mental Health Act 1987 before a District Court or a Magistrate and such a patient does not have sufficient mean to engage a legal practitioner then the District Court or Magistrate shall assign a legal practitioner to represent him at the expense of the State.

The above provisions clearly indicate that the Act does not spell out much on Human Rights, nor does it covers neglect or cruelty to mental patient sustained in families or alternate system of care like magicians, healers and quacks. The Mental Health Act 1987 also does not spell out any enforceable right of the mentally sick to minimum standard of care and treatment. The Good faith clause (Section 92) dispenses with accountability of the government or its servants for any negligence in the care and treatment of inmates of asylums. The provision for legal aid to the mentally sick (Section 91) restricts the facility to proceedings before a District Court or a Magistrate. The Act is silent on the right to legal aid and counselling at all stages together with the facility of approaching the High Court or the Supreme Court.

The Mental Health Act also by its definition of mentally sick persons excludes from its regime the mentally retarded. It also does not differentiate between the various degrees of mental sickness that calls for specialized care and treatment. Nevertheless, it permits the commitment to hospitals of the criminal mentally sick. It makes no special provision for their care, treatment and discharge. Beside the above, there is no provision for compensating those wrongfully incarcerated or negligently treated or victimized in any manner by misuse of powers under the Act. Another significant shortcoming in this context is that there is no right to rehabilitation of those mentally sick discharged after being found fit,

It is submitted that it is a matter of great regret that judiciary in India was given opportunities in number of public interests litigations filed and which were relating to inmates of mentally sick patients, but it didn't dare to enumerate the human rights of mentally sick patients. On the aspect of judicial intervention, the Supreme Court concerning the management of mental hospitals decided the following cases-

1. In B.R. Kapoor v. Union of India and PUCL v. Union of India, both relating to functioning of the hospitals for mental diseases, Shahdara, Delhi.
2. R.C. Narayan v. State of Bihar and the order dated 11.11.97 the case concerning the Ranchi Mental Asylum.
3. Supreme Court Legal Aid Committee v. State of MP where the Supreme Court intervened to improve the working of the Gwalior Mental Asylum.

The subject of health falls under the concurrent list in the Indian Constitution empowering both the centre and states to introduce measures together with the authority to legislate. The Mental Health Act 1987 is civil rights legislation with a focus on regulating standards in mental health institutions. There are serious questions over the effectiveness of this Act in ensuring protection to person's property and management of persons covered.

A perusal of the above referred cases clearly revel that till recently several mentally sick persons were consigned to jails and those living in mental health institutions were no better off, as the conditions both in prisons and in mental institutions were far below the stipulated standards. Sheela Barse v. Union of India concerned the detention of non-criminal mentally sick persons in the jails of West Bersal. The appalling conditions in which they were held was noted by the Supreme Court which observed that admission of non-criminal mentally sick persons to jails is illegal and unconstitutional.

Similarly in Chandan Kumar v. State of West Bersal the Supreme Court heard of the inhuman conditions in which mentally sick persons were held in mental hospital at mankaundi in the District of Hooghli. The Court denounced this practice and ordered the cessation of the practice of tying up the patients who wee unruly or not physically controllable with iron chains and ordered medical treatment for these patients. Nevertheless on August 6th 2001 the indifference of state and private authorities resulted in the tragic death of 26 patients in Erwadi as they were tied to their beds when fire engulfed the building. Following this tragedy the National Human Rights Commission of India(NHRC) advised all the Chief Ministers to submit a certificate stating no person with mental sickness are kept chained in either government and private institutions.

The NHRC is mandated under section 12 of the protection of Human Rights Act 1993 to visit government run mental hospital to study the living conditions of inmates and make recommendation thereon. In 1997 project quality assurance in Mental Health Institutions was initiated to analyze the conditions in general persisting in 37 government run mental hospitals and departments. The findings of this study confirm that mental hospitals in India are still being managed and administered on a custodial mode of care. Characters sized by prison like structure with high walls, watch towers, fenced wards and locked cells. Mental Hospitals are like detention centres where persons with mental sickness are kept caged in order to protect society from the danger their existence poses.

The above discussion has clearly pointed out that each of these cases reached the Supreme Court at different point of times through public litigation. Nevertheless, in these cases, there was no mention of the rights of the inmates to minimum standards of care and treatment. Nevertheless, the cases have demonstrated the need for continued judicial monitoring in order to ensure that the state acts in accordance with the statute and the Constitution.

FORENSIC PSYCHIATRY

Forensic psychiatry is a sub-specialty of psychiatry. It encompasses the interface between law and psychiatry. Some practitioners of forensic psychiatry have taken extra training in that specific area. An expanding area of competence assessment is informed consent, which manifests itself in issues ranging from the right to refuse treatment to the right to receive high-cost treatment. The informed-consent model is being adapted for other issues as well, such as the competence of mentally sick or mentally retarded persons to consent to sexual relations in or out of institutions. Meanwhile, the seemingly straightforward question of competence to give informed consent has taken on depth and complexity with the recognition of selective competence. For instance, a patient whose competence is impaired at the affective level by bipolar disorder may incompetently refuse treatment with lithium even while being able to recite accurately the risks and benefits of the drug. In a manic state, the possibility of needing the medication may not 'feel real' to the patient. While depressed, the patient may feel too dispirited and worthless to apply the information he possesses.

This recognition that informed consent is not an easy matter prompts reconsideration of what constitutes an adequate informed-consent process. If a person's whole capacities need to be engaged for competent consent to be given, then merely having the patient sign a form is insufficient. Such pro forma informed consent minimally addresses the cognitive dimension, but does not bring about the kind of deep understanding on the patient's part that calls for affective as well as cognitive engagement. Indeed, signing a long checklist of improbable risks can reduce affective competence by arousing unrealistic feelings either of helplessness and dread or of certainty and control. If, instead, the patient is to make a truly informed, competent choice, the doctor must engage in an ongoing informed-consent process, creating an alliance with the patient around the need to make decisions in the face of uncertainty. The forensic psychiatrist, versed in both the affective and cognitive components of decision making, increasingly will be called on to determine whether such a process has occurred.

PTSD; INDICATOR OF SPECIFIC IMPAIRMENTS OF COMPETENCE

Since Post-Traumatic Stress Disorder (PTSD) became an officially recognized psychiatric diagnosis in 1980, it has brought about revolutionary changes in the relationship between psychiatry and the law. In criminal law, variants of PTSD such as battered-woman syndrome have bolstered defences ranging from diminished capacity to self-defence. Crime victims have used PTSD to press their claims for strict sentencing of the offender and for compensation. In civil law, PTSD provides a reliable diagnostic class, which comprises physical signs and symptoms, and an identifiable proximate cause for numerous forms of psychic damage. These comprise traumas resulting from rape, incest, sexual abuse by therapists, sexual or other workplace harassment, and physical injury caused by negligence (e.g., automobile accidents). Not only can PTSD be a major element of damages in cases of physical injury, but PTSD itself has (in varying proportions) physical as well as affective and cognitive manifestations.

Nonetheless, there is an underlying complexity to PTSD that belies its image (in the eyes of cynics) as a neat package in which all manner of damage claims can be wrapped with black-and-white ribbon and an expensive price tag. For instance, the alleged traumatic event may not have occurred. Or the symptoms may be misattributed to an actual traumatic event to avoid the memory of an even more traumatic event.

Thus, a false memory may, by way of displacement, feed off a real experience.

Contrary to the popular stereotype, a diagnosis of PTSD does not signify a easy ascription of causality to one event. Properly understood, PTSD results from an interaction between environmental stress (the traumatic event) and preexisting capacities. People are vulnerable in different degrees to different kinds of trauma on the basis of their past experience. The effects of the trauma depend not only of the intensity of the stressor, but also on the feelings of isolation and helplessness the person associates with that class of event. The evaluee may, on occasion, malinger, exaggerate, or misattribute such symptoms, but it is also possible that the evaluee will deny, minimize, or discount the symptomatology by way of attempting to control the underlying distress as well as the shame secondary to experiencing it.

This complex understanding of PTSD amounts to a rediscovery of psychoanalytic insight. Even as psychodynamic psychiatry is losing out in the clinical marketplace to drug therapy and cost-containment, its interweaving of the several strands of past and present personal history is finding receptive ears in at least some courtrooms. Much depends on the judge as well as on the ideological climate and available resources in a given jurisdiction. The complex narrative of a life history is a story that the courts both want to hear and resist hearing. Whether forensic psychiatrists are given the wherewithal to tell this story in full depends on the ability of public defenders to argue for, and the willingness of underfunded, overworked courts to allocate, sufficient funds to mount an adequate defence. A foundation for vigorous advocacy and ample allocation has been laid by a U.S. Supreme Court decision that calls for the federal and state governments to furnish adequate medical care for people in their custody. The degree to which this standard will be applied to forensic evaluations will be decided on a state-by-state and case-by-case basis.

If the severity of PTSD depends on prior vulnerabilities, traumatic stress in turn creates future vulnerabilities. That is, some capacities can be diminished under stress or as a consequence of stress. In this way, PTSD may be an underlying factor in diminished capacity or selective impairment of competence. An individual may function well in a non-conflictual, non-stressful area (e.g., work), but not in a conflictual, stressful area (e.g., family life). These are the sorts of patterns that the forensic psychiatrist traces.

Evaluees can attempt to fake, malinger, or exaggerate PTSD symptomatology, but the sensitive evaluator, working over time to accomplish a thoroughgoing contextual understanding, can normally distinguish the fraudulent from the genuine. Such a differentiation involves a deep understanding of the evaluee, beginning with a developmental history, inventory of characteristic ways of coping with stress and distress, and an understanding of the overall life course. The evaluator must also take into account the possible effects of prior traumas on the reliability of the victim/witness. Though standardized tests may be helpful in this regard, they are no substitute for an extended forensic psychiatric evaluation.

As noted above, not only faking, but its opposite number – repression, denial, or other avoidance of reliving the traumatic stress – can be a diagnostic pitfall. One of the capacities impaired by PTSD may indeed be the capacity to see a connection between the symptoms and the stressor. Especially in cases of sexual abuse in therapy, courts have begun to begun to toll the statute of restrictions only from the time when the plaintiff became aware of this connection (i.e., of the damage resulting from the trauma), rather than from the time when the trauma occurred. Forensic psychiatrists will need to continue to raise the consciousness of the courts concerning this principle, as well as to make the assessments essential to apply it on a case-by-case basis.

a. Affect: Just as the clinician is aware of transference and countertransference, the evaluator needs to observe the feelings of both parties in the interview. In this case the woman being interviewed initially displayed severe anger, which eventually gave way to sadness. The evaluator felt this sadness as well.

b. Boundaries: The evaluee made numerous attempts to come closer to the interviewer physically and to inquire into his personal life. Her initiation of boundary crossings provided a clue as to what might have happened between her and the defendant therapist.

c. Credibility: The evaluee spoke easily about her experience with the therapist in question. She had more difficulty verbalizing her feelings of frustration and loss over the disappointments she had suffered, after a promising start, in her personal and professional life.

d. Damages: The patient had suffered intense disabilities in many areas of functioning. Therapy with a number of clinicians, culminating in the one she was suing, had brought about little or no improvement. The examiner noted the underlying sense of despair.

Guided by these observations, the evaluator was able to establish a working (although not therapeutic) alliance with the evaluee – this in spite of the fact that he had been retained by the opposing party in the lawsuit. This working alliance gave the evaluee the emotional strength to take responsibility for her inner reality. She remembered that the alleged sexual contact with her therapist had not occurred. She and the therapist had exchanged hugs, but she now saw that her interpretation of these gestures as sexual reflected her deep wish to be taken care of by the therapist and her disappointment that this wish couldn't be simply and straightforwardly gratified. Following this forensic psychiatric examination, she withdrew her legal action.

ACTS RELATED TO NARCOTIC AND PSYCHOTROPIC SUBSTANCES AND ILLEGAL DRUG TRAFFICKING

THE NARCOTIC DRUGS AND PSYCHOTROPIC SUBSTANCES ACT, 1985

A significant number of young people in their productive lives fall pray to drugs and endanger their lives. They are illegally procuring them with very high cost from bad elements of the society. Drug traffic is also associated with many crimes that is why legal regulation was sought.

The Act provides stringent control and regulation of operations relating to narcotic drugs and psychotropic substances. It extends to the whole of India. The Act defines Addict, Cannabis-Charas, Ganja, Coca-derivatives and plant, opium, illicit traffic (i.e. cultivating cocoa or opium, manufacturing, possessing, sale, purchase, transportation, concealment, use or consumption, import or export, etc). The Act provides power to the Central government to add to or omit the list of psychotropic substances, to take measures for preventing and combating abuse of and illicit traffic of narcotic drugs.

There is a Consultative Committee to advise the Central Government for the implementation of this Act. The Narcotics Commissioner look after the production of opium. The cocoa plant and cocoa leaves can be used in the preparation of flavouring agents with the permission of central government. For import of any such drugs required import certificate. No person shall engaged in or control any trade in which a narcotic drug or psychotropic substance is obtained from outside India and supplied to any person staying outside India.

Any officer of Gazette rank of the Department of Central Excise, Narcotics, Customs, Revenue intelligence or any other department of the Central Government or of the Border Security Force but superior in rant to a peon, sepoy, or a constable, is empowered to search, seize, or arrest any person who is engaged in dealing, sale, manufacturing narcotics, or psychotropic substances or helping other person for the same. Any violation of the Act is punishable with rigorous imprisonment for a term which shall not be less than ten years but which may extend to twenty years and shall also be liable to fine which shall not be less than one lakh rupees but which may extend to two lakh rupees.

The NDPS Act 1985 sets out the statutory framework for Drug Law Enforcement in India. The main elements of the control regime mandated by the Act are as follows

a. The cultivation, production, manufacture, possession, sale, purchase, transportation, warehousing, consumption, inter-State movement, transshipment and import and export of narcotic drugs and psychotropic substances is prohibited except for medical or scientific purposes and in accordance with the terms and conditions of any license permit or authorization given by the Government. (Section 8)

b. The Central Government is empowered to regulate the cultivation production, manufacture, import, export, sale, consumption, use etc of narcotic drugs and psychotropic substances. (Section 9).

c. State Governments are empowered to permit and regulate possession and inter-State movement of opium, poppy straw, the manufacture of medicinal opium and the cultivation of cannabis excluding hashish. (Section 10).

d. All person in India are prohibited from engaging in or controlling any trade whereby narcotic drugs or psychotropic substances are obtained outside India and supplied to any person outside India except with the previous authorisation of the Central Government and subject to such conditions as may be imposed by the Central Government. (Section 12).

e. The Central Government is empowered to declare any substance, based on an assessment of its likely use in the manufacture of narcotics drugs and psychotropic substances as a controlled substance. (Section 9-A).

f. Assets derived from drugs trafficking are liable to forfeiture (Chapter V-A).

g. Both the Central Government and State Governments are empowered to appoint officers for the purposes of the Act. (Sections 4, 5 and 7).

The NDPS Act is in effect a comprehensive code not only for the control and regulation of Narcotics Drugs and Psychotropic Substances, but also for the control of selected chemicals - commonly known as precursors - which can be used in the illicit manufacture of narcotic drugs and psychotropic substances, as well as for the investigation and forfeiture of drug related assets.

Enforcement

Given India's size and the federal nature of our polity, a number of agencies both at the Centre and in the States have been empowered to enforce the provisions of the Act. These agencies include the department of Customs and Central Excise, the Directorate of Revenue Intelligence, the Central Bureau of Narcotics, the Central Bureau of Investigation and the Border Security Force at the Central level and State Police and Excise Departments at the State level.

The Union Ministries of Social Justice and Empowerment and Health are responsible for the demand reduction aspects of drug law enforcement, which broadly covers health-care and the deaddiction, rehabilitation, and social reintegration of addicts.

Section 4(3) of the Act envisages the creation of a Central Authority to coordinate the activities of the various Central and State agencies involved in drug law enforcement, to implement India's obligations under various international conventions, and to coordinate with international organizations and authorities in foreign countries in the prevention and suppression of the illicit traffic in narcotic drugs and psychotropic substances. In terms of this provision, the Narcotics Control Bureau was set up by the Central Government in 1986 with the broad remit to coordinate drug law enforcement nationally.

The empowerment of a large number of agencies under the NDPS Act ensures that India's drug laws are enforced effectively on the ground. The NCB basically functions as national coordinator international liaison and as the nodal point for the collection and dissemination of intelligence. This system assures coordinated implementation within the parameters of a broad national strategy.

Investigative Procedures

Chapter V of the NDPS Act (Sections 41 to 68) sets out the powers as well as the procedures for the investigation of offences under the Act. This Chapter empowers officers duly authorized by the Central Government or a State Government to issue warrants, to enter and search premises, to stop and search conveyances, to seize narcotic drugs and psychotropic substances, to take statements and to arrest persons suspected of having committed an offence, punishable under the Act. The power to issue search and arrest warrants, has in terms of Section 41 been vested both in Magistrates as well as in especially designated (Gazetted) officers of the Central and State Governments.

This is designed to ensure both timely and effective action in response to any information and to obviate the need for judicial satisfaction each time a warrant is required to be issued. In addition, both the Central and the State Governments are authorized to entrust any Officer duly empowered under the Act with the powers of an Officer-in-charge of a Police Station for the investigation of offences under the Act. It needs to be noted however, that while the powers to search, seize, arrest etc., are inherent in the Act, all these are subject to both the substantive and procedural safeguards mandated by the Code of Criminal Procedure, in relation, inter-alia, to the presence of independent witnesses at a search, the drawing up of search lists or panchanamas, and the constitutional obligation to produce an arrested person before a Judge within 24 hours etc.

Licit Opium Cultivation

Section 8 of the NDPS Act, inter-alia, prohibits the cultivation of the opium Poppy except for medical and scientific purposes and in accordance with the terms and conditions of a license, permit or authorization given by the Government. Section 9, inter-alia, empowers the Central Government to permit and regulate the cultivation of the opium poppy such cultivation only being on account of the Central Government. Section 5 requires the Central Government to appoint a Narcotics Commissioner who shall exercise all powers and perform all functions relating to the superintendence of the cultivation of the opium poppy and the production of opium. India is the largest licit producer of opium in the world, which is both exported as well as used by the domestic pharmaceutical industry. The licit cultivation of opium in India is regulated and controlled by the Narcotics Commissioner of India in terms of the provisions of Sections 8, 9 and 5 of the NDPS Act. The Central Government announces an opium policy each year which sets out the terms and conditions subject to which licenses for the cultivation of opium shall be given, the areas where cultivation shall be allowed, the prices at which the opium crop shall be purchased by the Government and the minimum qualifying yield for a license in the ensuing crop year. The crop cycle runs from October to May. Based on this policy, the Narcotics Commissioner of India issues licenses to individual cultivators for specified tracts of land. The key elements of the licit opium control regime in India are as follows:

i. Opium can be cultivated only on fields specifically licensed for the purpose.

ii. The entire crop must be tendered to the Central Government at prices fixed by the Government.

iii. Failure to tender the minimum qualifying yield can disentitle the cultivator to a license in the following crop season.

These policy controls are backed by strict enforcement on the ground which include the measurement of fields, periodical crop surveys and physical checks to prevent diversion. Failure to tender the entire yield to the Government is treated as a serious offence and any cultivator who embezzles or otherwise illegally disposes of the opium produced by him, is in terms of section 19 of the Act, punishable with rigorous imprisonment for a term of between 10 to 20 years and a fine which shall not be less than Rs.100,000/- but which may extend to Rs.200,000/-.

Special Provisions Relating to Forfeiture of Property

A new Chapter, Chapter V-A, was introduced into the Act in May 1989 to provide for the investigation, freezing, seizure and forfeiture of property derived from or acquired through illicit trafficking in narcotic drugs and psychotropic substances. This Chapter prohibits any person from holding any property derived from drugs trafficking and authorizes officers empowered under the Act to investigate, identify and seize such property.

The Chapter also sets out a quasi- judicial procedure for the forfeiture of such property consequent to which it shall vest in the Central Government. Chapter V-A, does not however, constitute a comprehensive code against the laundering of the proceeds of drugs trafficking, in that it is limited to the forfeiture of drug related assets, but does not establish the laundering of the proceeds of drug trafficking or the act of dealing in such proceeds as a punishable criminal offence. This lacuna will however, be catered for when the Money Laundering Bill, which is presently in Parliament is enacted into law.

Offences and Penalties

Chapter IV, (Sections 15 to 40) sets out the penalties for offences under the Act. These offences are essentially related to violations of the various prohibitions imposed under the Act on the cultivation, production, manufacture, distribution, sale, import and export etc. of narcotic drugs and psychotropic substances. All these offences are triable by Special Courts and the punishments prescribed range from imprisonment from 10 to 20 years for first offences to 15 to 30 years for any subsequent offences together with monitory fines.

In addition to persons directly involved in trafficking narcotic drugs and psychotropic substances, any person who finances trafficking or harbors a person involved in trafficking, or abets, or is a party to a criminal conspiracy, including a criminal conspiracy to commit an offence outside India is also liable to the same scale of punishments. The Act was amended in May 1989 to mandate the death penalty for second offences relating to contraventions involving more than certain quantities of specified narcotic drugs and psychotropic substances.

The Act, however, makes a distinction between possession for personal consumption and trafficking, the punishment for the former being limited to between six months and one year only. The application of this provision is subject to the following two qualifications:

i. The quantity of the drug involved in the offence should be a small quantity as specified by the Central Government.

ii. The onus is on the accused to establish that the drug in question was meant for personal consumption and not for sale, distribution etc

Precursor Control

The 1998 U.N. Convention against Illicit Traffic in Narcotic Drugs and Psychotropic Substances to which India is a signatory, requires Parties to impose controls over the manufacture, internal distribution and import and export of chemicals which can be used in the illicit manufacture of narcotic drugs and psychotropic substances. In order to implement India's obligations under this Convention, the NDPS Act was amended in 1998 in order to empower the Central Government to declare any substance as a controlled substance and to regulate its manufacture, import and export etc. (Section 9-A). Violations relating to such substances were established as criminal offences punishable with imprisonment for upto 10 years (Section 25-A). In 1993, the Government of India promulgated the NDPS

(Regulation of Controlled Substances) Order, to regulate the manufacture, distribution etc., of any substance declared to be a "Controlled Substance".

In exercise of its powers under the Act, the Central Government has so far notified Acetic Anhydride, which is used in the processing of opium into heroin, N-Acetylanthranilic acid which is used in the illicit manufacture of Methaqualone and Ephedrine and Pseudoephedrine which are used in the illicit manufacture of Amphetamine type stimulants as controlled substances.

NARCOTIC DRUGS AND PSYCHOTROPIC SUBSTANCES (AMENDMENT) ACT 2001

An Act further to amend the Narcotic Drugs and Psychotropic Substances Act, 1985. BE it enacted by Parliament in the Fifty-second Year of the Republic of India as follows:

Short title and commencement.

1. Short title and commencement.-(1) This Act may be called the Narcotic Drugs and Psychotropic Substances (Amendment) Act, 2001.
2. It shall come into force on such date as the Central Government may, by notification in the Official Gazette, appoint; and different dates may be appointed for different provisions of this Act, and any reference in any provision to the commencement of this Act shall be construed as a reference to the coming into force of that provision.

Amendment of section 1. 2. Amendment of section 1.-In the Narcotic Drugs and Psychotropic Substances Act, 1985 (61 of 1985) (hereinafter referred to as the principal Act), in section 1, in sub-section (2), after the words "whole of India", the following shall be inserted, namely: "and it applies also- (a) to all citizens of India outside India; (b) to all persons on ships and aircrafts registered in India, wherever they may be".

Amendment of section 2. 3. Amendment of section 2.-In section 2 of the principal Act,- (a) for clause (i), the following clause shall be substituted, namely: '(i) "addict" means a person who has dependence on any narcotic drug or psychotropic substance;'; (b) clause (viia) shall be relettered as clause (viid) and before clause (viid) as so relettered, the following clauses shall be inserted, namely: '(viia) "commercial quantity", in relation to narcotic drugs and psychotropic substances, means any quantity greater than the quantity specified by the Central Government by notification in the Official Gazette; (viib) "controlled delivery" means the technique of allowing illicit or suspect consignments of narcotic drugs, psychotropic substances, controlled substances or substances substituted for them to pass out of, or through or into the territory of India with the knowledge and under the supervision of an officer empowered in this behalf or duly authorised under section 50A with a view to identifying the persons involved in the commission of an offence under this Act; (viic) "corresponding law" means any law corresponding to the provisions of this Act;'; (c) after clause (xxiii), the following clause shall be inserted, namely: '(xxiiia) "small quantity", in relation to narcotic drugs and psychotropic substances, means any quantity lesser than the quantity specified by the Central Government by notification in the Official Gazette.'.

Amendment of section 7A. 4. Amendment of section 7A.-In section 7A of the principal Act, for sub-sections (2) and (3), the following sub-sections shall be substituted, namely: "(2) The Fund shall be applied by the Central Government to meet the expenditure incurred in connection with the measures taken for- (a) combating illicit traffic in narcotic drugs, psychotropic substances or controlled substances; (b) controlling the abuse of narcotic drugs and psychotropic substances; (c) identifying, treating, rehabilitating addicts; (d) preventing drug abuse; (e) educating public against drug abuse; and (f) supplying drugs to addicts where such supply is a medical necessity. The Central Government may constitute a Governing Body as it thinks fit to advise that Government and to sanction money out of the said Fund subject to the limit notified by the Central Government in the Official Gazette.".

Insertion of new section 8A. 5. Insertion of new section 8A.-After section 8 of the principal Act, the following section shall be inserted, namely: '8A. Prohibition of certain activities relating to property derived from offence.-No person shall- (a) convert or transfer any property knowing that such property is derived from an offence committed under this Act or under any other corresponding law of any other country or from an act of participation in such offence, for the purpose of concealing or disguising the illicit origin of the property or to assist any person in the commission of an offence or to evade the legal consequences; or (b) conceal or disguise the true nature, source, location, disposition of any property knowing that such property is derived from an offence committed under this Act or under any other corresponding law of any other country; or (c) knowingly acquire, possess or use any property which was derived from an offence committed under this Act or under any other corresponding law of any other country.'.

Substitution of new sections for sections 15 to 18. 6. Substitution of new sections for sections 15 to 18.-For sections 15 to 18 of the principal Act, the following sections shall be substituted, namely: "15. Punishment for contravention in relation to poppy straw.- Whoever, in contravention of any provisions of this Act or any rule or order made or condition of a licence granted thereunder, produces, possesses, transports, imports inter-State, exports inter-State, sells, purchases, uses or omits to warehouse poppy straw or removes or does any act in respect of warehoused poppy straw shall be punishable,- (a) where the contravention involves small quantity, with rigorous imprisonment for a term which may extend to six months, or with fine which may extend to ten thousand rupees, or with both; (b) where the contravention involves quantity lesser than commercial quantity but greater than small quantity, with rigorous imprisonment for a term which may extend to ten years, and with fine which may extend to one lakh rupees; (c) where the contravention involves commercial quantity, with rigorous imprisonment for a term which shall not be less than ten years but which may extend to twenty years, and shall also be liable to fine which shall not be less than one lakh rupees but which may extend to two lakh rupees: Provided that the court may, for reasons to be recorded in the judgment, impose a fine exceeding two lakh rupees. 16. Punishment for contravention in relation to coca plant and coca leaves.-Whoever, in contravention of any provision of this Act or any rule or order made or condition of licence granted thereunder, cultivates any coca plant or gathers any portion of a coca plant or produces, possesses, sells, purchases, transports, imports inter-State, exports inter-State or uses coca leaves shall be punishable with rigourous imprisonment for a term which may extend to ten years, and with fine which may extend to one lakh rupees. 17. Punishment for contravention in relation to prepared opium.-Whoever, in contravention of any provision of this Act or any rule or order made or condition of licence granted thereunder, manufactures, possesses, sells, purchases, transports, imports inter-State, exports inter-State or uses prepared opium shall be punishable- (a) where the contravention involves small quantity, with rigorous imprisonment for a term which may extend to six months, or with fine which may extend to ten thousand rupees, or with both; or (b) where the contravention involves quantity lesser than commercial quantity but greater than small quantity, with rigorous imprisonment for a term which may extend to ten years, and with fine which may extend to one lakh rupees; or (c) where the contravention involves commercial quantity, with rigorous imprisonment for a term which shall not be less than ten years but which may extend to twenty years, and shall also be liable to fine which shall not be less than one lakh rupees but which may extend to two lakh rupees: Provided that the court may, for reasons to be recorded in the judgment, impose a fine exceeding two lakh rupees. 18. Punishment for contravention in relation to opium poppy and opium.-Whoever, in contravention of any provision of this Act or any rule or order made or condition of licence granted thereunder, cultivates the opium poppy or produces, manufactures, possesses, sells, purchases, transports, imports inter-State, exports inter-State or uses opium shall be punishable,- (a) where the contravention involves small quantity, with rigorous imprisonment for a term which may extend to six months, or with fine which may extend to ten thousand rupees, or with both; (b) where the contravention involves commercial quantity, with rigorous imprisonment for a term which shall not be less than ten years but which may extend to twenty years, and shall also be liable to fine which shall not be less than one lakh rupees which may extend to two lakh rupees: Provided that the court may, for reasons to be recorded in the judgment, impose a fine exceeding two lakh rupees; (c) in any other case, with rigorous imprisonment which may extend to ten years and with fine which may extend to one lakh rupees.".

Amendment of section 20. 7. Amendment of section 20.-In section 20 of the principal Act, in clause (b), for sub-clauses (i) and (ii), the following sub-clauses shall be substituted, namely: "(i) where such contravention relates to clause (a) with rigorous imprisonment for a term which may extend to ten years, and shall also be liable to fine which may extend to one lakh rupees; and (ii) where such contravention relates to sub-clause (b),- (A) and involves small quantity, with rigorous imprisonment for a term which may extend to six months, or with fine which may extend to ten thousand rupees, or with both; (B) and involves quantity lesser than commercial quantity but greater than small quantity, with rigorous imprisonment for a term which may extend to ten years, and with fine which may extend to one lakh rupees; (C) and involves commercial quantity, with rigorous imprisonment for a term which shall not be less than ten years which may extend to twenty years and shall also be liable to fine which shall not be less than one lakh rupees but which may extend to two lakh rupees: Provided that the court may, for reasons to be recorded in the judgment, impose a fine exceeding two lakh rupees.".

Substitution of new sections for sections 21 to 23. 8. Substitution of new sections for sections 21 to 23.-For sections 21 to 23 of the principal Act, the following sections shall be substituted, namely: "21.

Punishment for contravention in relation to manufactured drugs and preparations.-Whoever, in contravention of any provision of this Act or any rule or order made or condition of licence granted thereunder, manufactures, possesses, sells, purchases, transports, imports inter-State, exports inter-State or uses any manufactured drug or any preparation containing any manufactured drug shall be punishable,- (a) where the contravention involves small quantity, with rigorous imprisonment for a term which may extend to six months, or with fine which may extend to ten thousand rupees, or with both; (b) where the contravention involves quantity, lesser than commercial quantity but greater than small quantity, with rigorous imprisonment for a term which may extend to ten years, and with fine which may extend to one lakh rupees; (c) where the contravention involves commercial quantity, with rigorous imprisonment for a term which shall not be less than ten years but which may extend to twenty years, and shall also be liable to fine which shall not be less than one lakh rupees but which may extend to two lakh rupees: Provided that the court may, for reasons to be recorded in the judgment, impose a fine exceeding two lakh rupees. 22.

Punishment for contravention in relation to psychotropic substances.-Whoever, in contravention of any provision of this Act or any rule or order made or condition of licence granted thereunder, manufacturers, possesses, sells, purchases, transports, imports inter-State, exports inter-State or uses any psychotropic substance shall be punishable,- (a) where the contravention involves small quantity, with rigorous imprisonment for a term which may extend to six months, or with fine which may extend to ten thousand rupees, or with both; (b) where the contravention involves quantity, lesser than commercial quantity but greater than small quantity, with rigorous imprisonment for a term which may extend to ten years, and with fine which may extend to one lakh rupees; (c) where the contravention involves commercial quantity, with rigorous imprisonment for a term which shall not be less than ten years but which may extend to twenty years, and shall also be liable to fine which shall not be less than one lakh rupees but which may extend to two lakh rupees: Provided that the court may, for reasons to be recorded in the judgment, impose a fine exceeding two lakh rupees. 23. Punishment for illegal import into India, export from India or transhipment of narcotic drugs and psychotropic substances.-Whoever, in contravention of any provision of this Act or any rule or order made or condition of licence or permit granted or certificate or authorisation issued thereunder, imports into India or exports from India or tranships any narcotic drug or psychotropic substance shall be punishable,- (a) where the contravention involves small quantity, with rigorous imprisonment for a term which may extend to six months, or with fine which may extend to ten thousand rupees, or with both; (b) where the contravention involves quantity, lesser than commercial quantity but greater than small quantity, with rigorous imprisonment for a term which may extend to ten years, and with fine which may extend to one lakh rupees; (c) where the contravention involves commercial quantity, with rigorous imprisonment for a term which shall not be less than ten years but which may extend to twenty years, and shall also be liable to fine which shall not be less than one lakh rupees but which may extend to two lakh rupees: Provided that the court may, for reasons to be recorded in the judgment, impose a fine exceeding two lakh rupees.".

Substitution of new section for section 25. 25. Substitution of new section for section 25.-For section 25 of the principal Act, the following section shall be substituted, namely: "25. Punishment for allowing premises, etc., to be used for commission of an offence.-Whoever, being the owner or occupier or having the control or use of any house, room, enclosure, space, place, animal or conveyance, knowingly permits it to be used for the commission by any other person of an offence punishable under any provision of this Act, shall be punishable with the punishment provided for that offence.".

Substitution of new section for section 27. 10. Substitution of new section for section 27.-For section 27 of the principal Act, the following section shall be substituted, namely: "27. Punishment for consumption of any narcotic drug or psychotropic substance.-Whoever consumes any narcotic drug or psychotropic substance shall be punishable,- (a) where the narcotic drug or psychotropic substance consumed is cocaine, morphine, diacetyl-morphine or any other narcotic drug or any psychotropic substance as may be specified in this behalf by the Central Government by notification in the Official Gazette, with rigorous imprisonment for a term which may extend to one year, or with fine which may extend to twenty thousand rupees, or with both; and (b) where the narcotic drug or psychotropic substance consumed is other than those specified in or under clause (a), with imprisonment for a term which may extend to six months, or with fine which may extend to ten thousand rupees, or with both.".

Amendment of section 30. 11. Amendment of section 30.-In section 30 of the principal Act, for the words, figures and brackets "section 15 to section 25 (both inclusive) and from the circumstances of the case", the words, figures and letter "sections 19, 24 and 27A and for offences involving commercial quantity of any narcotic drug or psychotropic substance and from the circumstances of the case" shall be substituted.

Substitution of new section for section 31. 12. Substitution of new section for section 31.-For section 31 of the principal Act, the following section shall be substituted, namely:

"31. Enhanced punishment for offences after previous conviction: 1. If any person who has been convicted of the commission of, or attempt to commit, or abetment of, or criminal conspiracy to commit, any of the offences punishable under this Act is subsequently convicted of the commission of, or attempt to commit, or abetment of, or criminal conspiracy to commit, an offence punishable under this Act with the same amount of punishment shall be punished for the second and every subsequent offence with rigorous imprisonment for a term which may extend to one-half of the maximum term of imprisonment, and also be liable to fine which shall extend to one-half of the maximum amount of fine. 2. Where the person referred to in sub-section (1) is liable to be punished with a minimum term of imprisonment and to a minimum amount of fine, the minimum punishment for such person shall be one-half of the minimum term of imprisonment and one-half of the minimum amount of fine: Provided that the court may, for reasons to be recorded in the judgment, impose a fine exceeding the fine for which a person is liable. 3. Where any person is convicted by a competent court of criminal jurisdiction outside India under any corresponding law, such person, in respect of such conviction, shall be dealt with for the purposes of sub-sections (1) and (2) as if he had been convicted by a court in India.".

Amendment of section 31A. 13. Amendment of section 31A.-In section 31A of the principal Act,-

(a) in sub-section (1),- (i) for the words, figures, brackets and letter "section 15 to section 25 (both inclusive) or section 27A", the words, figures and letter "section 19, section 24, section 27A and for offences involving commercial quantity of any narcotic drug or psychotropic substance" shall be substituted;

(ii) in sub-clause (a), in the Table, in column (2), against entry (viii), for the figures and word "1,500 grams", the words "lesser of the quantity between the quantities given against the respective narcotic drugs or psychotropic substances mentioned above forming part of the mixture" shall be substituted;

(b) in sub-section (2), for the words, figures, brackets and letter "section 15 to section 25 (both inclusive), section 27A, section 28 or section 29", the words, figures and letter "section 19, section 24 or section 27A and for offences involving commercial quantity of any narcotic drug or psychotropic substance" shall be substituted.

Insertion of new section 32B. 14. Insertion of new section 32B.- After section 32A of the principal Act, the following section shall be inserted, namely: "32B. Factors to be taken into account for imposing higher than the minimum punishment.-Where a minimum term of imprisonment or amount of fine is prescribed for any offence committed under this Act, the court may, in addition to such factors as it may deem fit, take into account the following factors for imposing a punishment higher than the minimum term of imprisonment or amount of fine, namely: (a) the use or threat of use of violence or arms by the offender; (b) the fact that the offender holds a public office and that he has taken advantage of that office in committing the offence; (c) the fact that the minors are affected by the offence or the minors are used for the commission of an offence; (d) the fact that the offence is committed in an educational institution or social service facility or in the immediate vicinity of such institution or faculty or in other place to which school children and students resort for educational, sports and social activities; (e) the fact that the offender belongs to organised international or any other criminal group which is involved in the commission of the offence; and (f) the fact that the offender is involved in other illegal activities facilitated by commission of the offence.".

Substitution of new section for section 36A. 15. Substitution of new section for section 36A.-For section 36A of the principal Act, the following section shall be substituted, namely:

'36A. Offences triable by Special Courts.-(1) Notwithstanding anything contained in the Code of Criminal Procedure, 1973 (2 of 1974),- (a) all offences under this Act which are punishable with imprisonment for a term of more than three years shall be triable only by the Special Court constituted for the area in which the offence has been committed or where there are more Special Courts than one for such area, by such one of them as may be specified in this behalf by the Government; (b) where a person accused of or suspected of the commission of an offence under this Act is forwarded to a Magistrate under sub-section

(2) or sub-section (2A) of section 167 of the Code of Criminal Procedure, 1973 (2 of 1974), such Magistrate may authorise the detention of such person in such custody as he thinks fit for a period not exceeding fifteen days in the whole where such Magistrate is a Judicial Magistrate

and seven days in the whole where such Magistrate is an Executive Magistrate:

Provided that in cases which are triable by the Special Court where such Magistrate considers- (i) when such person is forwarded to him as aforesaid; or (ii) upon or at any time before the expiry of the period of detention authorised by him, that the detention of such person is unnecessary, he shall order such person to be forwarded to the Special Court having jurisdiction; (c) the Special Court may exercise, in relation to the person forwarded to it under clause (b), the same power which a Magistrate having jurisdiction to try a case may exercise under section 167 of the Code of Criminal Procedure, 1973 (2 of 1974), in relation to an accused person in such case who has been forwarded to him under that section; (d) a Special Court may, upon perusal of police report of the facts constituting an offence under this Act or upon complaint made by an officer of the Central Government or a State Government authorised in this behalf, take cognizance of that offence without the accused being committed to it for trial.

(2) When trying an offence under this Act, a Special Court may also try an offence other than an offence under this Act with which the accused may, under the Code of Criminal Procedure, 1973 (2 of 1974), be charged at the same trial.

(3) Nothing contained in this section shall be deemed to affect the special powers of the High Court regarding bail under section 439 of the Code of Criminal Procedure, 1973 (2 of 1974), and the High Court may exercise such powers including the power under clause (b) of

sub-section (1) of that section as if the reference to "Magistrate" in that section included also a reference to a "Special Court" constituted under section 36.

(4) In respect of persons accused of an offence punishable under section 19 or section 24 or section 27A or for offences involving commercial quantity the references in sub-section (2) of section 167 of the Code of Criminal Procedure, 1973 (2 of 1974) thereof to "ninety days", where they occur, shall be construed as reference to "one hundred and eighty days": Provided that, if it is not possible to complete the investigation within the said period of one hundred and eighty days, the Special Court may extend the said period up to one year on the report of the Public Prosecutor indicating the progress of the investigation and the specific reasons for the detention of the accused beyond the said period of one hundred and eighty days.

(5) Notwithstanding anything contained in the Code of Criminal Procedure, 1973 (2 of 1974), the offences punishable under this Act with imprisonment for a term of not more than three years may be tried summarily.'.

Substitution of new section for section 36D. 16. Substitution of new section for section 36D.-For section 36D of the principal Act, the following section shall be substituted, namely:

"36D. Transitional provisions.-(1) Any offence committed under this Act on or after the commencement of the Narcotic Drugs and Psychotropic Substances (Amendment) Act, 1988 (2 of 1989), which is triable by a Special Court shall, until a Special Court is constituted under section 36, notwithstanding anything contained in the Code of Criminal Procedure, 1973 (2 of 1974), be tried by a Court of Session.

(2) Where any proceedings in relation to any offence committed under this Act on or after the commencement of the Narcotic Drugs and Psychotropic Substances (Amendment) Act, 1988 (2 of 1989) are pending before a Court of Session, then, notwithstanding anything contained in sub-section (1), such proceeding shall be heard and disposed of by the Court of Session: Provided that nothing contained in this sub-section shall affect the power of the High Court under section 407 of the Code of Criminal Procedure, 1973 (2 of 1974) to transfer any case or class of cases taken cognizance by a Court of Session under sub-section (1).".

Amendment of section 37. 17. Amendment of section 37.-In section 37 of the principal Act, in sub-section (1), in clause (b), for the words "a term of imprisonment of five years or more under this Act", the words, figures and letter "offences under section 19 or section 24 or section 27A and also for offences involving commercial quantity" shall be substituted.

Amendment of section 39. 18. Amendment of section 39.-In section 39 of the principal Act, in sub-section (1), after the words and figures "under section 27", the words "or for offences relating to small quantity of any narcotic drug or psychotropic substance" shall be inserted.

Substitution of new sections for sections 41 to 43. 19. Substitution of new sections for section 41 to 43.-For sections 41 to 43 of the principal Act, the following sections shall be substituted, namely:

'41. Power to issue warrant and authorisation.-(1) A Metropolitan Magistrate or a Magistrate of the first class or any Magistrate of the second class especially empowered by the State Government in this behalf, may issue a warrant for the arrest of any person whom he has reason to believe to have committed any offence punishable under this Act, or for the search, whether by day or by night, of any building, conveyance or place in which he has reason to believe any narcotic drug or psychotropic substance or controlled substance in respect of which an offence punishable under this Act has been committed or any document or other article which may furnish evidence of the commission of such offence or any illegally acquired property or any document or other article which may furnish evidence of holding any illegally acquired property which is liable for seizure or freezing or forfeiture under Chapter VA of this Act is kept or concealed.

(2) Any such officer of gazetted rank of the departments of central excise, narcotics, customs, revenue intelligence or any other department of the Central Government including the para-military forces or the armed forces as is empowered in this behalf by general or special order by the Central Government, or any such officer of the revenue, drugs control, excise, police or any other department of a State Government as if empowered in this behalf by general or special order of the State Government if he has reason to believe from personal knowledge or information given by any person and taken in writing that any person has committed an offence punishable under this Act or that any narcotic drug or psychotropic substance or controlled substance in respect of which any offence under this Act has been committed or any document or other article which may furnish evidence of the commission of such offence or any illegally acquired property or any document or other article which may furnish evidence of holding any illegally acquired property which is liable for seizure or freezing or forfeiture under Chapter VA of this Act is kept or concealed in any building, conveyance or place, may authorise any officer subordinate to him but superior in rank to a peon, sepoy or a constable to arrest such a person or search a building, conveyance or place whether by day or by night or himself arrest such a person or search a building, conveyance or place.

(3) The officer to whom a warrant under sub-section (1) is addressed and the officer who authorised the arrest or search or the officer who is so authorised under sub-section (2) shall have all the powers of an officer acting under section 42. 42. Power of entry, search, seizure and arrest without warrant or authorisation.-(1) Any such officer (being an officer superior in rank to a peon, sepoy or constable) of the departments of central excise, narcotics, customs, revenue intelligence or any other department of the Central Government including para-military or armed forces as is empowered in this behalf by general or special order by the

Central Government, or any such officer (being an officer superior in rank to a peon, sepoy or constable) of the revenue, drugs control, excise, police or any other department of a State Government as is empowered in this behalf by general knowledge or information given by any person and taken down in writing that any narcotic drug, or psychotropic substance, or controlled substance in respect of which an offence punishable under this Act has been committed or any document or other article which may furnish evidence of the commission of such offence or any illegally acquired property or any document or other article which may furnish evidence of holding any illegally acquired property which is liable for seizure or freezing or forfeiture under Chapter VA of this Act is kept or concealed in any building, conveyance or enclosed place, may between sunrise and subset,- (a) enter into and search any such building, conveyance or place; (b) in case of resistance, break open any door and remove any obstacle to such entry; (c) seize such drug or substance and all materials used in the manufacture thereof and any other article and any animal or conveyance which he has reason to believe to be liable to confiscation under this Act and any document or other article which he has reason to believe may furnish evidence of the commission of any offence punishable under this Act or furnish evidence of holding any illegally acquired property which is liable for seizure or freezing or forfeiture under Chapter VA of this Act; and (d) detail and search, and, if he thinks proper, arrest any person whom he has reason to believe to have committed any offence punishable under this Act:

Provided that if such officer has reason to believe that a search warrant or authorisation cannot be obtained without affording opportunity for the concealment of evidence or facility for the escape of an offender, he may enter and search such building, conveyance or enclosed place at any time between sunset and sunrise after recording the grounds of his belief.

(2) Where an officer takes down any information in writing under sub-section (1) or records grounds for his belief under the proviso thereto, he shall within seventy-two hours send a copy thereof to his immediate official superior. 43. Power of seizure and arrest in public place.-Any officer of any of the departments mentioned in section 42 may- (a) seize in any public place or in transit, any narcotic drug or psychotropic substance or controlled substance in respect of which he has reason to believe an offence punishable under this Act has been committed, and, along with such drug or substance, any animal or conveyance or article liable to confiscation under this Act, any document or other article which

he has reason to believe may furnish evidence of the commission of an offence punishable under this Act or any document or other article which may furnish evidence of holding any illegally acquired property which is liable for seizure or freezing or forfeiture under Chapter VA of this Act; (b) detain and search any person whom he has reason to believe to have committed an offence punishable under this Act, and if such person has any narcotic drug or psychotropic substance or controlled substance in his possession and such possession appears to him to be unlawful, arrest him and any other person in his company. Explanation.-For the purposes of this section, the expression "public place" includes any public conveyance, hotel, shop, or other place intended for use by, or accessible to, the public.'.

Amendment of section 44. 20. Amendment of section 44.-In section 44 of the principal Act, after the words "psychotropic substance", the words "or controlled substance" shall be inserted.

Amendment of section 49. 21. Amendment of section 49.-In section 49 of the principal Act, after sub-section (4), the following sub-sections shall be inserted, namely:

"(5) When an officer duly authorised under section 42 has reason to believe that it is not possible to take the person to be searched to the nearest Gazetted Officer or Magistrate without the possibility of the person to be searched parting with possession of any narcotic drug or psychotropic substance, or controlled substance or article or document, he may, instead of taking such person to the nearest Gazetted Officer or Magistrate, proceed to search the person as provided under section 100 of the Code of Criminal Procedure, 1973 (2 of 1974).

(6) After a search is conducted under sub-section (5), the officer shall record the reasons for such belief which necessitated such search and within seventy-two hours send a copy thereof to his immediate official superior.".

Insertion of new section 50A. 23. Insertion of new section 50A.- After section 50 of the principal Act, the following section shall be inserted, namely: "50A. Power to undertake controlled delivery.-The Director General of

Narcotics Control Bureau constituted under sub-section (3) of section 4 or any other officer authorised by him in this behalf, may, notwithstanding anything contained in this Act, undertake controlled delivery of any consignment to- (a) any destination in India; (b) a foreign country, in consultation with the competent authority of such foreign country to which such consignment is destined, in such manner as may be prescribed.".

Amendment of section 53. 24. Amendment of section 53.-In section 53 of the principal Act,-

(a) in sub-section (1), for the words "or Border Security Force", the words "or any other department of the Central Government including para-military forces or armed forces" shall be substituted;

(b) in sub-section (2), after the word "excise", the words "or any other department" shall be inserted.

Substitution of new section for section 54. 25. Substitution of new section for section 54.-For section 54 of the principal Act, the following section shall be substituted, namely: "54. Presumption from possession of illicit articles.-In trials under this Act, it may be presumed, unless and until the contrary is proved, that the accused has committed an offence under this Act in respect of- (a) any narcotic drug or psychotropic substance or controlled substance; (b) any opium poppy, cannabis plant or coca plant growing on any land which he has cultivated; (c) any apparatus especially designed or any group of utensils especially adopted for the manufacture of any narcotic drug or psychotropic substance or controlled substance; or (d) any materials which have undergone any process towards the manufacture of a narcotic drug or psychotropic substance or controlled substance, or any residue left of the materials from which any narcotic drug or psychotropic substance or controlled substance has been manufactured, for the possession of which he fails to account satisfactorily.".

Amendment of section 60. 26. Amendment of section 60.-In section 60 of the principal Act,-

(a) for sub-section (1), the following sub-section shall be substituted, namely:

"(1) Whenever any offence punishable under this Act has been committed, the narcotic drug, psychotropic substance, controlled substance, opium poppy, coca plant, cannabis plant, materials, apparatus and utensils in respect of which or by means of which such offence has been committed, shall be liable to confiscation.";

(b) in sub-sections (2) and (3), after the words "psychotropic substance", wherever they occur, the words "or controlled substances" shall be inserted.

Amendment of section 61. 27. Amendment of section 61.-In section 61 of the principal Act, for the words "narcotic drug or psychotropic substance", the words "narcotic drug, psychotropic substance or controlled substance" shall be substituted.

Amendment of section 62. 28. Amendment of section 62.-In section 62 of the principal Act, for the words "narcotic drug or psychotropic substance", the words "narcotic drug, psychotropic substance or controlled substance" shall be substituted.

Amendment of section 63. 29. Amendment of section 63.-In section 63 of the principal Act,-

(a) in sub-section (2), in the second proviso, after the words "psychotropic substance", the words "controlled substance" shall be inserted; (b) sub-section (3) shall be omitted.

Substitution of new section for section 64A. 30. Substitution of new section for section 64A.-For section 64A of the principal Act, the following section shall be substituted, namely: "64A. Immunity from prosecution to addicts volunteering for treatment.-Any addict, who is charged with an offence punishable under section 27 or with offences involving small quantity of narcotic drugs or psychotropic substances, who voluntarily seeks to undergo medical treatment for de-addiction from a hospital or an institution maintained or recognised by the Government or a local authority and undergoes such treatment shall not be liable to prosecution under section 27 or under any other section for offences involving small quantity of narcotic drugs or psychotropic substances: Provided that the said immunity from prosecution may be withdrawn if the addict does not undergo the complete treatment for de-addiction.".

Amendment of section 68A. 31. Amendment of section 68A.-In section 68A of the principal Act, in sub-section (2),- (i) in clause (a), for the word "five", the word "ten" shall be substituted; (ii) after clause (c), the following clause shall be inserted, namely: "(cc) every person who has been arrested or against whom a warrant or authorisation of arrest has been issued for the commission of an offence punishable under this Act with imprisonment for a term of ten years or more, and every person who has been arrested or against whom a warrant or authorisation of arrest has been issued for the commission of a similar offence under any corresponding law of any other country;"; (iii) in clauses (d), (e) and (f), after the word, brackets and letter "clause (c)", the words, brackets and letters "or clause (cc)" shall be inserted.

Amendment of section 68B. 32. Amendment of section 68B.-In section 68B of the principal Act, in clause (g), in sub-clause (i), for the words "illicit traffic", the words "the contravention of any provisions of this Act" shall be substituted.

Amendment of section 68C. 33. Amendment of section 68C.-In section 68C of the principal Act, in sub-section (2), for the proviso, the following proviso shall be substituted, namely: "Provided that no property shall be forfeited under this Chapter if such property was acquired, by a person to whom this Act applies, before a period of six years from the date he was arrested or against whom a warrant or authorisation of arrest has been issued for the commission of an offence punishable under this Act or from the date the order or detention was issued, as the case may be.".

Amendment of section 68E. 34. Amendment of section 68E.-In section 68E of the principal Act, for sub-section (1), the following sub-section shall be substituted, namely:

"(1) Every officer empowered under section 53 and every officer-in-charge of a police station shall, on receipt of information is satisfied that any person to whom this Chapter applies holds any illegally acquired property, he may, after recording reasons for doing so, proceed to take all steps necessary for tracing and identifying such property.".

Amendment of section 68-I. 36. Amendment of section 68-I.-In section 68-I of the principal Act, after sub-section (3), the following proviso shall be inserted, at the end, namely: "Provided that no illegally acquired property of any person who is referred to in clause (cc) of sub-section (2) of section 68A or relative of a person referred to in that clause or associate of a person referred to in that clause or holder of any property which was at any time previously held by a person referred to in that clause shall stand forfeited.".

Amendment of section 68-O. 37. Amendment of section 68-O.-In section 68-O of the principal Act, in sub-section (1), for the words "Any person aggrieved by an order of the competent authority", the words, brackets, figures and letter "Any officer referred to in sub-section (1) of section 68E or any person aggrieved by an order of the competent authority" shall be substituted.

Insertion of new section 68Z. 38. Insertion of new section 68Z.-After section 68Y of the principal Act, the following section shall be inserted, namely:

"68Z. Release of property in certain cases.-(1) Where the detention order of a detenu is set aside or withdrawn, properties seized or frozen under this Chapter shall stand released.

(2) Where any person referred to in clause (a) or clause (b) or clause (cc) of sub-section (2) of section 68A has been acquitted or discharged from the charges under this Act or any other corresponding law of any other country and the acquittal was not appealed against or when appealed against, the appeal was disposed of as a consequence of which such property could not be forfeited or warrant of arrest or authorisation of arrest issued against such person has been withdrawn, then, property seized or frozen under this Chapter shall stand released.".

Amendment of section 76. 39. Amendment of section 76.-In section 76 of the principal Act, in sub-section (2), after clause (c), the following clause shall be inserted, namely: '(ca) the manner in which "controlled delivery" under section 50A is to be undertaken;'.

Amendment of section 77. 40. Amendment of section 77.-In section 77 of the principal Act, for the portion beginning with the words "Every rule made under this Act" and ending with "shall be laid, as soon as may be, after it is made or issued", the following shall be substituted, namely: "Every rule made under this Act by the Central Government and every notification or order issued under clause (viia), clause (xi), clause (xxiiia) of section 2, section 3, section 7A, section 9A and clause (a) of section 27 shall be laid, as soon as may be, after it is made or issued".

Application of this Act to pending cases.

41. Application of this Act to pending cases.-(1) Notwithstanding

anything contained in sub-section (2) of section 1, all cases pending before the courts or under investigation at the commencement of this Act shall be disposed of in accordance with the provisions of the principal Act as amended by this Act and accordingly, any person found guilty of any offence punishable under the principal Act, as it stood immediately before such commencement, shall be liable for a punishment which is lesser than the punishment for which he is otherwise liable at the date of the commission of such offence: Provided that nothing in this section shall apply to cases pending in appeal.

(2) For the removal of doubts, it is hereby declared that no act or omission on the part of any person shall be punishable as an offence which would not have been so punishable if this Act has not come into force.

ADMISSION AND DISCHARGE PROCEDURES

Following are the rules and procedure for admission and discharge of a psychiatric patient in a hospital:

- The patient must be suffering from a major mental sickness.
- The patient normally has a chronic mental sickness, although the current episode may be an acute exacerbation of the sickness.
- Community based facilities have been utilized first and found not adequate to the need, or don't exist in the area of the state where the patient is found.
- A longer hospitalization is anticipated than what is normally considered for short-term acute care.
- The severity of the sickness makes management and treatment at Hospital the most reasonable alternative.
- Dangerousness or violence of behaviour factors makes management and treatment at Hospital the most reasonable alternative.
- The patient's needs may be best met by a specialized treatment program only available at Hospital.
- Referrals are made based on the availability of bed allocation for each Community Mental Health Centre (CMHC).
- If a CMHC wishes to loan or sell a bed to another mental health centre, the appropriate approval forms are signed through the Admissions Office.
- The referred individual is an established client of a community mental health centre and has been referred by that centre. The referred individual may also be committed to another state institution, and meet the criteria for inter-institutional transfer.
- The patient may be either voluntary or meet the criteria for civil commitment.
- Hospital considers any applicant who does not meet the above criteria as ineligible for admission. Additionally, the following circumstances or additions may render referred ineligible/ inappropriate for admission:
- Referrals with a primary problem of substance abuse, alcohol or drugs, will not normally be eligible for admission.

- Exceptions can be made where life threatening circumstances may exist if hospitalization is not provided.
- Patients with exceptional medical problems requiring physical care beyond the reasonable capability of Hospital are not eligible for admission. This restriction comprises patients with highly contagious infections or diseases that would normally call for isolation facilities, highly technical procedures, and extensive man-power. These are screened through the pre-admission process and it is expected that whenever possible, the referring agency screens the patients for such medical problems as those stated.
- RN contacts medical services provider to notify of the admission.
- If the patient is taken directly to the admitting unit at the time of arrival campus.
- Receiving unit RN contacts the admitting doctor at the time of arrival to indicate the patient is present and to report the current condition of the patient.
- If the proposed admitting doctor accepts the admission, the doctor gives an order to the RN to admit the patient, specifying the time of notification as the time of admission.
- The doctor may defer other admission orders such as diet, level, etc. to a time later in the day of admission.
- The unit RN records the order to admit, noting the time ordered for the admission.
- RN calls medical services provider to notify of admission.
- Medical records or information technology are contacted if ADT is unavailable.

ROLE AND RESPONSIBILITIES OF NURSE

Psychiatric mental health nurses work in a variety of hospital and community settings. During recent years in the growth of health services in the world, much emphasis has been placed on the "expanding role" of the nurse. Psychiatric nursing is a speciality area within the field of nursing. Traditionally, the function of the nurses was to furnish care and comforts as they carried out specific nursing function, but changes in nursing of the day have expanded the role to comprise increased emphasis on health promotion and sickness-prevention, as well as concern for the client as a whole. Tremendous changes has happened in all specialities of nursing together with psychiatric nursing. The role shift of psychiatric nursing and mental health care are be influenced by factors like economics, financing of health care, information technology, managed behavioural health care, the psychobiologic shift, accountability in practice, and mental health research.

GROWTH OF PSYCHIATRIC NURSING ROLES

A role is a set of expected and actual behaviours linked with a position in a social structure -Hardy & Hardy (1988). A role is the sum total of expected behaviours the behaviours expected from a person who occupies a specific position and status in a social pattern. The function of psychiatric nurse expanded after World War II. The discovery of psychiatric nursing theory and practice by Hildegard Peplau gave impetus to the advanced practice in psychiatric nursing. Several of the nursing roles are taken up by other new professionals, like activity therapists. But new roles are emerging for psychiatric nursing. Some of the new roles for psychiatric nurses in US are entrepreneur, manager, clinician, educator and researcher. Depending on the state laws, nurses are practicing psychotherapy and prescribing medicines to uncomplicated patients in US.

TRADITIONAL ROLES OF NURSING

Contemporary nursing calls for that the nurse possess knowledge and skills in different areas.

- Caregiver, Communicator, Educator/teacher, Manager, Advocate, Leader, Counsellor, Researcher, Career Growth

EXPANDED AND EXTENDED ROLES OF NURSE

Expanded function of nurse is the one that the nurse assumes by virtue of education and experiences. It goes beyond the traditional nursing roles with additional responsibilities.

- Clinician, Nurse researcher, Nurse Administrator/Manger, Nurse Educator, Advanced Practice Nurse (APN), Nurse practitioner, Clinical Nurse Specialist (CNS), School health nurse, Critical care nurse, Family nurse practitioner, Trauma nurse specialist.

The concept of extended roles means to reach out. The function of the nurse needs change along with that of other health professional which means that the knowledge and skills of nurse needs to be broadened. Extended nursing facilities are those agencies which provides variety of services for the patient of all age groups which may be a part of hospital or institution or a separate institution may be proprietary or non-proprietary.

- Nurse entrepreneurs, Nurse anaesthetist, Nurse Informatics, Palliative care nurse/Hospice care nurse, Nurse Oncologist, Nurse Prescriber, Infection control nurse, Nurse endoscopist

Expanded and extended roles of psychiatric nurse

The expansion of nursing role can be perceived in two ways.

First, the expansion is within the realm of medical knowledge and linked skills are required for the treatment and care of those who are sick, both acute and chronic. This role shares most of the characteristics of the replacement function, as the expansion is based on increasing the medical knowledge and skills of the nurse so that her understanding of the pathological processes, diagnosis, and treatment closely parallels that of the medical person. Though the medical facets are favoured in expanding the role in the direction of replacement, nursing has attempted to attend also to the psychological and social components which persist in each specific sickness situation like in psychiatric nursing.

Second, the expanded role for nursing is being enacted in primary care settings where emphasis is on the growth and maintenance of family health. This expansion of the nurse's role is viewed as complemental in that it does not replace that of other health professionals, but adds another dimension to health care service. It is an expansion of nursing into areas of need which are unmet and unfulfilled at this time; it is also an expansion of the core of what nursing basically is.

Expanded care role for the most part involves

1. The elements of normal nursing roles like
   - Psychiatric assessment
   - Patient and carer education
   - Basic psychotherapeutic practices
2. Advanced practice roles
   - Psychiatric diagnoses
   - Prescribing single emergency doses
   - Modifying doses of wide ranging psychotropic medication
   - Autonomy in admission and discharge

VARIOUS ROLES OF PSYCHIATRIC NURSES

Primary nurse/RN or novice: Primary nurse is responsible for the individual client's nursing care, whether in t he community or in hospital.

In the UK, the term psychiatric nurse has now for the most part been replaced with mental health nurse. In the US, at the basic level psychiatric health nurses are registered nurses (RNs) with baccalaureate degree who demonstrate skills beyond the beginning RN or novice to the speciality.

Ward manager/sister: The ward sister has the central responsibility of for integrating and strengthening interprofessional relationships and communication.

Psychiatric/Mental Health Clinical Nurse Specialists (PMHCNS): The Psychiatric Mental Health Clinical Nurse Specialist is an Advanced Practice Registered Nurse who specializes in psychiatric nursing care issues of children, adolescents and adults who have mental health and substance abuse disorders. The nurse is an expert in providing nursing care in a speciality area of work, for instance child and adolescent psychiatry or HIV and AIDS counselling, based on authoritative knowledge and expert skills.

Mental health nurse practitioner (MHNP): Mental Health Nurse Practitioner, also known as Psychiatric Nurse Practitioner, works in a primary care facility, out-patient mental health clinic or in a hospital or community health centre. MHNPs assess and furnish care for patients who have psychiatric disorders, medical mental conditions or substance abuse problems. They are licensed to furnish emergency psychiatric services, psychosocial and physical assessment of their patients, treatment plans, and to continually manage patient care. They may also serve as consultants or as educators for families and staff; nevertheless, the MHNP has a greater focus on psychiatric diagnosis, together with the differential diagnosis of medical disorders with psychiatric symptoms, and on medication treatment for psychiatric disorders. The function of the nurse practitioner has been described as the apex of nursing practice. Such a statement has significant implications for the professional status of nursing in its own right.

Nurse Therapist: First develop in Maudsley Hospital in London, where nurse trained in psychotherapy techniques. The nurse specialist is recognized as a trained and skilled independent practitioner, who diagnoses, prescribes and caries out treatment for clients in hospital and community settings. The nurse therapist may be private practice nurse.

Nurse Manager: Nurse manager work less directly with clients, but has the responsibility to furnish nursing leadership to ensure that an appropriate therapeutic milieu is maintained. A key responsibility is the support and growth of nurses representing nursing views to senior managers. Nurse manager plays a significant role in negotiating and allocating nursing resources within clinical directorates.

Nurse researcher: The function of nurse has expanded with increase in complexity of skills required. Investigates problems to improve nursing care and to further define and expand the scope of nursing practice. Nurse researcher may be employed in an academic setting, hospital, or independent professional/community service agency. Minimum educational requirement-doctoral degree, with master's in nursing.

Nurse Educator/Health Educator: Nurse educators work in educational institutions, staff growth dept. of healthcare agencies, client education dept(teach the disabled/sick and their families about care to furnish at home). Nurse educator need experience in clinical practice to furnish with practical skills and theoretical knowledge. Call for Graduate degree in nursing and an additional education in the educational process, several hold doctorate/advanced degree in nursing, education, administration etc.

Community Mental Health Nurse or CMHN: DeInstitutionalization in the 1960's gave birth to the community mental health services and community mental health nurses. The focus of community mental health programs are primary, secondary and tertiary prevention of mental sickness. The community mental health nurse provides psychiatric home care. Nursing services for the patient with active psychiatric sickness comprises complete assessment, performing venipuncture for medication or liver function monitoring, providing Psychoeducation and conducting psychotherapy. They may also specialise in areas such as drug and alcohol rehabilitation, or child and adolescent mental health.

Psychiatric consultation-liaison nurse/liaison mental health nurse: Nurses practicing in this subspecialty are in an advanced practice role. In addition to direct care of patients/families, psychiatric consultation-liaison nurses (PCLN) also function in consultative, collaborative, and educative relationships with nurses and other health care providers to improve their knowledge and skills in addressing the biopsychosocial facets of care. PCLNs may practice in several settings: hospitals, rehabilitation facilities, long term care facilities, home care, and clinics. The psychiatric nurse liaison provided consultation to nurses and attending doctors who were providing care to patients with a medical/psychiatric illnesses.

Forensic psychiatric nurses: The word forensic pertains to legal proceedings. When forensics is applied in the context of health care it refers especially to that area of law applied in the criminal justice system.

Forensic psychiatric nursing is a relatively new branch of nursing under the broader term of mental health care. Forensic nursing is the application of the forensic facets of health care combined with the bio-psycho-social education of the registered nurse in the scientific investigation and treatment of trauma, and or death of victims and perpetrators of violence, criminal activity, and traumatic accidents.

Forensic nurse is "a nurse who provides care of victims of traumatic injuries and catastrophic accidents, assessment and treatment of perpetrators of crime and violence, and the families of both". The people whom forensic psychiatric nurses care for have been charged with an offence under criminal law and are thus ensconced in the criminal justice system and may be pre- or post-sentencing.

SUBSPECIALTIES OF FORENSIC NURSING

Clinical forensic nursing: The application of the forensic facets of health care in the scientific investigation and treatment of trauma and or death or related medicolegal issues to living patients or those whose death is pronounced upon arrival or during trauma treatment.

Forensic correctional nursing: The provision of biopsychosocial nursing care to persons who have been charged or convicted of a crime.

Forensic ER nursing: The awareness and provision of forensic facets of care provided to all patients by nurses who practice in Emergency rooms.

Forensic geriatric nursing: The application of nursing knowledge to the provision of care and concern to aging persons with regards to any legal or human rights issues of abuse and/or neglect or exploitation.

Forensic legal nurse consulting: Registered nurses who use their clinical knowledge and expertise to assist attorneys with their cases in any context where law and medicine overlap. They fit under the broad umbrella of forensic nursing and are the one group of forensic nurses whose expertise is used mainly in civil, rather than in criminal cases.

Forensic mental health nursing: The application of nursing knowledge and provision of psychiatric rehabilitative care to persons who have interfaced in some way with the criminal justice system, and as a result of that interface, have been judicially designated mentally sick and in need of psychiatric evaluation and/or treatment.

Forensic investigator nursing (death or medical examiner nurse): The application of nursing knowledge in the investigation of any medicolegal death. Medicolegal deaths comprise any unexpected or violent death. Wherever the cause of death is unclear or even remotely suspicious, the medical examiner must investigate.

Forensic examiner nursing: Furnish an incisive examination and evaluation of trauma, related to sexual assault, and other types of impersonal violence. Serves as a liaison between the health care institution, legal agencies, and court of law.

Sexual assault nursing - (clinician or examiner): A registered nurse who has been specifically trained to furnish complete care to sexual assault survivors. She is normally certified by her local institution after completing a training program of approximately 40 hours. Demonstrated competence in conducting a complete evidential examination is also required.

ROLE OF PSYCHIATRIC NURSES: INDIAN CONTEXT

History reveals, as early in fourth century AD, during the period of Emperor Ashoka, hospitals with 15 beds for mentally sick with two male and two female nurses.

- The function of the nurses was to administer herbal medication to psychiatric patients in addition to meeting their basic needs.
- In India the function of psychiatric nurse is for the most part confined to institutional care.
- There are developments in the form of community mental health care role and nurse educator role.
- Nurses with experience in mental health care or having special training in psychiatry with diploma or masters degree work in community mental health programs.

REFERENCES

Chamberlin, J. (1998). Citizenship rights and psychiatric disability. Psychiatric Rehabilitation Journal, 21(4), 405–408.

Dickinson, D. (1997). Ethical issues in long-term psychiatric management. Journal of Medical Ethics, 23, 300–304.

Felthous, A. R. (1999). The clinician's duty to protect third parties. Psychiatric Clinics of North America, 22(1), 49–61.

Kennedy-Swartz, J. (2000). The ethics of instinct: Trust your gut but use your head. American Journal of Nursing, 100(4), 71–72.

King, E. C. (1984). Affective education in nursing: A guide to teaching and assessment. Rockville, MD: Aspen Systems.

Niveau, G., & Kelley-Puskas, M. (2001). Psychiatric disorders and fitness to drive. Journal of Medical Ethics, 27, 36–39.

Roberts, L. W., Battaglia, J., & Epstein, R. S. (1999). Frontier ethics: Mental health care needs and ethical dilemmas in rural communities. Psychiatric Services, 50(4), 497–503.

Rolef, T. L., & Egendorf, L. (Eds.) (2000). Mental illness: Opposing viewpoints. San Diego: Greenhaven Press, Inc.

15

Community Mental Health Nursing

Community Mental Health Nursing encompasses an identification and treatment of those problems that occur as a result of human reactions to an actual or potential menace posed to a person's mental health. This branch of nursing have developed into a specialized area of practice, employing the use of various theories about human behaviour and the learned skill of therapeutic intervention. Mental health care providers have met numerous challenges in their effort to furnish a vision of wellness for those with mental sickness and to increase public awareness of its existence. Historically, the journey to furnish this humane and therapeutic approach to those with mental alterations has been a difficult one.

GROWTH OF COMMUNITY MENTAL HEALTH SERVICES

Before the advent of psychotherapeutic drugs, which are now used extensively in the treatment of mental health issues, the available options for control of symptoms were few. Those with bizarre behaviour were considered outcasts of society and harboured in asylums for the remainder of their lives. Several of the more violent patients were referred to as "lunatics," and they frequently became a spectacle for public viewing. The first institution for the mentally sick was opened in London as the Bethlehem Royal Hospital in 1247.

During the Renaissance, in the early 1400s, there was a growing interest in what let to various abnormal behaviours. An early classification of depression, neurosis, mania, and psychosis was developed by scholars and doctors as per the behaviours they saw. In spite of the increased interest in what caused these situations, the care given to those with the mental disorders didn't improve.

Around the middle of the nineteenth century, we begin to see a change in perspective toward the care provided to those with mental sickness. Dorothea Dix, a nineteenth-century schoolteacher started to question the treatment of both prisoners and the mentally sick. She started a tireless effort to expose these conditions and provoke legislation to help in the construction of mental hospitals with standard for care.

During the late nineteenth and early twentieth centuries, training programs for nurses were created and provided an option for those interested in caring for the sick. There was also an increasing social awareness of the problems that related to mental sickness. Though the need for trained nurses was recognized, caring for the insane was not seen as a fit occupation for women.

During the twentieth century a slow component of psychiatric nursing was included in all nursing curricula. The well-known National Mental Health Act of 1946 was the first legislation to furnish funds for research, advanced nursing degree programs, and improved community service for the mentally sick. In 1955 the Joint Commission on Mental Sickness and Health was established to conduct a study on the guidelines used by mental institutions to furnish care for their patients.

NATIONAL MENTAL HEALTH PROGRAMME

Current mental health practice in the country is regulated by the National Mental Health Programme (1982) (NMHP). The main objectives of the NMHP are: (i) to ensure availability and accessibility of minimum mental health care for all in the foreseeable future, especially to the most vulnerable and underprivileged sections of the population; (ii) to encourage application of mental health knowledge generally health care and in social growth; (iii) to promote community participation in the mental health service growth and to stimulate efforts towards self- help in the community.

As such, the NMHP is in tune with the Alma Ata Declaration. More importantly, we must also see it as being in line with the politics of health policies in the emerging (third) world order organised mainly by the WHO, with nation states by-and-large relinquishing their welfare functions to private enterprises or to community practice. The salient features of the community package of the NMHP are: (i) tying up mental health care with the existing general health infrastructure, such as the public health centres and the district hospitals, and training the existing staff, (ii) tying up mental health care with already existing community growth programmes and promoting culture friendly cures. Although the NMHP says nothing specific about the use of purely medical techniques like drug therapy and electroconvulsive therapy, it seems to imply that it favours non- invasive techniques of treatment. The NMHP states: 'There is good evidence to say that about 15- 20% of all patients who seek help generally health services both in developed and developing countries, do so for emotional and psychosocial problems. Current medical methods of dealing with these problems by unnecessary investigations and costly medicines are not only inadequate and ineffective but produce widespread frustration to both the seeker and the provider of these health services'.

The NMHP also has a place for the practitioners of the Indian systems of medicine, who should play their 'unique role in the discipline of health. The agenda of the NMHP is then to humanise mental health practice by articulating the 'proper' mental health principles, that is, the principles of community care.

The NMHP has been proclaimed a historical landmark document in our national health policy. Given the fact that we didn't have any document at all till 1982 on mental health policy, this proclamation is excusable. Community care philosophy, which the NMHP embodies, is probably also a more humane alternative for the mentally sick to the highly restrictive and regulative mental hospital services. Nevertheless, the NMHP is at best ineffective, and at worst it promotes the dehumanised models of cure that it explicitly rejects.

MENTAL HEALTH PRACTICE

Mental health practice, like other types of social practices, can be used as tools of social control, because practitioners implicitly or explicitly resource social stereotypes to assess, diagnose and cure. The criteria of cure, such as 'socialisation', 'adjustment', 'becoming socially useful', 'inner happiness' etc., frequently contain moral assumptions, preferred social values and stereotypes. Broverman et. al. showed that psychiatric practice is informed by 'highly consensual norms' about gender stereotypes. Their study showed that the notions of mental health the professionals used were 'more influenced by the greater social value of masculine stereotypic characteristics than by the lesser valued feminine stereotypic characteristics'. Later studies in the West showed that this trend is probably changing. For instance, clinicians are now reported to show positive attitudes towards homosexuals. Nevertheless, the West has had a long history of feminist and anti- psychiatric dissent and effective social planning altering mainstream consciousness, which we have not had. Till studies are initiated, we can only conjecture about how professionals' attitude would colour their psychiatric evaluations, and consequently, the treatment options for their patients. I have found it useful to go over some of our own psychiatric journals to obtain some insights about possible biases in professional practice.

All interpersonal negotiations in social practice must inevitably involve the use of stereotypes, increasing one's vulnerability to social control. Choosing to cope with the system of health is already to accept the possibilities and liabilities of such control. This is even more descriptive of health systems that seek to modify human behaviour. But whether one retains one's dignity within the system depends on the power one has in these negotiations.

The degree of choice one has over what happens to one within the mental health systems arguably reduces with psychotherapy, psychopharmacology, electroconvulsive therapy and psychosurgery, in that order. One has very little lay information about the changes linked with drug use and other body techniques. Often, one experiences irremediable bodily changes, such as tardive dyskinesia, occurring with long term use of neuroleptics or anti- psychotics. The shock of having to cope with a pair of abruptly crippled limbs can be an added trauma to someone already suffering from a intense mental sickness. The sense of betrayal one feels at not having been informed before by her physician of the likely consequences of the drugs she has been utilizing is understandable.

NEED FOR STUDIES

Studies abroad show that the marginalised and the vulnerable (especially women) are more likely to be given more prescriptions for psychoactive drugs. We have no comparable studies of psychoactive drug use patterns in our country. Such a study is a dire need. Prescriptions for drugs may have more to do with the stereotypes that the psychiatrist is processing in his dealings with the patient, rather than any 'objective' knowledge about the healing potential of chemicals.

ELECTRO-CONVULSIVE THERAPY

The use of ECT or 'shock therapy', as it is frequently called, has gone up by 20 times in the last twenty years, as per one study done at KEM Hospital, Bombay. Studies show that ECT is what everybody wants, the professionals as well as the 'close relatives' of the mentally sick. Boral, Bagchi and Nandi reported that an overwhelming 70% of relatives of patients favoured ECT treatment, and an equally large 75% of relatives favoured drug treatment, as against 77% of relatives who were doubtful about the efficiency of psychotherapy. Professionals will swear by the humaneness of the treatment and maintain that it has no long term adverse effects. But cognitive deficits have been consistently linked up with ECT use. And even professionals will admit that the administration of ECT in the country is far from humane. Agarwal in an editorial note, wrote that surveys in the West showed 'remarkable deficiencies' in the administration of ECT. Agarwal warns that 'as a developing country, the situation in India is bound to be more disappointing'. Murthy cautions soberingly against the widespread and unconditional use of ECT in the case of depression and suicide.

Even if one grants that the knowledge base we have on ECT justifies its use, the ethical basis of ECT depends upon how closely the practical conditions of administering ECT conform to several standards of medical care; whether clear diagnostic criteria are practised (not just prescribed in the treatment manuals) in the use of the treatment; and whether informed consent is obtained, and whether such consent comprises information about possible cognitive deficits following ECT. Agarwal, above, in listing the problems about abuse of ECT techniques in the country, notes that the question of patient's consent is rarely looked into by practitioners. The problem, here, as with the prescriptions and use of drugs, is that no information is available.

The NMHP commits itself to non- invasive cures by resourcing 'proper' principles of community care. But it does not specify policies for the use of the medical cures. While the policy prescribes generally terms the administrative structure of mental health care through the community, it remains silent on the nature of 'proper' principles and practices. Does the silence on these issues imply a sanction of these widely practised medical cures?

MENTAL HEALTH CARE FOR ALL

The NMHP promises 'availability and accessibility of mental health care for all'. Nevertheless, it prioritises epilepsy, mental retardation and psychoses. This prioritisation takes away all the promised benefits of the policy. These debilities are what are called 'intense' illnesses. Studies show that intense illnesses in the community is of the order of 1%. The frequency of epilepsy, MR and psychoses is probably less than this. There is nevertheless, a whole range of psychological problems (developmental, psycho-social, etc.) which contribute to the other 10 to 15% recorded as morbidity rate in Indian communities. Especially among the vulnerable sections of society, such as the elderly, the women, people in cultural or geographic transition, disaster struck people, the divorced, widowed, etc., the morbidity rate of the common mental disorders is very high. Thus the NMHP limits itself to only a very small target population by prioritising the intense mental disorders.

More significantly, the use of the medical models- drug therapy or ECT for cure is almost inevitable in the case of these sickness. In treating psychotic disorders, mental retardation or epilepsy, a practitioner is almost never called upon to invent non- invasive techniques or forms of psychotherapy. If drug use or ECT can be justified at all, it is justified all the more easily in the case of these endogenous types of mental disorders than other common types. So while the NMHP seems to pledge its philosophy on the side of non- invasive and community close techniques, it prioritises illnesses in such a way that the use of medical models of cure is inevitable.

There are of course economic reasons for the studied ineffectiveness of the NMHP to serve community needs. Covertly adopting the medical model ensures that no additional resources are spent on mental health. The very terms of the NMHP state this quite emphatically.

NMHP APPROACHES

The NMHP has been designed to have the following approaches:

- Integration of the mental health care service with the existing general health services;
- To utilise the existing infrastructure of health services and also to deliver the minimum mental health care services;
- To furnish appropriate task oriented training to the existing health staff;
- To link mental health services with the existing community growth programme.

The design of the programme is such that we make do with existing infrastructure and personnel, ensuring that no extra expenditure is incurred in implementing the mental health programme. The medical practitioners can be 'trained' to address mental health issues also, and also the PHC staffers. Psychotherapy, which works in the more frequent common disorders, calls for expert training, institutional and organisational investments. If the state wanted to implement the mental health policy in principle, it would call for to spend much more than if it simply linked up mental health with existing health facilities. This attitude to minimize resources spent on mental health care is completely consistent with the recent trends of the dimunition of state funding for health care generally.

Thus, while the NMHP openly proclaims a community care philosophy, it works by prioritisations which will ensure that the medical model will persist, also ensuring that no additional costs will be expended for mental health care. By remaining silent on the nature of treatment options to be made available in community care, it does not call into question or debate the widespread medical models of mental health cure.

INSTITUTIONALIZATION VERSUS DEINSTUTIONALIZATION

Even if physicians of prior generations had understood the essentially biological nature of mental health nursing, it is unclear that they would have had much to offer patients in the way of effective therapy beyond the segregation and physical restraints that characterized institutionalization prior to the advent of the modern pharmaceutical industry. In the Middle Ages, mentally sick people were integrated into society and labeled as holy fools or just fools - these persons were tolerated with amusement. Segregation and institutionalization was reserved for those with leprosy. In the 17th century, nevertheless, as leprosy waned in Europe, the stigma attached to leprosy evidently transferred to mental sickness, and people with schizophrenia gradually became seen as a menace to society. As a result, they were socially and physically excluded from society in the first insane asylums, or maintained by families who would have for the most part regarded them as social embarrassments. Thus, the cultural climate concerning madness changed from one of amusement or disinterest to one of fear. This history is documented in author Michele Foucault's book, "Madness and Civilization". The tradition of institutionalizing schizophrenic people has persisted in developed countries ever since.

Hospitals such as Bethlem Royal (popularly known as 'Bedlam') and Bellevue became known for their specialization in and care for the mentally sick; they were early psychiatric facilities. Patient conditions in these institutions were poor, nevertheless. The physical treatments hospital staff employed to control patients would be considered abusive by today's standards. Patients were placed in strait-jackets, neglected, isolated from other people, or forced to endure primitive electroshock therapy, insulin coma or (in some cases) lobotomy.

Popularized by Walter Freeman, an American neurologist of the early twentieth century, lobotomy involved the surgical destruction of the frontal cortex of patients' brains. Lobotomy had the effect of calming several formerly agitated patients, but it accomplished this feat by destroying the very part of patients' brains responsible for judgment, emotional control, and personality. It was not a humane procedure, and thankfully it was for the most part discontinued and discredited by mid-century as more effective drug therapies and refined shock therapies became available.

Mental healthcare experienced a revolution at the mid-point of the twentieth century with the availability of the first anti-psychotic medications. For the first time, schizophrenic patients could experience partial symptom relief rather than simply being restrained or tranquilized. In this heady environment, a social movement came into being with the goal of deinstitutionalizing the mentally sick. This movement found expression in critical state and federal supreme court decisions supporting patient rights. Numerous state hospitals were shut down as a result, and formerly institutionalized patients were released to live in society with the aid of the newly created community mental health centres (CMHCs) built in most communities as a result of the 1963 US Federal Community Mental Health Centres Construction Act. The noble goals of deinstitutionalization have been for the most part accomplished, but the follow through has not been well supported; a condition we hope is remedied in coming years, but which seems unlikely to occur any time soon.

MODEL OF PREVENTIVE PSYCHIATRY: LEVELS OF PREVENTION

Mental illnesses are among the leading causes of disability worldwide. Thus, psychiatrists should put all their effort to decrease the mental health "epidemic" in the society, by preventive and health promotion programs. Health promotion intervention implies better understanding of the multidimensional origin of mental sickness and acceptance of the mentally sick, both from their family and their social environment. Traditional sickness-based clinical treatment should be broadened to a complete, multidimensional approach to clinical care, based upon positive attitudes and reduction of persisting skepticism regarding the possibility of cure. Combining sickness-focused treatment with health promotion interventions and strengthening positive mental health such as life skills, would decrease psychological distress, improve quality of life, i.e. self-esteem, mastery of one's life, life satisfaction, competence and psychological adjustment. It would break the spiral of stress, increase psychobiological immunity, and reduce in-patient treatment and stigmatization of mental diseases.

Primary, secondary and tertiary prevention should be only parts of the whole, influencing each other, and not artificial fragments. Thus, national and international programs on the protection and promotion of mental health should be complete because these activities are mutually interwoven and pervaded. It is of utmost importance for prevention and treatment to be continuously led by demystification of psychiatric disease, investment into healthy potentials of the patient, as well as by structuring the life of the patients and focusing on health rather than disease.

Nevertheless, in spite of the dictum of traditional wisdom that prevention is better than treatment, as well as the growing body of evidence-based preventive programs that have shown their efficacy, preventive psychiatry is still neglected and marginalized.

Following are the recommendations for the preventive Psychiatry:

- Psychiatrists should be actively involved in prevention and health promotion, exercising not overt but covert leadership. They should collaborate with other mental health professionals, but also with people and agencies indirectly involved with mental health (universities, teachers, clergy, administrators, government, police, journalists and practically every sector of the community).
- Member societies should influence policy makers to develop complete national preventive programs, that would be of benefit to mental health professionals, governmental and non-government agencies, consumers and the general public. Member societies should be involved in national task forces on prevention and growth of systems of mental health care services, based on the concept of community care. In preparing national programs, providers and consumers should co-operate.
- There should be a continuous follow-up of the needs and determination of priority needs of each community regarding mental health problems. Determination of resources at the disposal of each community in the implementation of preventive programs is also needed.
- Networks of services covering the needs of the population should be created. Links should also be developed between national and international preventive programs. Cooperation between member societies and exchange of information and experience should be encouraged.

- A continuous education and training of the primary care staff, social services, professionals and paraprofessionals should be stimulated. Special attention should be paid to the training of undergraduate and postgraduate students, where prevention of mental health problems should be part of the regular curriculum.
- Special attention should be paid to dissemination of information on prevention to the patients, families and population at large, through special programs and with the aid of mass media.
- Research on the efficacy of preventive programs is very significant. There should be a continuing growth and rapid translation into practice of the scientific evidence base for preventive programs. Both scientific research and consensual experience should guide this process.
- Legal and other regulations should be adjusted to offer support to preventive programs and facilitate their implementation, with maximally possible protection of mental patients. Member societies should offer aid in this significant task.
- The programs of prevention of mental disorders and mental health protection and promotion should be incorporated in programs of promotion of health generally as well as in the program of socio-economic growth of the country as a whole.
- Collaboration with other agencies is vital, together with voluntary ones. Taking into consideration that mental health is a fundamental right, the patients should be active participants in the process of prevention. The involvement of the service users is extremely significant in helping to determine policy and practice.

PRIMARY, SECONDARY, TERTIARY LEVELS

PRIMARY PREVENTION

- It is estimated that in several countries one third to one half of all mental disorders could be averted by primary prevention measures These measures should be aiming at improvement of mental health of the population at large, promotion of positive mental health, and protection of sub-groups at higher danger of developing mental disorders.
- Identification of high-risk groups should be a significant aim of preventive psychiatry, as well as applying adequate strategies

to these groups at all developmental stages, which should comprise the following: early stage care, before delivery; healthy start of life; high-quality parenting; care for the children of mentally sick or addicted parents; mental health promotion in schools; upholding of family cohesion (with close cooperation of psychiatrists and family physicians); prevention at the work place; life skill education of the population; prevention in old age, etc.

- Extensive and rapid socio-economic changes in several countries are followed by numerous factors, which exert their damaging effects on health generally and especially on the mental health of the population. Non-developed societies as well as societies in transition undergoing social and economic upheavals should be helped by developed countries in implementation of preventive programs.
- Natural and man-made disasters are unfortunately frequent, and far from eradicated, especially the latter. Wars, terrorism, growing violence in several countries, made the life of several populations extremely difficult. Experienced psychological trauma may have several psychiatric consequences, together with acute stress reactions and posttraumatic stress disorders, psychosomatic disorders, and increased morbidity and mortality of somatic disorders. Late and serious consequences of man-made disasters can cause a spiral of violence and transgenerational transmission of trauma. Though the population at large is exposed to the effect of damaging agents, some population groups are especially endangered, such as children, the elderly, incomplete families, unemployed, the poor, migrants, etc. These groups at risk call for intensive programs of prevention. Thus, a systematic education of health care workers and their associates in the discipline of disaster psychiatry should be given priority. There is a necessity of preparing national programs for prevention and mitigation of psychosocial consequences of disasters.

SECONDARY PREVENTION

- Early recognition and effective management of mental disorders, especially at the level of primary health care, is necessary to prevention. Primary care physicians must be adequately trained in mental health matters. Appropriate guidelines like the WHO ICD-10 Primary Care Guidelines and other aids, together with screening procedures, may be helpful in this context. Local task forces on prevention, should undertake a continuous education, in cooperation with universities and policy makers.

- Treatment and prevention of several disorders (depression, eating disorders, personality disorders, substance abuse, etc.) with high public health significance, i.e. deleterious effects on the immediate (micro) and wider (macro) environment should be part of extensive community programs.
- Public awareness should be raised in early detection of symptoms and need for a prompt intervention. Primary care physicians, staff of medical and other services, the patients and their families, and community at large should learn how to recognize mental disorders.
- Dissemination of information is useful for health promotion. The education of staff members and nonprofessional caregivers concerning life stresses, which are likely to act as precipitating events for relapse, is of importance.
- Services should involve users to ensure that support is relevant to their needs as they see them. Self-advocacy and self-help schemes may enable service users to help one another. Partnership in treatment, instead of passivity should be encouraged. The traditional paternalistic attitude should be overcome and sharing encouraged.

TERTIARY AND QUATERNARY PREVENTION

Most mental disorders call for a prompt application of rehabilitation measures from the very initiation of treatment. Tertiary prevention services, aiming at reducing disability produced by mental health disorders must be developed in adequate numbers. Rehabilitation should have highly set goals. It should increase competence of the patients and creative reintegration into community. Families and all other community factors should be engaged in the successful implementation of rehabilitation. Community-based care, i.e. maintaining the patient in the most natural environment should be stimulated.

Quaternary prevention is necessary because mental illnesses may have deleterious effects upon the family and community at large. And whilst destigmatization is related to all phases of prevention, it should be part of special programs, covering the public, the families and the professionals. In this significant aspect of prevention, the WPA task forces and sections should be actively involved and should collaborate closely with member societies.

It is widely accepted that a multidimensional (i.e. a biopsychosocial) approach is essential in psychiatry. International collaboration, harmonization, integration and unification of preventive and treatment models are among the key words of contemporary psychiatry. Nevertheless, they are only theoretical labels for a large part of the world. "Health for All" is a wonderful dictum that is unfortunately an utopian goal for several psychiatric communities. Prevention and health promotion are most significant, but complex tasks. They are difficult to carry out in several countries with more demanding priorities, determined by socioeconomic problems or adverse conditions like violence, war, or sanctions. Several of them don't have the means to obtain even the cheapest medication for psychiatrically sick patients. Psychiatrists in these countries are sharing adversities with their patients; they are frequently burnt out and deprived of possibilities of participating at the international professional scene. The capability to apply preventive and treatment models varies as a function of several factors involving economic growth, professional resource availability, national priorities and the specific culture. Globalization should comprise understanding and aid to nondeveloped countries. Unless these countries are helped, psychiatry and international organizations will remain elitistic and their accepted goals and intentions will only be declarations without a wider impact.

MENTAL HEALTH AGENCIES

The function of voluntary sector within the health and welfare sectors has always been extensive though not always highly visible. In some cases the absence of a voluntary agency would mean that these services would have to be provided by government. With increasing demands on existing government provided services, and a reluctance or an inability on the part of government to furnish more services, the nongovernment voluntary sector in India appears to be expanding in amount and range of service provision.

India, the second most populated country of the world with a population of 1.027 billion, is a country of contrasts. It is characterized as one of the world's largest industrial nations, yet most of the negative characteristics of poor and developing countries define India too. The population is predominantly rural, and 36% of people still live below poverty line. There is a continuous migration of rural people into urban slums creating major health and economic problems. India is one of the pioneer countries in health services planning with a focus on primary health care. Improvement in the health status of the population has been one of the major thrust areas for social growth programmes in the country. Nevertheless, only a small percentage of the total annual budget is spent on health. Mental health is part of the general health services, and carries no separate budget. The National Mental Health Programme serves practically as the mental health policy. Recently, there was an eight-fold increase in budget allocation for the National Mental Health Programme for the Tenth Five-Year Plan (2002-2007). India is a multicultural traditional society where people visit religious and traditional healers for general and mental health related problems. Nevertheless, wherever modern health services are available, people do come forward. India has a number of public policy and judicial enactments, which may impact on mental health. These have tried to address the issues of stigma attached to the mental illnesses and the rights of mentally sick people in society. A large number of epidemiological surveys done in India on mental disorders have demonstrated the prevalence of mental morbidity in rural and urban areas of the country; these rates are comparable to global rates. Though India is well placed as far as trained manpower generally health services is concerned, the mental health trained personnel are quite limited, and these are mostly based in urban areas.

Considering this, growth of mental health services has been linked with general health services and primary health care. Training opportunities for various kinds of mental health personnel are gradually increasing in various academic institutions in the country and recently, there has been a major initiative in the development of private psychiatric services to fill a vacuum that the public mental health services have been slow to address. A number of non-governmental organizations have also initiated activities related to rehabilitation programmes, human rights of mentally sick people, and school mental health programmes. In spite of all these efforts and progress, a lot has still to be done towards all facets of mental health care in India in respect of training, research, and provision of clinical services to promote mental health in all sections of society.

Following are the Mental Health Institutes of India:

- All India Institute of Medical Sciences (AIIMS), Delhi
- Central Institute of Psychiatry, Ranchi, Bihar
- Morarji Desai National Institute of Yoga, Delhi

- National Institute of Mental Health & NeuroSciences (NIMHANS), Bangalore
- Vidya Sagar Institute of Mental Health and Neurosciences (VIMHANS), Delhi
- IHBAS Mental Hospital, Shahdara, Delhi
- National Institute of Rehabilitation Training And Research, Cuttack, Orissa
- North Eastern Indira Gandhi Regional Institute of Health and Medical Sciences, Shillong, Meghalaya
- Sher-i-Kashmir Institute of Medical Sciences, Srinagar
- Bus Sada Mental Hospital (Hospitals/Mental - Ernakulam)
- Cochin Mental Health Centre (Hospitals/Mental - Ernakulam)
- Kusumagiri Mental Health Centre (Hospitals/Mental - Ernakulam)
- Kusumagiri Mental Health Centre (Hospitals/Mental - Ernakulam)
- Sri Guru Teg Bahadur Hospital, Amritsar
- T.B. Sanatorium (T.B.& Chest Diseases Hospital) Amritsar
- Punjab Government Dental College and Hospital, Amritsar
- Govt. Hospital for Mental Care, Waltair, Vishakhapatnam, Andhra Pradesh
- Govt. Hospital for Mental Care, Hyderabad, Andhra Pradesh
- L.G.B. Institute of Mental Health, Tezpur, Assam
- Ranchi Institute of Neuro Psychiatry and Allied Sciences, Ranchi, Bihar
- Central Institute of Psychiatry, Kanke, Ranchi, Bihar
- Devis Institute of Neuro-psychiatry, Kanke, Ranchi, Bihar
- Mental Hospital, Institute of Psychiatry and Human Behaviour, Altinho, Panaji, Goa
- Mental Hospital, Outside Delhi Gate, Shahibag Road, Ahmedabad, Gujrat
- Mental Hospital, Karelibag, Baroda
- Kasturba Mental Hospital, Kalawada, Rajkot
- B.M. Institute of Mental Health, Ahmedabad

- Govt. Hospital for Psychiatric Diseases, Jammu & Kashmir
- National Institute of Mental Health & Neuro Sciences, Bangalore, Karnataka
- Mental Hospital, Dharwar, Karnataka
- Mental Health Centre, Peroorkada, Thiruvanthapuram, Kerala
- Govt. Mental Hospital, Thrissur, Kerala
- Govt. Mental hospital, Kozhikode, Kerala
- Mental Hospital, Indore, Madhya Pradesh
- Mental Hospital, Gwalior, Madhya Pradesh
- Central Mental Hospital, Yervada, Pune, Maharshatra
- N, M. Mental Hospital, Thane, Maharshtra
- Mental Hospital, Chhindwara Road, Nagpur, Maharshtra
- Mental Hospital, Ratnagiri, Nagpur, Maharshtra
- Kripamayee Institute for Mental Health P.O.Wanleswadi, Distt. Sangli, Miraj, Maharashtra
- Meghalaya Institution of Mental Health & Neurological Science (MIMHANS)

Mawlai, Shillong, Meghalaya

- Mental Hospital, Aradura Hills, Kohima, Meghalaya
- Mental Health Institute, S.C.B. Medical College Hospital, Cuttack, Meghalaya
- Punjab Mental Hospital, Amritsar, Punjab
- Mental Hospital, (Psychiatric Centre), Jodhpur, Rajasthan
- Mental Hospital (Psychiatric Centre), Jaipur, Rajasthan
- Institute of Mental Health, Kilpauk Chennai, Tamil Nadu
- Mental Hospital, Agra, Uttar Pradesh
- Mental Hospital, Bareilly, Uttar Pradesh
- Mental Hospital, Varanasi, Uttar Pradesh
- Noor Manzil, Psychiatric Centre, Lucknow, Uttar Pradesh
- Mental Observation Ward, Bhawanipur, Kolkata, West Bengal
- Hospital for Mental Diseases, Gobra Road, Kolkata, West Bengal
- Lumbini Park Mental Hospital, Kolkata, West Bengal
- Dutta Nagar Mental Health Centre, Kolkata, West Bengal

- Calcutta & Mankundu Mental Hospital, Kolkata, West Bengal
- Sarkarpol Mental Hospital, Kolkata, West Bengal
- Mental Hospital, Murshidabad, West Bengal
- Institute of Human Behaviour & Allied Sciences, Dilshad Garden, Delhi

MENTAL HEALTH NURSING ISSUES FOR SPECIAL POPULATION

CHILDREN MENTAL HEALTH NURSING

Child abuse is a blanket term for four types of child mistreatment: physical abuse, sexual abuse, emotional abuse, and neglect. In several cases children are the victims of more than one type of abuse. The abusers can be parents or other family members, caretakers such as teachers and babysitters, acquaintances (together with other children), and (in rare instances) strangers.

Nursing staff and allied health professionals can assist in the treatment of child abuse by being aware of physical symptoms and emotional reactions caused by abuse or neglect. During the diagnosis and treatment phase, nursing staff and allied health professionals can help patients and perpetrators by providing appropriate educational materials, and referrals to community and individual supportive programs.

WOMEN MENTAL HEALTH NURSING

Men and women have different mental health needs; some psychiatric disorders have been noted to be 'gender specific'. The greatest differential between men and women is seen in the prevalence of depression, anxiety disorders and eating disorders. Women are more likely to disclose their emotional distress and seek help for it. They are twice as likely to refer themselves for psychiatric treatment, take on the sick role and define their problems in mental health terms. An understanding of these theories enables mental health nurses to understand that treatment outcomes and services delivery must reflect the fundamental differences in the etiology, manifestation and presentation of women's mental health problems.

ELDERLY VICTIMS OF VIOLENCE AND ABUSE

The world health organization defines violence as the intentional use of physical force or power, threatened or actual, against oneself, another person or against a group or community, which either results in or has a high likelihood of resulting in injury, death, psychological harm, mal-growth or deprivation. Caring for frail elders can be difficult and stressful. Elders who are mentally or physically impaired are especially needy of special care that the family or caregiver is sick equipped to furnish. Both skills and resources in the form of family or financial support may be lacking. Increased stress and poor coping combine to lead to stress. The more impaired and dependent the elder, the greater the likelihood of maltreatment.

Elder maltreatment can be compared with child maltreatment regarding the dependent situation of the victim. Elders who are abused are frail and frequently mentally or physically impaired. They have a special relationship with and are dependent on a family member or caregiver. Elders are also at risk for financial or material exploitation.

Such abuse is in general classified into the following classes:

- Physical abuse - the infliction of pain or injury, physical coercion, or physical or drug induced restraint.
- Psychological or emotional abuse - the infliction of mental anguish.
- Financial or material abuse - the illegal or improper exploitation or use of funds or resources of the older person.
- Sexual abuse - non-consensual sexual contact of any kind with the older person.
- Neglect - the refusal or failure to fulfil a care-giving obligation. This may or may not involve a conscious and intentional attempt to inflict physical or emotional distress on the older person.

HANDICAPPED

The Mental Health Registered Nurse works in Mental Health hospitals, clinics and health care facilities or community based medically intensive training homes. The employee must maintain a sympathetic and understanding attitude toward mentally sick, developmentally or physically disabled, and physically sick patients. The Mental Health Registered Nurse works with unpredictable, potentially combative, residents who may be dangerous to themselves and others. They lift or move patients and equipment on a regular basis. There is frequent exposure to blood and body fluids. Some positions may be required to work overtime, on-call or rotating schedules or may be deployed to work in other than regularly allotted areas.

The mental health registered nurse has primary responsibility for providing nursing care to mentally sick, developmentally disabled and physically sick patients. They develop nursing care plans, delegate nursing care actions for specific patient needs and furnish clinical oversight for ancillary nursing staff. The Mental Health Registered Nurse is responsible to oversee and direct all medical and nursing procedures and the therapeutic environment for patients of a ward, home or unit for a designated shift. The duties listed below are not inclusive but characteristic of the type and level of work linked with this class. Individual positions may perform all or some combination of the duties listed below as well as other related duties.

- Preparation of Nursing Care Plan: Assess patient's psychological and physical condition, assess treatment needs, and develop nursing care plan. Carry out therapeutic treatments prescribed by the plan, delegating and assigning appropriate facets of care to ancillary nursing personnel. Assess patient's response to treatment and make changes to treatment, when indicated. Keep written records.
- Direct Patient Care: Observe and assess patients' physical and mental condition and behavioural changes (e.g., loss of appetite, depression, confusion, combativeness, etc.). Assess medication or food allergies and monitor patients' response and tolerance to medications. Carry out doctors' orders, verifying that there are no inadvertent errors. Initiate treatments as per nursing standards. Initiate emergency response activities or behavioural interventions, as required. Assist patients in daily living activities such as bathing, oral care and feeding. Coordinate all patient health services. Monitor and assess work of direct care nursing staff, together with certified nursing assistants (CNA's), certified medication assistants (CMA's) and licensed practical nurses (LPN's).
- Medications and Treatment: Verify doctors' orders. Counter sign transcriptions of doctors' orders on Medication Administration Reviews (MARS) and Treatment Administration Reviews (TARS) before carrying out the orders. Monitor the medication and document its effectiveness. Administer injectable medications and oversee or administer topical and oral medications as prescribed. Furnish treatments and various therapies and conduct tests to determine the effect of the prescribed treatment or therapy. Act as team leader during crisis with hands-on decision making responsibility till doctor or emergency medical team arrives. Assess individual's health

and security risk status for capability to partake in outings, school, etc. Partake in developing hospice plan, if essential. Form primary relationship with and furnish role modelling for selected patients. Spend time daily or weekly talking with patients personally and in groups. May furnish individual counselling, family education and group therapy.

- Documentation: Keep current and accurate legal written records, together with nursing care plans, treatment plans, progress notes, medications, case records of unusual incident reports involving patients.
- Patient and Staff Education: Educate patients and families about the sickness, medical or physical needs and how interventions and medications interrelate with the sickness. Teach patients daily living and self-management skills (e.g., communication, anger control, self esteem). Plan, organize, develop, and assess classes or group therapy in areas such as drug and alcohol abuse, human sexuality, and psychiatric rehabilitation.
- Monitor and help assess student nurses. Conduct in-service training for other staff members on new or specialized medical findings, procedures, or techniques. Train staff to hospice plan. Partake in interdisciplinary meetings with patients, family members, guardians and other nursing team members to plan scope of treatment for patients.
- Shift Responsibilities: Make patient and direct care staff assignments related to nursing and medical procedures and protocols. Schedule and oversee work to furnish quality patient care within scope of nursing practice. Solve problems with staff when possible or refer to supervisor. Assess LPN's, CMA's and CNA staff performance. Partake in training and orienting new employees. May partake in ward leadership meetings reviewing and discussing operational procedures designed to maintain, improve and improve a safe and therapeutic environment. Serve on nursing, program or hospital committees.
- Other Responsibilities: The Mental Health Registered Nurse has contact with patients on a daily basis to furnish care, and with patients' families to furnish support and answer questions regarding patients' condition and medical procedures. There is daily contact with doctors and nursing management to discuss

nursing issues and report changes in patients' conditions, with social workers, psychiatrists, psychologists, therapists and direct care staff to develop individual treatment plans for patients and with support personnel or community vendors to request test results, order supplies, and request special diets.

HIV/AIDS

Nurses and allied health professionals are likely to be the first medical contact for HIV-infected patients. Information obtained about the patient's signs and symptoms, lifestyle, and social behaviour must be documented by the medical staff. There has been recognition by researchers that behaviour that places a person at risk for other STDs increases the danger of HIV infection. Sexually-transmitted disease (STD) surveillance can furnish significant indicators of sites to which HIV infection may spread, as well as point to targets to which efforts to promote safe sexual behaviour should be aimed. Patient care activities, patient progress, and response to symptomatic or preventive therapies need to be documented by nurses. Medical record information is vital to continued research in the discipline. All information must be kept confidential and maintained in compliance with state and federal laws.

Education about HIV prevention has been proven cost-effective when compared with the rising cost of lifetime medical management of people with AIDS. Different types of preventive messages, skills, and support are needed to help reduce sexual and drug-related risks. Drug injectors should be educated about their high-risk behaviour. Drug counselling may help them stop using drugs or sharing needles. These persons need to be taught how to protect themselves from sexual transmission if their partners have ever been IV drug users and may have shared needles. Substance abuse is a major problem. The combination of substance abuse and sexual HIV transmission must be given serious attention. Substance abuse prevention and intervention are sorely lacking for users of morphine, cocaine, marijuana, and alcohol. These substances not only alter users' behaviour, but weaken their immune systems. This weakening may make them more susceptible to infection with HIV. Counselling and treatment should be available to those who abuse drugs and alcohol. They, too, are in need of aid in helping them stop using drugs and to help them prevent HIV infection.

Comprehensive health education programs need to be directed toward generation-specific behaviour and epidemiology. Programs for children and young adults should involve parents and educators. The most efficient programs begin training young people at an early age and are designed to promote healthy behaviours-such as exercising, eating healthy food, avoiding drug use, excessive alcohol consumption, smoking, and premature sexual activity.

REFERENCES

Burt, V. K., & Katzman, J. W. (2000). Impulse-control disorders not elsewhere classified. In B. J. Sadock & V. A. Sadock (Eds.), Comprehensive textbook of psychiatry, Vol. 2, (7th ed., pp. 1701–1713). Philadelphia: Lippincott Williams & Wilkins.

Davila, Y. R. (1990). Women and anger. Journal of Psychosocial Nursing, 37(7), 25–29.

Fava, M. (1997). Psychopharmacologic treatment of pathological aggression. Psychiatric Clinics of North America, 20(2), 427–451.

Flannery, R. B., Fisher, W., Kolodziej, K. K., & Spillane, M. J. (2000). Assaults on staff by psychiatric patients in community residences. Psychiatric Services, 51(1), 111–113.

Hughes, D. H. (1999). Acute psychopharmacological management of the aggressive psychotic patient. Psychiatric Services, 50(9), 1135–1137.

Kavoussi, R., Armstead, P., & Coccaro, E. (1997). The neurobiology of impulse aggression. Psychiatric Clinics of North America, 20(2), 395–403.

Lewis, M. L., & Dehn, D. S. (1999). Violence against nurses in outpatient mental health settings. Journal of Psychosocial Nursing, 37(6), 28–33.

Maier, G. J. (1996). Managing threatening behavior: The role of talk up and talk down. Journal of Psychosocial Nursing & Mental Health Services, 34(6), 25.

Bibliography

Adams, R. L., & Culbertson, J. L. (2000). Personality assessment: adults and children. In B. J. Sadock & V. A. Sadock (Eds.),

Adams, S. M., & Partee, D. J. (1998). Hope: The critical factor in recovery. Journal of Psychosocial Nursing, 36(4), 29-32.

Alonso, A. (2000). Group psychotherapy, combined individual and group therapy. In B. J. Sadock & V. A. Sadock (Eds.),

Andrews, M. M., & Boyle, J. S. (2003). Transcultural concepts in nursing care (4th ed.). Philadelphia: Lippincott Williams & Wilkins.

Auchus, M. P., Wood, K., & Kaslow, N. (1995). Exercise patterns of psychiatric patients admitted to a shortterm inpatient unit. Psychosocial Rehabilitation Journal, 18(3), 137-145.

Balzer Riley, J. W. (2000). Communications in nursing: Communicating assertively and responsibly in nursing (4th ed.). Philadelphia: Mosby.

Bandura, A. (1997). Insights: Self-efficacy. Harvard Mental Health Letter, 13(9), 4-6.

Benishek, L. A., & Lopez, F. G. (1997). Critical evaluation of hardiness theory: Gender differences, perception of life events, and neuroticism. Work & Stress, 11(3), 33-45.

Berne, E. (1964). Games people play. New York: Grove Press.

Bowsher, J. E., & Keep, D. (1995). Toward an understanding of three control constructs: Personal control, self-efficacy, and hardiness. Issues in Mental Health Nursing, 16(1), 33-50.

Buchanan, J. (1995). Social support and schizophrenia: A review of the literature. Archives of Psychiatric Nursing, 9(2), 68-76.

Campinha-Bacote, J. (2002). The process of cultural competence in the delivery of health care services: A model of care. Journal of Transcultural Nursing, 13(3), 181-184.

Caplan, G. (1964). Principles of preventive psychiatry. New York: Basic Books.

Carper, B. (1978). Fundamental patterns of knowing in nursing. Advances in Nursing Science, 13-23.

Casey, D. E., & Zorn, S. H. (2001). The pharmacology of weight gain with antipsychotics. Journal of Clinical Psychiatry, 62(suppl. 7), 4-10.

Castledine, G. (2002). Nurses' bedside manner: Is it deteriorating? British Journal of Nursing, 11(10), 723.

Chamberlin, J. (1998). Citizenship rights and psychiatric disability. Psychiatric Rehabilitation Journal, 21(4), 405-408.

Community Research Foundation. (2001). A communitybased program providing a successful alternative to acute psychiatric hospitalization. Psychiatric Services, 52(10), 1383-1385.

Crain, W. C. (1980). Theories of development: Concepts and application. Englewood Cliffs, NJ: Prentice-Hall, Inc.

Crouch, R. (2002). Communication is the key. Emergency Nurse, 10(3), 3-5.

Davila, Y. R. (1990). Women and anger. Journal of Psychosocial Nursing, 37(7), 25-29.

Deering, C. G. (1999). To speak or not to speak? Selfdisclosure with patients. American Journal of Nursing, 99(1), 34-39.

Glasser, W. (1965). Reality therapy: A new approach to psychiatry. New York: Harper & Row.

Hancock, C. (1998). How to decide about self-disclosure. Nursing, 98(3), 12-13.

Hewitt, J. (2002). A critical review of the arguments debating the role of the nurse advocate. Journal of Advanced Nursing, 37(5), 439-445.

Hyland, D. (2002). An exploration of the relationship between patient autonomy and patient advocacy: Implications for nursing practice. Nursing Ethics, 9(5), 472-482.

Juarbe, T. (1996). Puerto Ricans. In J. G. Lipson, S. L. Dibble, & P. A. Minarik (Eds.), Culture and nursing care: A pocket guide (pp. 222-238). San Francisco: USCF Nursing Press.

Kavoussi, R., Armstead, P., & Coccaro, E. (1997). The neurobiology of impulse aggression. Psychiatric Clinics of North America, 20(2), 395-403.

Kennedy, M. G. (1999). Cultural competence and psychiatric-mental health nursing. Journal of Transcultural Nursing, 10(1), 11.

King, E. C. (1984). Affective education in nursing: A guide to teaching and assessment. Rockville, MD: Aspen Systems.

Knapp, M., & Hall, J. (2002). Nonverbal behavior in human interaction (5th ed.). New York: Wadsworth.

Kohnke, M. F. (1982). Advocacy: What is it? Nursing and Health Care, 3(6), 314-318.

Kunyk, D., & Olson, J. K. (2001). Clarification of conceptualizations of empathy. Journal of Advanced Nursing, 35(3), 317-325.

Lamb, H. R., & Bachrach, L. L. (2001). Some perspectives on deinstitutionalization. Psychiatric Services, 52(8), 1039-1045.

Lamb, H. R., & Weinberger, L. E. (1998). Persons with severe mental illness in jails and prisons: A review. Psychiatric Services, 49(4), 483-492.

Lawson, W. B. (1996). The art and science of psychopharmacology of African Americans. Mt. Sinai Journal of Medicine, 63(5-6), 301-305.

Lewis, M. L., & Dehn, D. S. (1999). Violence against nurses in outpatient mental health settings. Journal of Psychosocial Nursing, 37(6), 28-33.

Low, J. (1996). The concept of hardiness: A brief but critical commentary. Journal of Advanced Nursing, 24, 588-590.

Maslow, A. H. (1954). Motivation and personality. New York: Harper & Row. National Alliance for the Mentally Ill (NAMI). (2002).

Mellow, J. (1986). A personal perspective of nursing therapy. Hospital and Community Psychiatry, 37(2), 182-183.

Miller, P. H. (1983). Theories of developmental psychology. San Francisco: W. H. Freeman & Co.

Millon, T. (Ed.). (1967). Theories of psychopathology. Philadelphia: W. B. Saunders.

Morley, W. E., et al. (1967). Crisis: Paradigms of intervention. Journal of Psychiatric Nursing, 5, 537-538.

Niveau, G., & Kelley-Puskas, M. (2001). Psychiatric disorders and fitness to drive. Journal of Medical Ethics, 27, 36-39.

Northouse, L. L., & Northouse, P. G. (1998). Health communication: Strategies for health professionals (3rd ed.). Stamford, CT: Appleton & Lange.

Puentas, W. J. (2000). Using social reminiscence to teach therapeutic communication skills. Geriatric Nursing, 21(6), 315-318.

Ries, R. (1997). Advantages of separating the triage function from the emergency service. Psychiatric Services, 48(6), 755-756.

Rogers, C. R. (1961). On becoming a person: A therapist's view of psychotherapy. Boston: Houghton Mifflin.

Schultz, J. M., & Videbeck, S. (2002). Lippincott's manual of psychiatric nursing care plans (6th ed.). Philadelphia: Lippincott Williams, & Wilkins.

Solomon, P., & Draine, J. (1995). Adaptive coping among family members of persons with serious mental illness. Psychiatric Services, 46(11), 1156-1160.

Sugarman, L. (1986). Life-span development: Concepts, theories and interventions. London: Methuen & Co., Ltd.

Sullivan, H. S. (1953). The interpersonal theory of psychiatry. New York: Norton.

Swearingen, L. (1987). Transitional day treatment: An individualized goal-oriented approach. Archives of Psychiatric Nursing, I(2), 104-110.

Szasz, T. (1961). The myth of mental illness. New York: Hoeber-Harper.

Tuck, I. (1997). The cultural context of mental health nursing. Issues in Mental Health Nursing, 18(3), 269-281.

Van Servellen, G. (1997). Communication skills for the health care professional: Concepts and techniques. Gaithersburg, MD: Aspen.

Viscott, D. (1996). Emotional resilience: Simple truths for dealing with the unfinished business of your past. New York: Harmony Books.

Wallace, L. (2002). More than good manners. Nursing 02, 33(7), 32.

Ware, N. C. (1999). Evolving consumer households. Psychiatric Rehabilitation Journal, 23(1), 3-10.

Ware, N. C., & Goldfinger, S. (1997). Poverty and rehabilitation in severe psychiatric disorders. Psychiatric Rehabilitation Journal, 21(1), 3-9.

Weaver, H. N., & White, B. J. (1997). The Native American family: Roots of resiliency. Journal of Family Social Work, 2(1), 67-79.

Weaver, R. L. (1996). Understanding interpersonal communication (7th ed.). New York: Harper-Collins College Publishers.

Index

A

Abdomen, 200

Abnormal, 40, 41, 42, 45, 77, 146, 147, 148, 245, 260

Action, 111, 195, 196, 197, 198, 204

Adaptation, 9, 12, 48, 275

Agreement, 14

Alcohol, 82, 195, 260, 273

Alcoholism, 200

Amphetamines, 196

Amygdala, 65

Application, 14, 18, 291, 329

Approaches, 10, 34

Assessment, 67, 71, 86, 144, 145, 164, 165, 187, 199, 200, 229, 233, 237, 254, 263, 264, 265

Ayurvedic Medicine, 127

B

Barbiturates, 196

Behaviour, 40, 41, 45, 58, 166, 200, 225, 230, 252, 353, 355

Biochemical, 161

Biological, 42, 44

Bipolar Affective Disorder, 154

Brain, 61, 62, 153, 247, 259, 260, 269

Bulimia Nervosa, 212, 226

C

Cancer, 81, 261

Children Mental Health Nursing, 355

Chronic Headaches, 78

Cocaine, 196

Cognition, 73, 85, 229

Cognitive-Behavioural Therapy, 219

Communication, 26, 91, 192, 193, 194, 205, 206, 242, 243, 249, 301, 362, 364

Community, 5, 31, 35, 36, 48, 86, 120, 129, 133, 134, 330, 335, 339, 341, 346, 350, 362, 363

Community Mental Health Nursing, 339

Contemplation, 204

Counselling, 5, 36, 37, 67, 86, 87, 121, 128, 166, 204, 205, 227, 228, 235, 236, 237, 254, 301, 334, 358, 359

CT Scan, 78, 79

D

Defences, 53, 55, 56, 57, 216

Delirium, 162, 273

Delusions, 135, 142, 155, 263, 264

Demographic, 39

Diagnosis, 67, 143, 161, 187, 199, 214, 216, 217, 222, 223, 227, 250, 263

Diseases, 29, 50, 182, 353, 354

Disorders, 10, 15, 43, 47, 50, 59, 60, 61, 129, 135, 137, 140, 153, 154, 166, 179, 182, 183, 195, 207, 208, 210, 215, 220, 221, 223, 224, 225, 231, 237, 238, 241, 242, 243, 245, 250, 251, 252, 259

Dissociation and Conversion Disorder, 181

Dizziness, 78

Drug, 16, 145, 192, 200, 235, 248, 260, 307, 308, 359

DSM-V, 43

Dysthymia, 157

E

Ego, 68

Electroconvulsive, 2, 130, 132, 154

Electroencephalogram, 82, 83, 235

Enforcement, 28, 308, 309

Environment, 40, 85

Epidemiology, 16

Etiology, 58, 141, 185, 198, 211, 214, 220, 223, 247, 261, 268, 355

F

Family, 24, 85, 148, 160, 166, 200, 205, 219, 229, 235, 262, 332, 364

Family Therapy, 219

Function, 1, 8, 13, 15, 25, 27, 37, 38, 39, 47, 48, 50, 51, 52, 53, 57, 59, 61, 75, 76, 81, 83, 114, 131, 136, 149, 164, 166, 168, 182, 186, 198, 232, 238, 242, 256, 264, 265, 269, 305, 331, 332, 333, 334, 335, 337, 351, 364

G

Gender, 39, 85, 210, 239, 361

Genetics, 85

Group Therapy, 219

H

Hallucinations, 82, 135, 136, 142, 263

Hallucinogens, 197

Handicapped, 356

Health, 1, 2, 3, 5, 8, 9, 10, 12, 13, 14, 15, 18, 22, 23, 24, 25, 26, 27, 28, 29, 30, 31, 32, 33, 34, 35, 36, 37, 38, 40, 41, 48, 49, 50, 51, 53, 59, 66, 67, 68, 71, 72, 84, 85, 87, 88, 98, 100, 101, 104, 107, 117, 118, 119, 120, 122, 125, 126, 127, 128, 129, 131, 132, 133, 134, 136, 139, 145, 146, 148, 153, 158, 160, 162, 163, 164, 173, 184, 186, 191, 193, 194, 207. 211, 213, 214, 224, 230, 231, 236,

237, 238, 239, 241, 245, 249, 252, 256, 257, 264, 270, 276, 277, 278, 289, 290, 296, 297, 298, 299, 302, 309, 330, 331, 332, 343, 344, 345, 346, 347, 348, 349, 352, 355, 356, 357, 359, 360, 361, 362, 363, 364

Height, 200

Helpseeking, 44

Hippocampus, 64

Hippocrates, 4

HIV/AIDS, 22, 359

Homeopathy, 29, 128

Hospitalization, 156, 218

Hypothalamus, 63

I

Id, 68

Illusions, 229, 263, 264

Inhalants, 198

International, 50, 182, 257, 298, 300, 351

Interviews, 217

K

Kidney Disease, 261

L

Limbic System, 62

Liver Disease, 261

M

Management, 17, 67, 95, 135, 153, 179, 195, 202, 207, 239, 241, 259, 271, 273, 282, 290

Mania Depression, 154

Marijuana, 197

Maturity, 57

Medications, 200, 220, 248, 357

Mental Disorder, 42

Mental Health Care, 33, 49, 338, 339, 343

Mood, 13, 41, 72, 118, 119, 135, 136, 141, 144, 145, 150, 153, 154, 155, 156, 157, 158, 160, 161, 162, 164, 165, 166, 167, 168, 169, 171, 173, 174, 176, 186, 187, 195, 196, 200, 216, 220, 226, 227, 232, 233, 241, 248, 250, 259, 261, 262, 271, 285

MRI Scan, 79

N

Naturopathy, 127

Negative Symptoms, 143

Neurological, 75, 79, 265, 354

Nicotine, 198

O

Observation, 43, 57, 354

Obsessive Compulsive Disorder, 182

Opiates, 197

P

Patient, 2, 3, 5, 6, 8, 11, 12, 13, 14, 19, 20, 32, 35, 36, 37, 38, 40, 44, 49, 58, 59, 67, 68, 69, 71, 72, 73, 75, 76, 77, 78, 79, 80, 81, 82, 83, 84, 86, 87, 88,

91, 92, 93, 94, 95, 96, 97, 98, 99, 100, 101, 105, 106, 107, 108, 109, 110, 111, 112, 113, 114, 115, 117, 120, 121, 122, 123, 124, 126, 128, 129, 130, 131, 133, 134, 144, 145, 146, 149, 151, 154, 162, 163, 164, 165, 166, 167, 168, 169, 170, 171, 172, 173, 174, 175, 176, 182, 184, 187, 190, 191, 192, 193, 201, 202, 203, 204, 205, 216, 217, 218, 227, 228, 230, 236, 238, 239, 254, 255, 262, 263, 265, 266, 267, 268, 269, 271, 272, 273, 274, 275, 276, 285, 286, 287, 289, 291, 292, 300, 301, 303, 304, 306, 330, 331, 332, 334, 335, 342, 346, 347, 350, 357, 358, 359, 360, 362

Personality, 39, 51, 54, 58, 60, 84, 187, 207, 208, 214, 215, 216, 218, 229, 236, 257, 361

PET Scan, 81

Phencyclidine, 197

Phobias, 180

Physical, 2, 44, 98, 115, 130, 132, 164, 198, 200, 221, 233, 234, 264, 273, 356

Positive Symptoms, 143

Post Traumatic Stress Disorder, 184

Practice, 1, 3, 5, 10, 11, 13, 14, 24, 26, 30, 31, 32, 36, 37, 38, 49, 66, 67, 68, 69, 71, 72, 87, 89, 91, 100, 101, 106, 120, 123, 126, 127, 128, 132, 183, 188, 193, 214, 232, 262, 263, 289, 302, 332, 333, 334, 335, 336, 339, 340, 341, 342, 348, 358, 362

Precontemplation, 204

Preparation, 81, 83, 204, 357

Primary Prevention, 348

Psychoanalytical Model, 68

Psychodynamics, 85

Psychopathology, 39, 60, 61, 214, 221, 224, 248, 261

Psychopharmacology, 118, 146

Psychotherapy, 2, 34, 120, 122, 166, 219, 229, 235, 344

Psychotic Disorders, 135

Q

Qualities, 101

R

Recovery, 17, 135

Relationships, 57

Resistance, 7, 26, 94, 95, 96, 108, 114, 190, 236, 266, 281, 324

S

Schizophrenia, 16, 17, 50, 59, 135, 137, 139, 140, 250, 272

Secondary Prevention, 349

Seizures, 78, 273

Sex, 59, 96, 115, 178, 200, 207, 208, 220, 221, 222, 231, 237, 337, 356

Skin, 200

Smoke, 197

Socioeconomic, 85, 159

Somatoform Disorders, 183
Speech, 73, 200, 243
Spiritual, 85, 133, 233
Stigma, 169, 297
Strokes, 78
Studies, 11, 29, 31, 32, 38, 39, 71, 118, 126, 127, 158, 159, 161, 162, 191, 204, 212, 227, 234, 235, 262, 271, 273, 341, 342
Suicide, 271
Superego, 68
Supportive, 122, 219

T

Therapy, 67, 121, 122, 123, 124, 128, 129, 130, 166, 202, 219, 225, 228, 306
Thyroid Disease, 261
Traditional Chinese Medicine, 126
Trauma, 85, 332
Treatment, 4, 44, 114, 117, 127, 128, 146, 147, 166, 187, 190, 191, 192, 199, 201, 203, 218, 220, 227, 235, 244, 254, 255, 267, 274, 350, 357

V

Vitamin Deficiency, 261

W

Weakness, 78
Weight, 69, 200, 233
Women Mental Health Nursing, 355